Peripheral Nerve Surgery

NEUROSURGERY BY EXAMPLE

Key Cases and Fundamental Principles

Series edited by: Nathan R. Selden, MD, PhD, FACS, FAAP

Volume 1: Peripheral Nerve Surgery, Wilson & Yang

Volume 2: Surgical Neuro-Oncology, Lonser & Elder

Peripheral Nerve Surgery

Edited by

Thomas J. Wilson, MD
Clinical Assistant Professor
Co-Director, Center for Peripheral Nerve Surgery
Department of Neurosurgery
Stanford University
Stanford, CA

Lynda J.-S. Yang, MD, PhD
Professor
Department of Neurosurgery
University of Michigan
Ann Arbor, MI

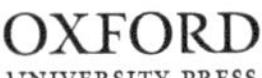

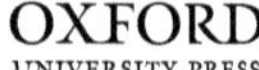

Oxford University Press is a department of the University of Oxford. It furthers the University's objective of excellence in research, scholarship, and education by publishing worldwide. Oxford is a registered trade mark of Oxford University Press in the UK and certain other countries.

Published in the United States of America by Oxford University Press
198 Madison Avenue, New York, NY 10016, United States of America.

CIP data is on file at the Library of Congress
ISBN 978–0–19–061712–7

Contents

Section 2: Peripheral Nerve Pain Syndromes

Section 3: Peripheral Nerve Tumors

Section 4: Peripheral Nerve Trauma

Series Editor's Preface

Dear Reader,

I am delighted to introduce this volume of *Neurosurgery by Example: Key Cases and Fundamental Principles*. Neurosurgical training and practice are based on managing a wide range of complex clinical cases with expert knowledge, sound judgment, and skilled technical execution. Our goal in this series is to present exemplary cases in the manner they are actually encountered in the neurosurgical clinic, hospital emergency department, and operating room.

In this volume, Drs. Thomas Wilson and Lynda Yang and their contributors share their extensive wisdom and experience with all major forms of peripheral nerve disease. The list of contributors reflects the increasingly multidisciplinary practice of peripheral nerve surgery. The cases presented in the volume are divided into four distinct areas of peripheral nerve pathology: entrapment and inflammatory neuropathies, peripheral nerve pain syndromes, peripheral nerve tumors, and peripheral nerve trauma. Each chapter contains a classic presentation of an important peripheral nerve disorder, guiding readers through the assessment and planning, decision-making, surgical procedure, aftercare, and complication management. "Pivot points" illuminate the changes required to manage patients in alternate or atypical situations.

Each chapter also presents pearls for the accurate diagnosis of, successful treatment of, and effective complication management for each clinical entity. These three focus areas will be especially helpful to neurosurgeons preparing to sit for the American Board of Neurological Surgery oral examination, which bases scoring on the three areas.

Finally, each chapter contains focused reviews of medical evidence and expected outcomes, which are helpful for counseling patients and setting accurate expectations. Rather than exhaustive reference lists, the authors provide lists of selected references recommended to deepen understanding.

The resulting volume provides a dynamic tour through the practice of peripheral nerve surgery, guided by some of the leading experts in North America and beyond. Additional volumes in the series will cover each subspecialty area of neurosurgery, using the same case-based approach and Board review features.

Nathan R. Selden, MD, PhD
Campagna Professor and Chair
Department of Neurological Surgery
Oregon Health & Science University
Portland, OR

Contributors

Hussam Abou-Al-Shaar, MD
College of Medicine
Alfaisal University
Riyadh, Saudi Arabia

Zarina S. Ali, MD, MS
Department of Neurosurgery
University of Pennsylvania
Philadelphia, PA, USA

Adam Bevan, MD, PhD
WUSTL Department of Neurosurgery
Washington University School of Medicine in St. Louis
St. Louis, MO, USA

Yarema B. Bezchlibnyk, MD, PhD
Department of Neurosurgery and Brain Repair
University of South Florida
Tampa, FL, USA

Lisa M. Block, MD
Resident
Department of Surgery
University of Wisconsin School of Medicine and Public Health
Madison, WI, USA

Nicholas Boulis, MD
Associate Professor
Department of Neurosurgery
Emory University
Atlanta, GA, USA

David L. Brown, MD
Professor
Section of Plastic Surgery
University of Michigan Medical School
Ann Arbor, MI, USA

Kevin Chan, MD, MSc
SHMG Orthopedics & Sports Medicine
Grand Rapids, MI, USA

Ron Ron Cheng, MD
Department of Neurosurgery
Medical University of South Carolina
Charleston, SC, USA

Srinivas Chiravuri, MD
Department of Anesthesiology
University of Michigan
Ann Arbor, MI, USA

Kevin C. Chung, MD, MSc
Professor of Surgery
Section of Plastic Surgery
Assistant Dean for Faculty Affairs
University of Michigan Medical School
Ann Arbor, MI, USA

Nora F. Dengler, MD
Department of Neurosurgery
Charité Universitätsmedizin Berlin
Berlin, Germany

Ashley Diaz
Department of Neurosurgery
Emory University
Atlanta, GA, USA

Rishi Dihr, MBChB
Royal National Orthopaedic Hospital NHS Trust
London, England, UK

Aaron G. Filler, MD, PhD, FRCS
Medical Director
Institute for Nerve Medicine
Santa Monica, CA, USA

Leandro Pretto Flores, MD, PhD
Chairman
Department of Neurosurgery
Hospital das Forças Armadas
Brasília, Distrito Federal, Brazil

Michael Fox, MD
Royal National Orthopaedic Hospital NHS Trust
London, England, UK

Nasa Fujihara, MD
Research Associate
Section of Plastic Surgery
Department of Surgery
University of Michigan Health System
Ann Arbor, MI, USA

Daniel Hafez, MD, PhD
Department of Neurosurgery
Washington University School of Medicine in St. Louis
St. Louis, MO, USA

Amgad S. Hanna, MD
Associate Professor
Department of Neurological Surgery
University of Wisconsin School of Medicine and Public Health
Madison, WI, USA

Kimberly S. Harbaugh, MD
Associate Professor
Department of Neurosurgery
Penn State Health
Hershey, PA, USA

Sandra Hearn, MD
Clinical Instructor
University of Michigan Health System
Department of Physical Medicine and Rehabilitation
Ann Arbor, MI, USA

Marie-Noëlle Hébert-Blouin, MD
Assistant Professor
Division of Neurology and Neurosurgery
McGill University
Montreal Neurological Hospital and Institute
Montreal, QC, Canada

Christian Heinen, MD
Department of Neurosurgery
University of Oldenburg Evangelisches
Krankenhaus Oldenburg, Germany

Gregory G. Heuer, MD, PhD
Department of Neurosurgery
University of Pennsylvania
The Children's Hospital of Philadelphia
Philadelphia, PA, USA

Jason H. Huang, MD
Texas A&M Health Science Center College of Medicine
Department of Neurosurgery
Baylor Scott & White Healthcare
Temple, TX, USA

Line G. Jacques, MD, MSc, FRCS(C)
Professor of Clinical Neurological Surgery
Chief of Peripheral Nerve and Pain Surgery
Department of Neurological Surgery
University of California, San Francisco
San Francisco, CA, USA

Orion Paul Keifer, Jr., MD, PhD
Department of Neurosurgery
Emory University School of Medicine
Atlanta, GA, USA

Hélène T. Khuong, MD
Division of Neurosurgery
Department of Neurological Sciences
Québec-Université Laval
Quebec, QC, Canada

Thomas Kretschmer, MD, PhD
Department of Neurosurgery
University of Oldenburg Evangelisches
Krankenhaus Oldenburg, Germany

Meghan E. Lark, BS
Research Associate
Section of Plastic Surgery
Department of Surgery
University of Michigan Health System
Ann Arbor, MI, USA

Pascal Lavergne, MD
Division of Neurosurgery
Department of Neurological Sciences
Québec-Université Laval
Quebec, QC, Canada

Angelo B. Lipira, MD, MA
Division of Plastic Surgery
University of Washington
Seattle, WA, USA

Daniel A. Lyons, MD
Resident
Section of Plastic Surgery
University of Michigan Medical School
Ann Arbor, MI, USA

Mark A. Mahan, MD
Department of Neurosurgery
Clinical Neurosciences Center
University of Utah
Salt Lake City, UT, USA

Andrés A. Maldonado, MD, PhD
Unfallklinik Frankfurt
Department of Plastic, Hand and Reconstructive Surgery
Frankfurt, Germany

Sethesh Mansinghani, BS
Texas A&M Health Science Center College of Medicine
Temple, TX, USA

Rajiv Midha, MD, MSc, FRCSC
Division of Neurosurgery
Department of Clinical Neurosciences and Hotchkiss Brain Institute
University of Calgary
Calgary, AB, Canada

Mustafa Nadi, MD
Division of Neurosurgery
Department of Clinical Neurosciences and Hotchkiss Brain Institute
University of Calgary
Calgary, AB, Canada

Russell A. Payne, MD
Department of Neurosurgery
Hershey Medical Center
Penn State College of Medicine
Hershey, PA, USA

Jared M. Pisapia, MD
Department of Neurosurgery
University of Pennsylvania
Philadelphia, PA, USA

Miriana Popadich, FNP
Nurse Practitioner
Department of Neurosurgery
University of Michigan
Ann Arbor, MI, USA

Xiaoming Qi, MD
Department of Neurosurgery
Baylor Scott & White Healthcare
Temple, TX, USA

Wilson Z. Ray, MD
Vice Chair
Department of Neurosurgery
Associate Professor in Neurosurgery & Biomedical Engineering
Associate Residency Program Director
Department of Neurological Surgery
Washington University School of Medicine
St. Louis, MO, USA

Elias B. Rizk, MD
Assistant Professor
Department of Neurosurgery
Pennsylvania State University
Hershey, PA, USA

A. Neil Salyapongse, MD
Department of Surgery
University of Wisconsin-Madison
Madison, WI, USA

Mariano Socolovsky, MD, PhD, IFAANS, IMCNS
Chairman, WFNS Peripheral Nerve Committee
Chief, Peripheral Nerve & Brachial Plexus Program
University of Buenos Aires School of Medicine
Staff Surgeon
British Hospital of Buenos Aires
Buenos Aires, Argentina

Robert J. Spinner, MD
Burton M. Onofrio MD Professor of Neurosurgery
Chair, Department of Neurosurgery
Mayo Clinic
Rochester, MN, USA

Rafael Torino, MD
Chief, Department of Neurosurgery
British Hospital of Buenos Aires
Past President, Argentine Association of Neurosurgery
Buenos Aires, Argentina

Raymond Tse, MD
Division of Plastic Surgery
Seattle Children's Hospital
University of Washington
Seattle, WA, USA

Abhay K. Varma, MD, MSCR
Department of Neurosurgery
Medical University of South Carolina
Charleston, SC, USA

Thomas J. Wilson, MD
Clinical Assistant Professor
Co-Director, Center for Peripheral Nerve Surgery
Department of Neurosurgery
Stanford University
Stanford, CA, USA

Christopher J. Winfree, MD, FACS
Department of Neurological Surgery
Columbia University Medical Center
New York, NY, USA

Stacy N. Wong, ACNP-C
Nurse Practitioner
Department of Neurological Surgery
University of California, San Francisco School of Medicine
San Francisco, CA, USA

Eric L. Zager, MD
Department of Neurosurgery
University of Pennsylvania
Philadelphia, PA, USA

Anna Zdunczyk, MD
Department of Neurosurgery
Charité Universitätsmedizin Berlin
Berlin, Germany

Section 1

Entrapment and Inflammatory Neuropathies

Median Neuropathy—Carpal Tunnel Syndrome

Meghan E. Lark, Nasa Fujihara, and Kevin C. Chung

1

Case Presentation

A 53-year-old woman presents to her primary care physician complaining of numbness, tingling, and pain in her hands that has worsened over the past year. Although she is right-hand dominant, she states that she experiences the majority of the numbness and intermittent pain in her left index and middle fingers. She also reports that she has been experiencing increased clumsiness as a result of decreased grip strength and has been feeling uncoordinated while performing fine motions with her left hand. She notes that her symptoms increase when she is sleeping or when her wrist is in a flexed position for a prolonged period of time and usually subside with active movement or shaking of the hands. She admits that she has tried to wear wrist splints and that they initially helped to alleviate her symptoms but recently have not provided relief. She does not report pain in her neck or pain radiating from her neck to her fingers. She adds that she does not have a history of hand trauma or surgery but does have controlled diabetes and a history of smoking. Examination of the left hand reveals pain and numbness that is localized to the median nerve distribution and mild thenar muscle wasting. She has full range of motion in both hands.

Questions

1. What is the likely diagnosis?
2. What is the most appropriate diagnostic modality?
3. What are the most important anatomic areas for the diagnostic workup? Why?
4. What is the appropriate timing of the diagnostic workup?

Assessment and Planning

The primary care physician suspects carpal tunnel syndrome (CTS) and attributes the patient's symptoms to compression of the median nerve by the flexor retinaculum. CTS is one of the most common hand disorders, with an incidence of nearly 50 cases per 1,000 people in the United States and a higher incidence among women.[1]

Disclosure: Research reported in this publication was supported by a Midcareer Investigator Award in Patient-Oriented Research (2K24 AR053120-06) to Dr. Kevin C. Chung. The content is solely the responsibility of the authors and does not necessarily represent the official views of the National Institutes of Health.

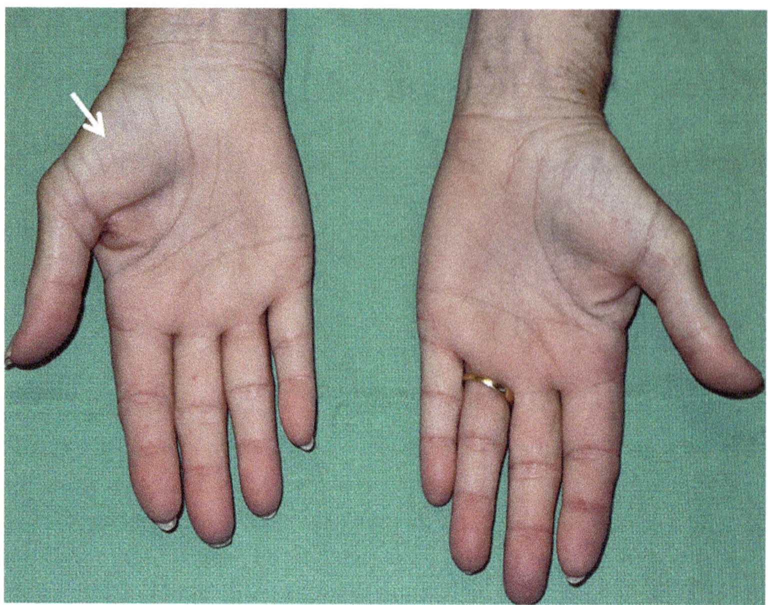

Figure 1.1. Photograph comparing the affected right hand (on left in photograph) and unaffected left hand (on right side of photograph) of a patient with carpal tunnel syndrome demonstrating thenar muscle wasting (arrow) in the affected hand.

Differential diagnoses include peripheral neuropathy, polyneuropathies, cervical radiculopathy, arthritis, pain syndromes, and vascular abnormalities. CTS can also present in combination with other nerve compression or tendon conditions, such as diabetes mellitus, Raynaud disease, thyroid disorders, nonspecific tenosynovial edema, rheumatoid tenosynovitis, trigger finger, and de Quervain disease. A detailed and careful evaluation of patient history, clinical examination tests, and laboratory tests can accurately diagnose CTS.

It is recommended that physicians utilize a variety of available diagnostic modalities to increase sensitivity and specificity of diagnosis.[2] Clinical provocative tests, including Phalen's test, a Tinel sign, and Durkan's carpal compression test, are used to assess for the presence of CTS in a clinical setting (Figure 1.1). These physical tests can locate a patient's numbness to specific nerves, but they are not reliable in assessing the severity of nerve compression.

After a clinical diagnosis of median nerve compression, an electrodiagnostic study can be performed to provide a confirmatory assessment of median nerve health and to determine the severity of injury. Nerve conduction studies (NCS) with electromyography (EMG) have been shown to identify carpal tunnel nerve compression with a high degree of accuracy and can classify the patient's CTS as mild, moderate, or severe, as well as help to rule out other diagnoses.[3] Although many classification systems exist, a common severity scale for CTS is shown in Table 1.1.[4–6] Most physicians apply a combination of patient history, one or more physical tests, and an electrodiagnostic study to arrive at a diagnosis of CTS and to determine the first course of treatment.

Table 1.1.
Severity Scale with Corresponding Nerve Conduction Study Values That Are Commonly Used in Electrodiagnosis of Carpal Tunnel Syndrome

Severity	Nerve Conduction Study Characteristics
Mild	• Normal distal motor latency (< 4.5 ms) • Slowing of median digit-wrist segment • Sensory nerve action potential amplitude below lower limit of normal
Moderate	• Distal motor latency > 4.5 ms • Abnormal median sensory latencies
Severe	• Prolonged median motor and sensory distal latencies with absence of median sensory nerve action potentials • In extreme cases, absence of thenar motor and sensory response

Oral Boards Review—Diagnostic Pearls

1. It is important for the clinician to focus on evaluating nerve health in the median distribution of the hand, which includes the thumb, index finger, middle finger, and radial half of the ring finger sensory distribution and the first and second lumbricals, opponens pollicis, abductor pollicis brevis, and flexor pollicis brevis for motor function.
2. Provocative tests
   a. Phalen's test: The patient's wrists are placed in flexion for 1 minute. If numbness occurs in the median nerve distribution, a positive test is indicated.
   b. Tinel sign: If symptoms occur during light percussion of the median nerve area, a positive test is indicated.
   c. Durkan's test: If symptoms occur during administration of pressure across the proximal palm for 30 seconds, a positive test is indicated.
3. NCS measure the speed of electricity conducting through the nerve and use EMG to quantify electrical activity of specific nerves on the innervated muscles. CTS diagnosis is confirmed if the distal median nerve sensory latency is greater than 3.5 milliseconds and motor latency is greater than 4.5 milliseconds.[7]
4. Patients with prolonged median nerve compression may present with thenar muscle atrophy on an affected hand (see Figure 1.1).
5. Nocturnal symptoms of burning and numbness are common to CTS; it is also common for patients to experience relief of CTS symptoms with shaking of the hand.

In the present case, a Tinel sign, Phalen's test, and EMG are chosen to evaluate the patient. Physical examination reveals a positive Tinel sign over the left median nerve at the carpal tunnel, as well as a positive Phalen's test. EMG results indicate severe median mononeuropathy of the patient's left wrist, characterized by mild denervation. The results are consistent with a diagnosis of CTS.

Questions

1. How do these findings influence treatment planning?
2. What is the most appropriate timing for intervention in this patient?
3. What is the appropriate treatment approach for this patient?

Decision-Making

In CTS management, in order to maximize the utility of noninvasive and cost-effective methods to relieve symptoms, nonsurgical treatment is typically recommended before surgical treatment. Patients presenting with mild or moderate symptoms are typically good candidates for nonsurgical treatment, such as splinting or steroid injection.[8]

In cases where the first selected nonsurgical treatment fails to alleviate symptoms within roughly 2 to 7 weeks, another nonsurgical treatment should be tried, assuming CTS continues to be the working diagnosis.[1] Failure of more than one conservative treatment may indicate a need for surgical intervention. There are numerous circumstances where early surgery is beneficial for the patient. For instance, if there is evidence of median nerve denervation paired with severe symptoms, the most effective treatment is prompt surgical intervention.[1] Additionally, patients may prefer early surgery and may choose to forgo nonsurgical treatments. Surgical treatment typically produces more effective results than conservative treatment and can be considered the most reliable method of treatment.[9]

In the present case, the patient had previously failed conservative treatment (splinting) and EMG results indicated severe CTS with mild median nerve denervation. These results, combined with the clinically observed thenar muscle wasting, suggest that the patient's CTS symptoms are severe and that the patient is a good candidate for surgery.

Surgical Procedure

Carpal tunnel release (CTR), the standard surgery for CTS, is the most common hand and wrist surgery performed in the United States.[1] The most important goal of CTR is complete division of the transverse carpal ligament comprising the roof of the carpal tunnel (Figure 1.2). CTR is an effective and safe surgery that has high patient-satisfaction scores and low complication rates.[1]

Open Carpal Tunnel Release (OCTR)

The patient is prepped for surgery in a supine position and the procedure is performed under tourniquet control (optional) in combination with local anesthesia. The surgeon should typically plan for a 3-cm incision that is centered on the radial border of the fourth metacarpal, with special care taken to ensure the incision line never crosses the wrist crease (see Figure 1.2). A "safe zone" can be created by drawing four intersecting lines to create a box:

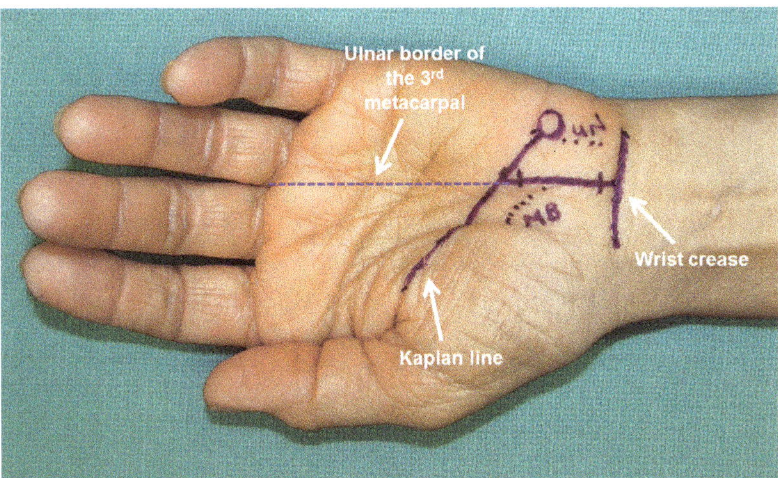

Figure 1.2. Intraoperative photograph showing the safe zone for the surgical incision for open carpal tunnel release. MB = motor branch (recurrent branch of the median nerve); UN = ulnar nerve.

1. Kaplan's cardinal line, starting at the base of the thumb and paralleling the palmar crease
2. A line across the wrist crease
3. A line perpendicular to the wrist crease from the webspace between digits 4 and 5
4. A line perpendicular to the wrist crease from the webspace between digits 2 and 3.

An important anatomic structure is usually at or near the four intersections of these lines: at the radial-distal intersection is the thenar motor branch, at the radial-proximal intersection is the palmar cutaneous branch, at the ulnar-distal intersection is the deep branch of the ulnar nerve, and at the ulnar-proximal intersection is the ulnar nerve and artery.

The first step of carpal tunnel exposure cuts through the fat layer of the wrist while using gauze to push the fat away and ensure complete visualization of the palmar fascia layer (Figure 1.3). Once the palmar fascia layer is exposed, it is important to center the hand and continue dissection of the palmar fascia until visualization of the transverse carpal ligament is achieved (Figure 1.4). Dissection of the fascia should be executed layer by layer until the surgeon notices a popping feeling of the transverse carpal ligament, indicating exposure of the carpal tunnel (Figure 1.5). Distal dissection of the transverse carpal ligament is then performed using scissors, with occasional lifting to ensure that the impeding distal transverse carpal ligament is not present. Proximal dissection of the ligament is carried out in a similar manner. The visualization of palmar fat indicates the transverse carpal ligament has been completely divided distally. Proximally, the division of the transverse carpal ligament should continue beyond the wrist crease, where it blends with the fascia of the forearm.

Endoscopic Carpal Tunnel Release (ECTR)

ECTR is a less invasive alternative to OCTR and has been shown to provide similar results. However, it is a more complicated procedure with a significant learning curve

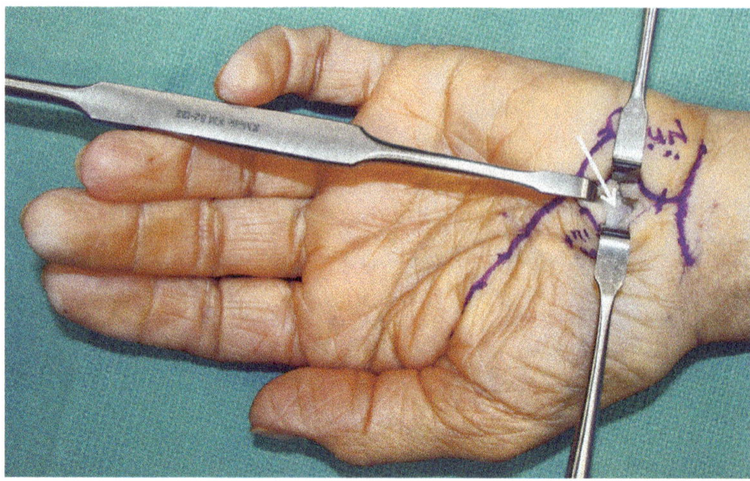

Figure 1.3. Intraoperative photograph showing the exposed palmar fascia (arrow) after the subcutaneous fat is dissected away.

and can be more costly if major complications occur, such as median nerve injury.[10] Therefore, the option of ECTR is dependent upon the surgeon's expertise, the patient's socioeconomic status, and the patient's preference.

ECTR incisions are designed to avoid disruption of the superficial fascia of the palm, and more importantly, to avoid cutting the sensory nerves in the palm that can lead to painful scars. Variation in portal technology requires either one or two small incisions. The ECTR prep is similar to the OCTR prep, and local anesthetic with tourniquet is used. A small transverse incision is made at the wrist crease, creating a hinged fascia flap for portal insertion. An additional small incision can be made distal to the first incision for a two-incision approach. After the proper incision is made, the

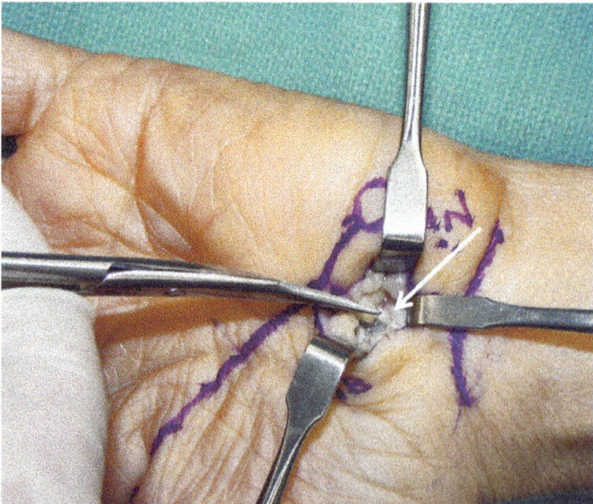

Figure 1.4. Intraoperative photograph showing the exposed transverse carpal ligament (arrow) after the palmar fascia is divided.

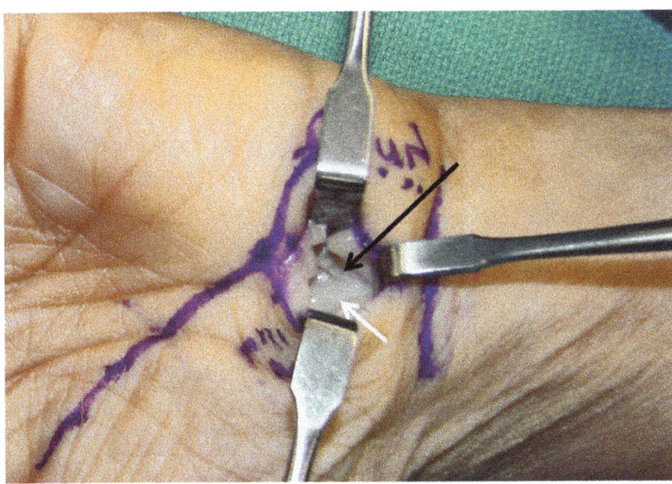

Figure 1.5. Intraoperative photograph showing the cut transverse carpal ligament (black arrow) and exposed median nerve (white arrow).

soft tissue is first freed by use of a dissector, with subsequent insertion of dilators to free space and to allow visualization for endoscopic knife placement. Once the distal border of the transverse carpal ligament is in view, the knife is introduced into the portal to begin distal-to-proximal division, with special care taken to prevent any nerve or tendon interposition. After complete division of the transverse carpal ligament is ensured by visualization of the fat pad, the endoscopic tools and tourniquet can be removed and the incision can be closed using methods similar to those in the OCTR technique.

Oral Boards Review—Management Pearls

1. Conservative treatment
   a. Splinting is best utilized for mild symptoms that may be experienced at night or during extended periods of rest. A carpal tunnel splint is an inexpensive and simple tool that provides wrist immobilization in a neutral position to decrease pressure and to enhance blood flow.
   b. Steroid injection provides maximum improvement of symptoms at 1 month but often does not produce permanent symptom alleviation, causing many patients to seek multiple injections or surgical treatment.
2. OCTR
   a. Careful planning includes measuring the distal part of the incision using a line between the base of the thumb and the pisiform.
   b. When the palmar fascia layer is exposed, and before dissection of the transverse carpal ligament, the hand must be centered to avoid cutting into Guyon's canal.
3. ECTR
   a. In ECTR, visualization is the most important factor in reducing the risk of nerve damage.

Pivot Points

1. If a patient presents with severe clinical findings and EMG results suggestive of CTS, prompt surgical management is recommended.
2. If poor visualization is encountered at any point in an ECTR procedure, the surgeon should be prepared to switch to the OCTR technique.

Aftercare

Postoperative wrist immobilization is not necessary after carpal tunnel surgery, as it has been shown to offer no benefit in patient outcomes. Additionally, restricted motion of the wrist after surgery may increase the risk of adhesions and stiffness, which could delay the patient's ability to return to work and other activities.[1] Also, there is limited and low-quality evidence suggesting a significant benefit of postoperative rehabilitation or therapy for CTR patients.[11]

Complications and Management

CTR is generally safe, provided that the surgeon understands the intricate anatomy during exposure and division of the transverse carpal ligament. When complications do occur, they can lead to treatment failure, patient dissatisfaction, and persistent symptoms.[12] Intraoperative complications typically include injury to branches of nerves, arteries, or tendons as a result of incorrect incision placement or excessive proximal or distal dissection. Complications arising from unintended injury to the common digital nerves, thenar branch, and palmar cutaneous branch may cause neuromas, persistent paresthesias, weakness of grip strength, and loss of hand function. Additionally, it is important to be mindful of nerve anatomy variations, such as a transligamentous course of the thenar branch of the median nerve, which occurs in approximately 23% of cases.

Postoperative complications are uncommon after CTR and could include infection, postoperative pain, or tendon problems. Postoperative pain is experienced at the site of the incision or at the thenar muscle and can increase with pressure or muscle use, which is commonly termed pillar pain. Pillar pain may occur as a result of swelling or instability of thenar insertions and should be treated with scar massage.

CTR may be considered a failure if symptom improvement is not experienced after 12 months.[1,12] Treatment failure can occur as a result of incomplete release, recurrent compression, or incorrect CTS diagnosis. The presence of diabetes and a smoking history may also contribute to a slower recovery or a higher recurrence rate. In some cases, persistent symptoms after surgical treatment indicate an incorrect CTS diagnosis, which should lead the surgeon to revisit alternative diagnoses.

Complication management should start with a detailed evaluation of the patient's preoperative and postoperative complaint history to identify the complication type. If the patient has persistent symptoms before and after surgery, it is likely that CTS was incorrectly diagnosed or incomplete release of the transverse carpal ligament has occurred. If the patient has relief of symptoms immediately after surgery, but symptoms recur in a delayed fashion, recurrent compression of the median nerve from scarring around the nerve or tenosynovitis within the flexor tendon sheath may require release of the carpal tunnel and extensive flexor tenosynovectomy.

> **Oral Boards Review—Complications Pearls**
>
> 1. Care must be taken to prevent excessive dissection in both the proximal and distal transverse carpal ligament sites. Overdissection distally may cause injury to the common digital nerves and thenar branch, whereas overdissection proximally may increase the risk of injury to the palmar cutaneous branch injury.
> 2. Incomplete release is the most common reason for reoperation in CTS patients, and it can occur at the distal end of the carpal ligament proper or at the flexor retinaculum, producing persistent CTS symptoms.
> 3. In cases with complications involving nerve compression, EMG can be a useful tool to gauge progression of worsening symptoms.

Evidence and Outcomes

Many different disease- and region-specific instruments have been used to assess outcomes of CTS treatment.[1] Disease-specific instruments, such as the Boston Carpal Tunnel Questionnaire, are the most responsive instruments to measure small differences in outcome and should be used for evaluating specific differences in outcome. Region-specific instruments, such as the Michigan Hand Outcomes Questionnaire (MHQ) and the Disabilities of the Arm, Shoulder, and Hand (DASH) questionnaire, are also responsive to CTS outcomes and may assess a wider outcome of CTS treatment on upper extremity health.

There are many publications about use of these instruments to assess the effectiveness of both nonoperative and operative treatments in alleviating CTS symptoms. For example, one randomized controlled trial investigated the efficacy of night splinting and found that splints improved symptoms in all patients and significantly reduced Boston Carpal Tunnel Questionnaire scores in patients compared to controls.[13] Corticosteroid injections have demonstrated similar therapeutic utility for short-term CTS management. A double-blinded, placebo-controlled trial compared patients receiving steroid injections beneath the transverse carpal ligament to control patients receiving placebo injections and found that steroid injections significantly improved patient satisfaction, median nerve conduction, and performance on functional assessments.[14] However, when the authors evaluated the steroid injection treatment group 18 months after initial injections, half of the patients experienced a return of symptoms and were referred for surgical release. These findings were mirrored in another study that compared splinting, splinting plus local steroid injection, and OCTR outcomes in patients 3 and 6 months after treatment.[15] In the study, the researchers found that patient satisfaction, EMG values, and Boston Carpal Tunnel Questionnaire scores improved similarly for all groups at the 3-month follow-up. Despite these improvements, at the 6-month visit, clinical and EMG values deteriorated for splinting and steroid treatments, whereas OCTR patients experienced continued improvement. The results of these studies suggest that, although splinting and corticosteroid injections can successfully improve symptoms and delay surgical treatment, surgery may be the best treatment for long-term CTS management.

References

1. Keith MW, Masear V, Chung KC, et al. American Academy of Orthopaedic Surgeons Clinical Practice Guideline on the treatment of carpal tunnel syndrome. *J Bone Joint Surg Am*. 2010;92:218–219.
2. Keith MW, Masear V, Chung KC, et al: American Academy of Orthopaedic Surgeons Clinical Practice Guideline on diagnosis of carpal tunnel syndrome. *J Bone Joint Surg Am*. 2009;91:2478–2479.
3. Priganc VW, Henry SM. The relationship among five common carpal tunnel syndrome tests and the severity of carpal tunnel syndrome. *J Hand Ther*. 2003;16:225–236.
4. Bland JD. A neurophysiological grading scale for carpal tunnel syndrome. *Muscle Nerve*. 2000;23:1280–1283.
5. Padua L, LoMonaco M, Gregori B, Valente EM, Padua R, Tonali P. Neurophysiological classification and sensitivity in 500 carpal tunnel syndrome hands. *Acta Neurol Scand*. 1997;96:211–217.
6. Stevens JC. AAEM minimonograph #26: the electrodiagnosis of carpal tunnel syndrome. American Association of Electrodiagnostic Medicine. *Muscle Nerve*. 1997;20:1477–1486.
7. Jablecki CK, Andary MT, So YT, Wilkins DE, Williams FH. Literature review of the usefulness of nerve conduction studies and electromyography for the evaluation of patients with carpal tunnel syndrome. AAEM Quality Assurance Committee. *Muscle Nerve*. 1993;16:1392–1414.
8. Ono S, Clapham PJ, Chung KC. Optimal management of carpal tunnel syndrome. *Int J Gen Med*. 2010;3:255–261.
9. Kim PT, Lee HJ, Kim TG, Jeon IH. Current approaches for carpal tunnel syndrome. *Clin Orthop Surg*. 2014;6:253–257.
10. Chung KC, Walters MR, Greenfield ML, Chernew ME. Endoscopic versus open carpal tunnel release: a cost-effectiveness analysis. *Plast Reconstr Surg*. 1998;102:1089–1099.
11. Peters S, Page MJ, Coppieters MW, Ross M, Johnston V. Rehabilitation following carpal tunnel release. *Cochrane Database Syst Rev*. 2016;2:CD004158.
12. Karl JW, Gancarczyk SM, Strauch RJ. Complications of carpal tunnel release. *Orthop Clin North Am*. 2016;47:425–433.
13. Manente G, Torrieri F, Di Blasio F, Staniscia T, Romano F, Uncini A. An innovative hand brace for carpal tunnel syndrome: a randomized controlled trial. *Muscle Nerve*. 2001;24:1020–1025.
14. Armstrong T, Devor W, Borschel L, Contreras R. Intracarpal steroid injection is safe and effective for short-term management of carpal tunnel syndrome. *Muscle Nerve*. 2004;29:82–88.
15. Ucan H, Yagci I, Yilmaz L, Yagmurlu F, Keskin D, Bodur H. Comparison of splinting, splinting plus local steroid injection and open carpal tunnel release outcomes in idiopathic carpal tunnel syndrome. *Rheumatol Int*. 2006;27:45–51.

Failed Carpal Tunnel Release—Recurrent Carpal Tunnel Syndrome

Christopher J. Winfree

2

Case Presentation

A 63-year-old, right-handed female, with no significant past medical history, presents with 6 months of right hand pain. The pain is worse at night and sometimes awakens her from sleep. She also notes numbness in the first three digits of her hand and clumsiness, manifesting as worsening handwriting and difficulty buttoning buttons. Physical examination is notable for median sensory deficits, sparing the palmar cutaneous division, and weakness of the abductor pollicis brevis muscle. Electrodiagnostic studies confirm a median neuropathy at the wrist. After a trial of nonoperative management, including splinting and steroid injections, the patient undergoes an uneventful, mini-open carpal tunnel release (CTR). She presents 1 month postoperatively with persistent pain in the hand.

Questions

1. What is the most common cause of persistent pain after CTR?
2. What are other, less common causes of persistent pain after CTR?
3. What are the best diagnostic tests to perform at this point?

Oral Boards Review—Diagnostic Pearls

1. The main differential diagnoses are insufficient decompression, scarring and re-entrapment, iatrogenic nerve injury, and a new pain syndrome.
2. The history, physical examination, electrodiagnostic tests, and imaging can help differentiate between the diagnostic considerations:
   a. Insufficient decompression/entrapment at a site not addressed by surgery
      i. Symptoms were never relieved by surgery and are similar to preoperative symptoms.
      ii. Postoperative physical examination findings are similar to preoperative findings.
      iii. Postoperative electrodiagnostic findings are similar to preoperative findings. More detailed studies, including inching studies or the addition of more muscles for electromyography, may reveal a site of entrapment at a different level than that addressed by surgery.

iv. Imaging may reveal signs of entrapment at a site not addressed by surgery or, in the case of inadequate decompression, may reveal only persistent changes in the affected nerve.

b. Scarring and re-entrapment
   i. Symptoms were relieved for several weeks after surgery but then recurred.
   ii. Postoperative physical examination findings are similar to preoperative findings.
   iii. Postoperative electrodiagnostic findings are roughly similar to preoperative findings.
   iv. Imaging reveals nerve abnormalities at the site of previous entrapment.

c. Iatrogenic nerve injury
   i. New postoperative symptoms of numbness or weakness occur that were not present preoperatively.
   ii. Postoperative physical examination finds new numbness or weakness that was not present preoperatively.
   iii. Postoperative electrodiagnostic studies find new conduction abnormalities or denervation changes.
   iv. If the images are of sufficiently high quality, they may reveal the location of the injury (e.g., neuroma-in-continuity or nerve transection).

d. New pain syndrome
   i. Postoperative pain is different from the preoperative pain, especially if the pain transcends the confines of the territory of the entrapped nerve.
   ii. Physical examination may reveal signs of an infection, hematoma, inflammatory process, regional pain syndrome, or another process.
   iii. Electrodiagnostic studies should rule out a new nerve injury. In the case of complex regional pain syndrome (CRPS) type II (CRPS-II), electrodiagnostic studies can confirm that a new nerve injury has contributed to the emergence of the new pain syndrome.
   iv. Imaging of the surgical site and nerve may reveal the presence of an infection, hematoma, fluid collection, inflammation, or another process.

Assessment and Planning

In this case, the history helps clarify the diagnosis. Detailed questioning reveals that the patient's symptoms were never relieved by the surgery and are essentially the same as preoperatively. This suggests that the nerve was insufficiently decompressed at the time of surgery. Large-scale meta-analyses have shown that the success rates after typical CTR are around 85%.[1,2] The most common cause of failure to improve after CTR is failure to completely divide the transverse carpal tunnel ligament at the time of surgery. In these cases, one would expect the patient to have persistent, similar symptoms after surgery. This patient does not report postoperative symptom relief, so there is no reason to think that scarring and re-entrapment are likely. Also, the patient does not report the emergence of any new problems, such as numbness, weakness, swelling, or wound drainage, so a new nerve injury, infectious process, or regional pain syndrome is unlikely to be present.

The physical examination corroborates the history in this case. Detailed neurologic examination reveals the same pattern of deficits the patient displayed preoperatively. This suggests that the same neurologic issue is present, rather than a new problem. When the examination reveals new deficits, a new nerve injury should be suspected. If additional findings are present, such as pain and/or allodynia that transcends the confines of the affected nerve distribution, swelling, color abnormalities, or temperature abnormalities, a regional pain syndrome may be present. In some cases, patients may be diagnosed with CRPS when specific clinical criteria are met and other causes are excluded.

In this case, electrodiagnostic studies reveal postoperative findings similar to those that were present preoperatively. This suggests that there is persistent nerve entrapment. There are no new conduction abnormalities or new denervation changes to suggest a new nerve injury. Electrodiagnostic studies are important in these cases and are typically performed in a delayed fashion when patients have persistent symptoms after nerve decompression. There are no guidelines to suggest when the studies should be performed. One rough guide is that axonal regrowth after entrapment injury occurs at a rate of approximately 1 inch per month. Thus, a minimum of 3 months will normally be required to get meaningful nerve conduction studies across a clinically useful nerve segment. However, earlier electrodiagnostics, ideally after the 3-week time point, may be useful if a new nerve injury is suspected, as denervation changes in the affected muscles normally manifest by then. In this case, electrodiagnostic studies were performed and included inching studies across the elbow and wrist. They revealed persistent slowing across the wrist and normal conduction across the elbow and forearm, thus ruling out a more proximal level of entrapment.

Given that persistent nerve entrapment is suspected, this patient undergoes a high-resolution diagnostic ultrasound of the median nerve at the operative site, as well as more proximally along the forearm and elbow to ensure that entrapment at a more proximal level was not missed. The study reveals nerve flattening and fascicular compression within the carpal tunnel and enlargement of the nerve proximal to the carpal tunnel. These data corroborate the electrodiagnostic studies. Imaging showed no evidence of an operative-site fluid collection, which suggests absence of an infection. Also, imaging revealed normal postoperative changes in the surrounding tissues, which suggests that no significant inflammatory process was present.

High-resolution diagnostic ultrasound and MR neurography are imaging modalities that can be useful for the diagnosis of persistent pain after nerve decompression.[3–6] Unfortunately, these studies are not available at all centers. In cases where these imaging modalities are not available, the surgeon must make educated decisions based on the available clinical and electrodiagnostic data. When these modalities are available, the imaging can show persistent flattening, fascicular compression, and/or hyperintensity at the site of entrapment. When a new nerve injury is present, imaging can reveal nerve transection, neuroma, and/or disordered fascicular architecture across the injured nerve segment.

Questions

1. Given the persistent nerve entrapment, what are the most appropriate nonsurgical treatment options at this point?
2. If nonsurgical treatment options are ineffective, are there appropriate surgical treatment options?
3. How does this treatment differ from the initial treatment plan?

Decision-Making and Surgical Procedure

In this case, the patient has persistent neuropathic pain in the hand, among her other symptoms. In the early postoperative period, it is appropriate to treat this neuropathic pain using oral medications. Anticonvulsants represent first-line agents for the treatment of neuropathic pain. Their use is generally straightforward, and although they can have some side effects, they tend to have few contraindications and drug–drug interactions. Antidepressants can be effective for neuropathic pain, but their administration can be more complicated, and they tend to have more drug–drug interactions and contraindications than the anticonvulsants. Baclofen, topical compounded medications, and other topical therapies, such as local anesthetic patches, are additional options for the treatment of neuropathic pain. Opioids may be used if the pain is sufficiently severe and is unrelieved by the neuropathic pain medications. All of these medications may be used alone or in combination to keep side effects to a minimum. Nerve blocks and/or cortisone injections may play a role as well.[7] In these cases, the treatment can get complicated, and it is reasonable to refer the patient to a dedicated pain management specialist for this phase of treatment. Physical and occupational therapy may also be employed at this point to assist in the relief of pain. It is appropriate to institute a brief trial (4–6 weeks) of nonoperative therapy before considering surgical treatment.

In the patient in the case presented here, the less invasive pain management strategies are ineffective. Thus, redo CTR is the recommended treatment option. The goal of the surgery is to completely divide the transverse carpal ligament from the palmar fat pad into the fascia of the distal wrist. A typical approach would be to reopen the original incision, extending the incision slightly proximally and distally to ensure visualization of the nerve proximal and distal to the previous exposure. A more extensile exposure is not required, as long as the nerve is sufficiently decompressed safely through the more limited exposure. If the initial operation was done endoscopically, then the second operation should be done in a mini-open fashion. The key to any reoperation is to address the reason for failure of the first operation, which is usually failure to completely divide the transverse carpal ligament.

Some surgeons utilize nerve wraps, vascularized flaps, or fat pad transfers for recurrent carpal tunnel syndrome, but the benefits of these techniques remain somewhat controversial.[8–10]

Oral Boards Review—Management Pearls

1. The goal is to completely decompress the median nerve across the carpal tunnel.
2. The original incision is used and may be extended as needed to ensure complete decompression of the nerve and to limit the risk of nerve injury.
3. Some surgeons utilize nerve wraps, vascularized flaps, or fat pad transfers for recurrent carpal tunnel syndrome, but the benefits of these techniques remain somewhat controversial.

Pivot Points and Complication Pearls

1. If the patient has evidence of a new nerve injury, then the injury must be treated accordingly.
   a. Nerve transections can be treated as soon as they are discovered; if acute, they may be amenable to direct repair, and, if they are delayed, they may be treated with neuroma excision and graft repair.
   b. Neuromas-in-continuity undergo exploration at the 3-month post-injury time point.
   c. Nonconducting neuromas-in-continuity undergo neuroma excision and graft repair, as needed.
   d. Painful sensory neuromas may undergo excision, along with burial of the proximal end into bone or muscle if repair is not feasible (e.g., if no distal stump can be found).
2. If the patient has evidence of an infection or some other process, then it should be treated accordingly.
   a. Infections are cultured and are treated with antibiotics and wound washout when a significant purulent collection requires drainage.
   b. Some inflammatory conditions may respond to a course of oral steroids.
   c. Poorly controlled diabetes, if present, should be brought under better control.
3. If the patient has evidence of a regional pain syndrome, it should be treated appropriately.
   a. CRPS-I should be treated with aggressive pain management strategies and physical therapy.
   b. CRPS-II, if present and confirmed by electrodiagnostic studies and/or nerve imaging, should be treated with nerve repair and simultaneous aggressive pain management strategies to avoid exacerbating the pain problem.
   c. Patients whose symptoms and signs do not fully satisfy the diagnostic criteria for CRPS should be offered aggressive pain management and physical therapy strategies, as if CRPS were present.
   d. Early and aggressive control of pain is associated with better outcomes than if the pain is undertreated.

Aftercare

In this case, the patient undergoes an uneventful redo mini-open CTR. At the time of surgery, a portion of undivided transverse carpal ligament is seen and divided. Aftercare is similar to that for the initial CTR.

Complications and Management

Unfortunately, any of the postoperative complications already mentioned can occur after reoperation. The risk of nerve injury is greater during redo CTR. The management and workup of any of these complications are the same as described above.

Evidence and Outcomes

The reoperation rate after CTR is approximately 10%.[11–15] Not surprisingly, the outcomes after redo CTR are worse than after a first decompression procedure, with persistent symptoms following revision surgery in 25% to 90% of patients.[16] A number of factors that are associated with poor outcomes after revision surgery have been identified, including the presence of intraneural fibrosis, severe preoperative sensory deficit, higher baseline pain, neuroma of the palmar cutaneous branch, cases associated with worker's compensation claims, and the number of previous surgeries.[17,18] Successful symptomatic relief with a diagnostic cortisone injection has been shown to predict success with revision surgery and may be a good screening test to determine surgical candidacy.[7] Some surgeons continue to favor decompression with vascularized flap coverage as opposed to repeat decompression alone, with some studies citing better outcomes.[19] This, however, remains controversial.

References

1. Sayegh ET, Strauch RJ. Open versus endoscopic carpal tunnel release: a meta-analysis of randomized controlled trials. *Clin Orthop Relat Res*. 2015;473:1120–1132.
2. Zuo D, Zhou Z, Wang H, et al. Endoscopic versus open carpal tunnel release for idiopathic carpal tunnel syndrome: a meta-analysis of randomized controlled trials. *J Orthop Surg Res*. 2015;10:12.
3. Cartwright MS, Hobson-Webb LD, Boon AJ, et al. Evidence-based guideline: neuromuscular ultrasound for the diagnosis of carpal tunnel syndrome. *Muscle Nerve*. 2012;46:287–293.
4. Fowler JR, Maltenfort MG, Ilyas AM. Ultrasound as a first-line test in the diagnosis of carpal tunnel syndrome: a cost-effectiveness analysis. *Clin Orthop Relat Res*. 2013;471:932–937.
5. Taghizadeh R, Tahir A, Stevenson S, Barnes DE, Spratt JD, Erdmann MW. The role of MRI in the diagnosis of recurrent/persistent carpal tunnel syndrome: a radiological and intra-operative correlation. *J Plast Reconstr Aesthetic Surg*. 2011;64:1250–1252.
6. Todnem K, Sand T. Neurography for diagnosing carpal tunnel syndrome [in Norwegian]. *Tidsskr Nor Laegeforen*. 2013;133:170–173.
7. Beck JD, Brothers JG, Maloney PJ, Deegan JH, Tang X, Klena JC. Predicting the outcome of revision carpal tunnel release. *J Hand Surg Am*. 2012;37:282–287.

8. Craft RO, Duncan SF, Smith AA. Management of recurrent carpal tunnel syndrome with microneurolysis and the hypothenar fat pad flap. *Hand (N Y)*. 2007;2:85–89.
9. Fusetti C, Garavaglia G, Mathoulin C, Petri JG, Lucchina S. A reliable and simple solution for recalcitrant carpal tunnel syndrome: the hypothenar fat pad flap. *Am J Orthop (Belle Mead NJ)*. 2009;38:181–186.
10. Soltani AM, Allan BJ, Best MJ, Mir HS, Panthaki ZJ. Revision decompression and collagen nerve wrap for recurrent and persistent compression neuropathies of the upper extremity. *Ann Plast Surg*. 2014;72:572–578.
11. Bande S, De Smet L, Fabry G. The results of carpal tunnel release: open versus endoscopic technique. *J Hand Surg Br*. 1994;19:14–17.
12. Cobb TK, Amadio PC. Reoperation for carpal tunnel syndrome. *Hand Clin*. 1996;12:313–323.
13. Concannon MJ, Brownfield ML, Puckett CL. The incidence of recurrence after endoscopic carpal tunnel release. *Plast Reconstr Surg*. 2000;105:1662–1665.
14. Kulick RG. Carpal tunnel syndrome. *Orthop Clin North Am*. 1996;27:345–354.
15. Stutz N, Gohritz A, van Schoonhoven J, Lanz U. Revision surgery after carpal tunnel release—analysis of the pathology in 200 cases during a 2 year period. *J Hand Surg Br*. 2006;31:68–71.
16. Steyers CM. Recurrent carpal tunnel syndrome. *Hand Clin*. 2002;18:339–345.
17. Djerbi I, Cesar M, Lenoir H, Coulet B, Lazerges C, Chammas M. Revision surgery for recurrent and persistent carpal tunnel syndrome: Clinical results and factors affecting outcomes. *Chir Main*. 2015;34:312–317.
18. Zieske L, Ebersole GC, Davidge K, Fox I, Mackinnon SE. Revision carpal tunnel surgery: a 10-year review of intraoperative findings and outcomes. *J Hand Surg Am*. 2013;38:1530–1539.
19. Soltani AM, Allan BJ, Best MJ, Mir HS, Panthaki ZJ. A systematic review of the literature on the outcomes of treatment for recurrent and persistent carpal tunnel syndrome. *Plast Reconstr Surg*. 2013;132:114–121.

Median Neuropathy—Pronator Teres Syndrome and Anterior Interosseous Neuropathy

Russell A. Payne and Kimberly S. Harbaugh

3

Case Presentation

A 38-year-old mason presents to the neurosurgery peripheral nerve clinic with a complaint of left-sided, dull, achy forearm pain with paresthesias over the thenar eminence, thumb, index and middle fingers, and radial surface of the palm. The symptoms were insidious in their onset and have persisted for several months. His pain and paresthesias are worsened when he extends the wrist or pronates the forearm. His medical history is unremarkable. He has not had recent trauma to the arm or forearm and he reports no recent illnesses or surgeries. Physical examination reveals no asymmetry or atrophy on inspection and no masses on palpation. Strength testing shows no overt weakness and there is no change in sensation to light touch, pinprick, or temperature on sensory examination. Phalen's test is negative. A Tinel sign is present at the antecubital fossa, and it reproduces the paresthesias in the hand. Electromyography and nerve conduction studies are unremarkable.

Questions

1. Which nerve is affected and what is its course?
2. Where is the site of nerve entrapment? What findings on physical examination help localize the area of involvement?
3. What are the classic areas of entrapment that can result in the syndrome in the case presented?
4. How is this syndrome distinguished from carpal tunnel syndrome (CTS) and anterior interosseous syndrome (AIS)?
5. What additional studies may be beneficial?

Assessment and Planning

After examination, the neurosurgeon suspects involvement of the median nerve (MN) proximal to the carpal tunnel.

The MN is formed by contributions from the medial and lateral cords. The lateral cord contribution carries sensory fibers, while the medial cord contribution carries motor fibers. These contributions meet and give rise to the MN on the surface of the brachial artery. The MN first runs lateral to the artery, crosses at the insertion of the deltoid, and runs medial to the artery while in the neurovascular bundle between the triceps and biceps muscles. At the elbow, the nerve travels on top of the brachialis muscle until it passes once more over the brachial artery and beneath the lacertus fibrosus (bicipital aponeurosis). It then provides innervation to the pronator teres muscle (PT) before passing between its superficial and deep heads. Next, it passes deep to the flexor digitorum superficialis muscle (FDS) and its fibrous ridge (sublimis bridge) to run between the FDS and flexor digitorum profundus muscle (FDP). Just after passing deep to the fibrous ridge of the FDS, about 5 to 8 cm distal to the medial epicondyle, the MN gives off its largest motor branch, the anterior interosseous nerve (AIN), from the radial side. The MN proper continues between the flexor muscles until it emerges from beneath the flexor tendons to enter the carpal tunnel. Importantly, about 3 cm proximal to the flexor retinaculum, the palmar cutaneous nerve arises from the MN to travel on the ulnar side of the flexor carpi radialis (FCR) tendon.

In this case, numbness over the radial three digits of the hand points to MN involvement somewhere along its course. The fact that there are paresthesias over the radial aspect of the palm points to involvement of the nerve proximal to the emergence of the palmar cutaneous branch of the MN. The pain in the proximal forearm and Tinel sign over the MN course in the antecubital fossa further serve to localize the area of entrapment to the region of the elbow. The surgeon diagnoses the patient with pronator syndrome (PS), which is compression of the MN proximal to the carpal tunnel.

There are several well-known areas of entrapment that can be present in PS, including the supracondylar process and ligament of Struthers (when present), the lacertus fibrosus, between the heads of the PT, and the fibrous ridge of the FDS muscle.[1–5] Other, less common causes have also been described, including the presence of anomalous muscles (e.g., Gantzer's muscle).[6,7]

PS, unlike CTS, does not present with nocturnal symptoms. On physical examination, it is distinguished from MN compression at the wrist by involvement of the palmar cutaneous branch of the MN, negative provocative maneuvers at the carpal tunnel (e.g., Durkan's compression test and Phalen's test), and the presence of a Tinel sign in the proximal forearm (and not at the carpal tunnel). Typically, with MN compression proximal to the wrist, there is increased pain upon palpation of the PT, as well as pain upon resisted elbow flexion, pronation of the forearm, and flexion of the middle finger. Weakness is not usually present on strength testing.

Involvement of the AIN results in pinch-grasp weakness between the thumb and index finger without sensory disturbance. Difficulty with pinch grasp results from flexion weakness of the distal phalanges of the thumb (flexor pollicis longus; FPL) and index finger (FDP). The AIN travels between the heads of the PT, continues on the surface of the FDP, and then travels on the volar surface of the interosseous membrane. It provides innervation to the FPL, radial portion of the FDP, and pronator quadratus (PQ). Though there are some terminal branches of the AIN that provide joint sensation, there are no branches that provide cutaneous innervation. Anterior interosseous neuropathy is distinguished from CTS and PS in that it does not affect the muscles of the thenar eminence and does not result in sensory abnormalities.

Whereas PS often is the result of nerve compression, AIS is most commonly attributable to neuralgic amyotrophy. Other causes include entrapment by muscles or tendinous attachments. Thrombosis of the ulnar collaterals or the anterior interosseous vessels has also been implicated. Supracondylar humeral fractures are a well-documented cause of AIN palsy in children but are not common in adults.[8] Tumors or mass lesions can lead to compression of the AIN, and penetrating injuries to the antecubital fossa may cause nerve transection.

Diagnostic studies in the evaluation of PS may include MR imaging or ultrasound evaluation of the nerve at the elbow. MR imaging is typically not helpful for diagnosis and management of PS and AIS; however, it can be used to rule out tendon rupture or mass lesion. A variety of mass lesions have been associated with PS, including ganglion cysts, lipomas, and schwannomas.[9–12] An X-ray of the distal humerus may be indicated to rule out the presence of a supracondylar process, which can be identified only on oblique radiographs.[4,13] Electrodiagnostic studies may be useful to exclude other diagnoses, such as CTS and cervical radiculopathy, but, because of the dynamic nature of PS, they are frequently normal (positive in 50% of patients with PS).[14] Therefore, a negative test should not be used to exclude the syndrome. When electrodiagnostics are positive, the affected muscles may exhibit fibrillations, sharp waves, abnormal latency, and/or abnormal compound motor action potentials. Unlike with cervical radiculopathy, with PS, sensory nerve action potentials may also be affected.

Oral Boards Review–Diagnostic Pearls

1. History and physical examination for the diagnosis of PS:
    a. Common presenting symptoms include pain in the volar forearm and paresthesias in the MN distribution, including the radial palm. Weakness is not usually present on motor examination.
    b. Specific provocative maneuvers can be used to help locate the area of entrapment:
        i. Pronation against resistance aggravates compression at the PT.
        ii. Elbow flexion against resistance with the forearm supinated worsens compression symptoms when entrapment is at the lacertus fibrosus.
        iii. Entrapment at the fibrous edge of the FDS is provoked by flexion of the proximal interphalangeal joint of the middle finger against resistance.
    c. Numbness and/or paresthesias in the distribution of the palmar cutaneous nerve help distinguish PS from CTS. An exception to this is when patients have already had carpal tunnel decompression with a palmar incision.
2. Physical examination for diagnosis of AIS:
    a. On physical examination, weakness of the FPL and FDP results in the inability to make an "OK" sign with the thumb and index finger (Kiloh-Nevin sign), due to the lack of flexion of the distal phalanx of the thumb and index finger.
    b. The lack of sensory involvement distinguishes AIS from PS and CTS.

3. It is important to rule out "upstream" causes of weakness, such as spinal nerve root involvement or brachial plexopathy. The nondermatomal distribution of pain, lack of neck pain, and normal triceps, brachioradialis, and biceps tendon reflexes help to separate the two.
4. A careful history is imperative. Pain for hours to days preceding flaccid paralysis is typical of neuralgic amyotrophy (i.e., Parsonage-Turner syndrome), whereas a history of the onset of pain in the antecubital fossa in someone performing repetitive upper extremity activities is more typical of PS.

Questions

1. What is the first-line treatment for PS?
2. What are the components of conservative therapy?
3. What is the treatment for PS or AIS should it be due to neuralgic amyotrophy?

Decision-Making

In most cases of PS, conservative management is the first-line treatment. Conservative treatment includes anti-inflammatory medications as well as limitation of the activities that cause or aggravate symptoms. When these measures fail to resolve symptoms, some have recommended immobilization using a long arm splint with the elbow flexed to 90°, the forearm in slight pronation, and the wrist slightly flexed.[4,15] The authors have not used splints in their patients.

Treatment for both PS and AIS is controversial, and there is no clear consensus. There are no randomized controlled trials assessing the role of surgery in these syndromes. There does seem to be an agreement in the literature that, in the absence of traumatic injury or a space-occupying lesion, a trial of conservative, nonsurgical management should be implemented. Duration of conservative treatment varies widely among authors. The rate of favorable response to a range of conservative therapies for PS has been reported to be approximately 50%, while symptom improvement after surgical decompression has been quoted to be as high as 77% to 92%.[3,14,16–21]

In the setting of neuralgic amyotrophy with AIN involvement, the mainstay of initial treatment should be conservative and not surgical, because the condition is usually self-limiting. However, there are surgeons who advocate surgical release if there is no improvement in 3 to 9 months, particularly if the etiology is not thought to be neuralgic amyotrophy, and there are some reports of delayed improvement after surgery.[22–26]

In the case presented, despite adhering faithfully to the conservative measures, the patient returns several months later with worsening symptoms. An X-ray of the elbow excludes the possibility of a supracondylar process. An MR image is acquired and no space-occupying lesion or tendon rupture is identified. The patient's examination findings remain consistent with MN compression at the level of the antecubital fossa.

In our practice, we look for signs of MN compression on clinical exam. We do acquire MR imaging and EMG studies. Many patients will have evidence of EMG changes, but it is not a prerequisite for surgery. MR imaging often will show a dense tendinous band adjacent to or compressing the nerve, which helps direct surgical intervention. In cases of Parsonage-Turner syndrome, it is our practice to monitor the patient for a minimum of 6 months to allow for spontaneous recovery. Surgical intervention is reserved for cases that show no improvement and have signs and symptoms of nerve compression.

Questions

1. What are the areas of potential entrapment, listed proximally to distally?
2. What is the most common site of entrapment in the forearm?
3. What is the prevalence of supracondylar processes in the general population?
4. At approximately what level does the AIN branch from the MN?
5. What muscles receive branches from the MN in the forearm?

Surgical Procedure

The goal of surgery should be to decompress the MN along its length in the antecubital fossa and forearm. The areas of potential entrapment include the ligament of Struthers, the lacertus fibrosus, the PT, and the fibrous ridge of the FDS. Several approaches have been advocated in the literature, including minimally invasive and endoscopic techniques.[19,21,27] We advocate the use of a lazy S incision in order to expose all possible areas of compression and to allow systematic evaluation of each of the sites.

A supracondylar process is rare; it has been reported in only about 0.7% to 2.7% of the population and allows for attachment of the ligament of Struthers. It accounts for only 0.5% of cases of MN entrapment at the elbow.[1,4,13]

The most common sites of entrapment in the forearm are the PT, the fibrous arch of the FDS, and finally the bicipital aponeurosis. The fibrous band of the PT can be found about 3 to 7.5 cm distal to the epicondylar line of the humerus. The fibrous arch of the FDS is found distal to the PT and can be as proximal as 6.5 cm distal to the epicondylar line of the humerus.

Care should be taken not to damage the muscular branches innervating the PT and FDS. The AIN and its branches to the FPL and the radial portion of the FDP should also be carefully preserved.

Procedure Details

1. A lazy S incision is centered over the antecubital fossa. Proximal to the elbow, it starts medially, crosses over the antecubital fossa, and ends over the radial surface of the forearm (Figure 3.1).
2. The skin is incised and dissection is carried down to the level of the overlying fascia and the lacertus fibrosus, which can be seen fanning out from the biceps tendon (Figure 3.2).
3. Proximal to the elbow, the MN can be identified under the fascia as it travels in the neurovascular bundle between the biceps and triceps muscles. It is in this location

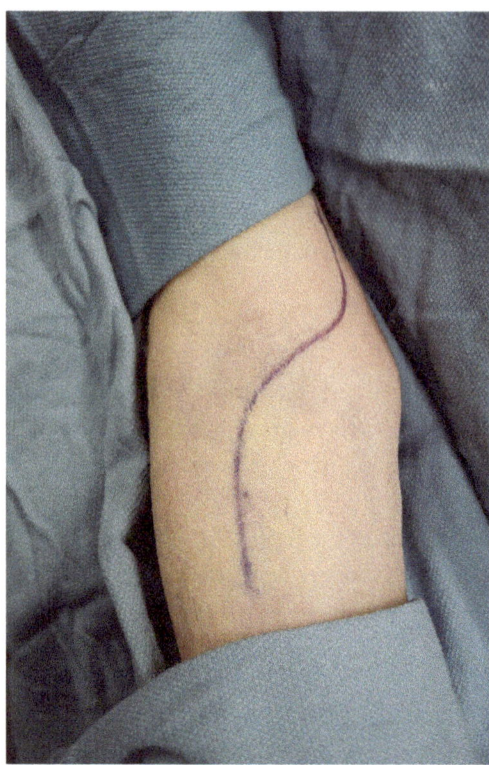

Figure 3.1. A lazy S incision is centered over the antecubital fossa. Proximal to the elbow, it starts medially, crosses over the antecubital fossa, and ends over the radial surface of the forearm.

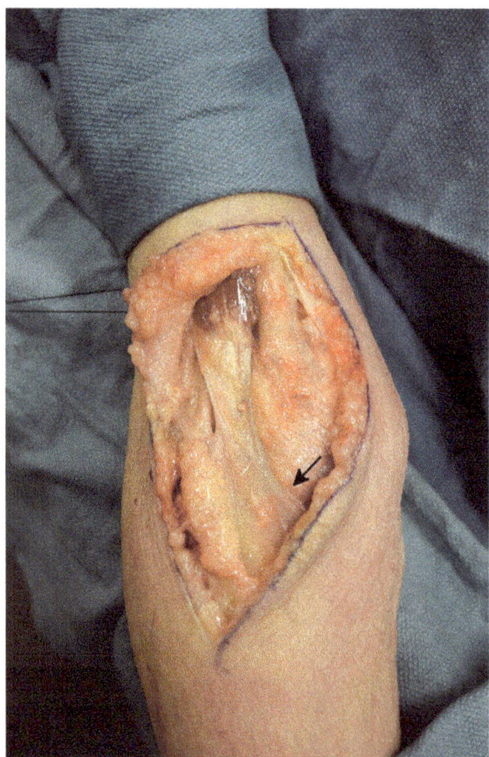

Figure 3.2. Exposure to the level of the fascia and lacertus fibrosus, seen fanning out from the biceps tendon (black arrow).

that, when present (although not present in this example), the ligament of Struthers can be identified and divided.

4. Once identified, the MN can be traced distally until it can be seen traveling under the lacertus fibrosus (Figure 3.3). The lacertus fibrosus can then be divided, while the biceps tendon is preserved.
5. After division of the lacertus fibrosus, the MN can be followed as it travels between the two heads of the PT. The MN then travels under the fibrous ridge of the FDS (Figure 3.4).
6. The fibrous ridge of the FDS can then be transected to reveal the branch point of the AIN from the MN proper, approximately 5 to 8 cm distal from the medial epicondyle (Figure 3.5).
7. The course of the MN is inspected for any other points of compression; once the surgeon is satisfied, the wound is copiously irrigated and is closed in layers.

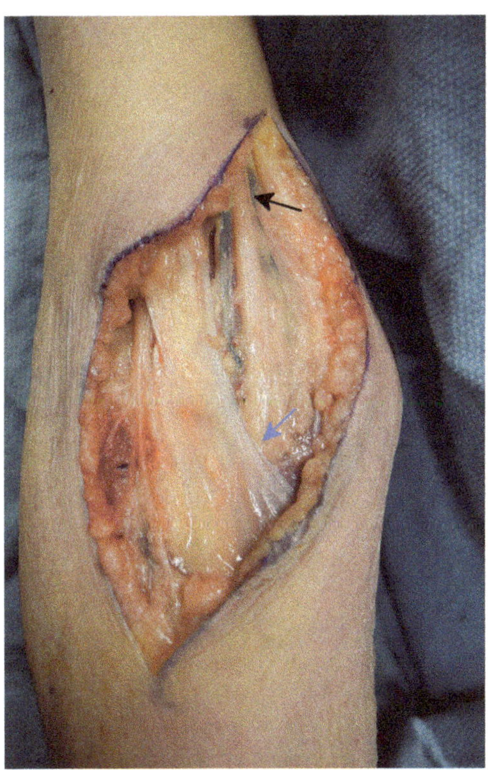

Figure 3.3. The median nerve (black arrow) can be identified under the fascia as it travels in the neurovascular bundle between the biceps and triceps muscles. The median nerve then courses distally, traveling under the lacertus fibrosus (blue arrow).

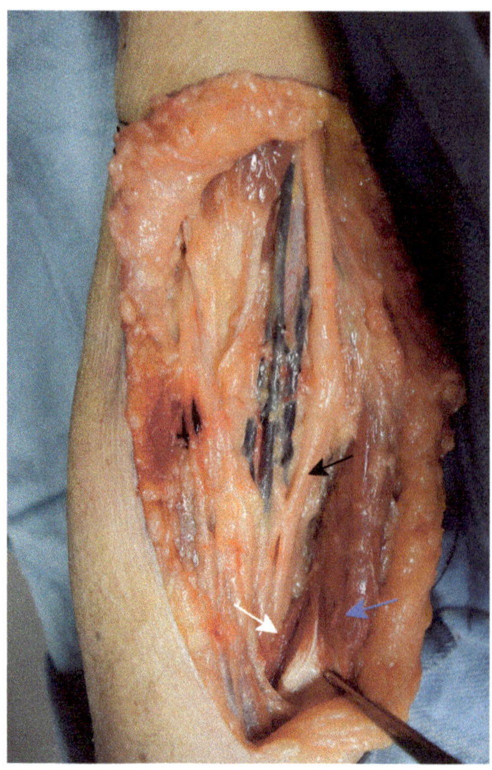

Figure 3.4. Exposure after opening of the lacertus fibrosus. The median nerve (black arrow) travels between the two heads of the pronator teres. The superficial head is shown retracted (blue arrow). The median nerve then travels under the fibrous ridge of the flexor digitorum superficialis muscle (white arrow).

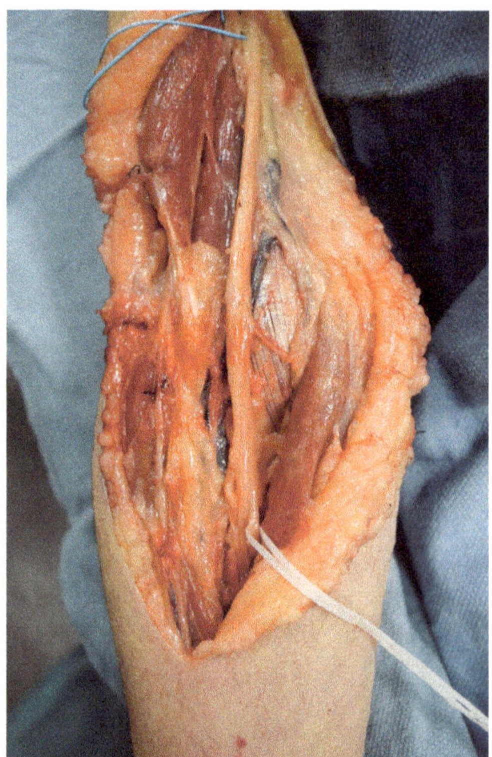

Figure 3.5. Exposure following transection of the fibrous ridge of the flexor digitorum superficialis muscle. The branch point of the anterior interosseous nerve (white loop) from the median nerve proper can be seen.

Oral Boards Review–Management Pearls

1. Although consensus does not exist concerning the duration of conservative therapy, it is generally accepted that a course of nonoperative therapy should be completed prior to considering surgery.
2. The goal of surgery is to identify areas of compression and to decompress the nerve. For this reason, it is necessary to visualize the MN along its course in the distal arm, antecubital fossa, and proximal forearm.

Pivot Points

1. PS is largely a clinical diagnosis and imaging studies should be obtained in the context of the larger clinical picture. Negative electrodiagnostic studies do not rule out PS.
2. PS must be distinguished from compression of the MN at the carpal tunnel (CTS) and from AIS.
3. Conservative measures are the mainstay of treatment initially and include the use of NSAIDs, behavior modification, and splinting.
4. When surgery is indicated, all potential areas of compression should be explored and decompressed, if necessary.

Aftercare

The incision is closed with interrupted absorbable sutures in the deep dermal layer, and a running subcuticular monofilament is used to further approximate the skin. Steri-Strips are placed over the top of the incision and a temporary bandage is worn over the incision for 48 hours and then is removed. The Steri-Strips are allowed to fall off on their own. Typically, the extremity is not immobilized, but a sling is used for comfort. Activities are restricted and lifting or strenuous activity involving the affected extremity is disallowed for 2 weeks.

In general, patients are not referred to physical therapy unless there are signs of motor weakness, significant functional impediment, or issues with range of motion or mobility.

We do not routinely repeat imaging or neurophysiologic testing during follow-up and instead rely on history and examination to assess improvements.

Complications and Management

Nerve injury is a rare but serious complication. In order to minimize the chance of injury to the MN and its muscular branches, proximal to distal dissection is carried out. In addition to protecting the MN, the surgeon should take care not to damage the other nerves in the region, which include the lateral antebrachial cutaneous nerve (LAC), the radial nerve (RN), and the ulnar nerve (UN). The LAC can be found lateral to the biceps tendon, where the nerve emerges between the brachialis and biceps muscles. The RN can be identified in the proximal and lateral portion of the exposure as it wraps around the lateral epicondyle and travels between the brachialis and brachioradialis muscles. The UN may be seen in the proximal and medial portion of the exposure after it pierces the medial intermuscular septum in the distal arm to travel posterior to the medial epicondyle.

Vascular injury is also a potential complication. The brachial artery runs just lateral to the MN in the antecubital fossa. The brachial artery bifurcates into the radial and ulnar arteries. The MN crosses over the proximal ulnar artery. Given their close proximity, these vessels may be accidentally damaged during exposure and decompression of the MN. If the AIN is decompressed, care should be taken not to damage the anterior interosseous artery, which runs along with it.

Infection is a potential complication in all peripheral nerve surgeries. The authors give preoperative prophylactic antibiotics for all of these cases and schedule follow-up within 1 to 2 weeks to assess the wound.

Oral Boards Review—Complications Pearls

1. In order to avoid nerve branch injury during exposure and decompression of the MN, start proximally and work distally.
2. It is important to be aware of other nerves that may enter into the surgical field, including the LAC, the RN, and the UN.
3. The MN and its branches are intimately associated with several vascular structures in the region of the antecubital fossa, including the brachial artery, the ulnar artery, and the anterior interosseous artery. Understanding the anatomic relationship of the MN to these structures will help prevent accidental injury.

Evidence and Outcomes

There are no randomized controlled trials evaluating the evidence for surgical versus nonsurgical therapy for treatment of PS. Furthermore, several different surgical approaches have been reported in the literature but have not been meticulously compared. The majority of the evidence for treatment of PS relies on case series and other retrospective analyses.

In general, there seems to be a consensus in the literature that PS should be treated conservatively initially for a period of weeks to months. In most studies, the reported response rate varies between 50% and 70%.[3,27,28] Nonsurgical treatment may include anti-inflammatory medications, immobilization, lifestyle or work modification, ultrasound therapy, and/or physical therapy.

Surgery is generally reserved for patients who do not respond to conservative management. Surgical strategies are varied. Some authors recommend an incision spanning the antecubital fossa (which the authors prefer) so that a full dissection can be carried out and all potential areas of compression can be evaluated. Others recommend more minimally invasive approaches, with targeted decompression.[19,21,27]

Taken together, the surgical literature, although lacking high-quality evidence, is fairly homogeneous with regard to surgical success rates. In the majority of studies, improvement or complete resolution of symptoms is reported in at least 75% of cases, including in studies involving more minimally invasive approaches.[3,14,17–21] Overall, there is support in the literature for surgical decompression in patients who do not respond to conservative therapy. Outcomes, though varied, are generally very good.

References

1. al-Qattan MM, Husband JB. Median nerve compression by the supracondylar process: a case report. *J Hand Surg Br.* 1991;16:101–103.
2. Eversmann W. *Operative Hand Surgery.* 3rd ed. New York, NY: Churchill Livingstone; 1993.
3. Johnson RK, Spinner M, Shrewsbury MM. Median nerve entrapment syndrome in the proximal forearm. *J Hand Surg Am.* 1979;4:48–51.
4. Koo JT, Szabo RM. Compression neuropathies of the median nerve. *J Am Soc Surg Hand.* 2004;4:156–175.
5. Smith RV, Fisher RG. Struthers ligament: a source of median nerve compression above the elbow. Case report. *J Neurosurg.* 1973;38:778–779.
6. al-Qattan MM. Gantzer's muscle. An anatomical study of the accessory head of the flexor pollicis longus muscle. *J Hand Surg Br.* 1996;21:269–270.
7. Dellon AL. Musculotendinous variations about the medial humeral epicondyle. *J Hand Surg Br.* 1986;11:175–181.
8. Vincelet Y, Journeau P, Popkov D, Haumont T, Lascombes P. The anatomical basis for anterior interosseous nerve palsy secondary to supracondylar humerus fractures in children. *Orthop Traumatol Surg Res.* 2013;99:543–547.
9. Afshar A. Pronator syndrome due to schwannoma. *J Hand Microsurg.* 2015;7:119–122.
10. Blagg R, Rockwell WB. Symptomatic elbow ganglion causing pronator syndrome. *Plast Reconstr Surg Glob Open.* 2014;2:e109.
11. Murphy SM, Browne K, Tuite DJ, O'Shaughnessy M. Dual pathology proximal median nerve compression of the forearm. *J Plast Reconstr Aesthetic Surg.* 2013;66:1792–1794.
12. Valbuena SE, O'Toole GA, Roulot E. Compression of the median nerve in the proximal forearm by a giant lipoma: A case report. *J Brachial Plex Peripher Nerve Inj.* 2008;3:17.
13. Ivins GK. Supracondylar process syndrome: a case report. *J Hand Surg Am.* 1996;21:279–281.
14. Hartz CR, Linscheid RL, Gramse RR, Daube JR. The pronator teres syndrome: compressive neuropathy of the median nerve. *J Bone Joint Surg Am.* 1981;63:885–890.
15. Presciutti S, Rodner CM. Pronator syndrome. *J Hand Surg Am.* 2011;36:907–909.
16. Johnson RK, Spinner M. *Median Nerve Compression in the Forearm: The Pronator Tunnel Syndrome.* Thorofare, NJ: Slack; 1989.
17. Olehnik WK, Manske PR, Szerzinski J. Median nerve compression in the proximal forearm. *J Hand Surg Am.* 1994;19:121–126.
18. Stal M, Hagert CG, Englund JE. Pronator syndrome: a retrospective study of median nerve entrapment at the elbow in female machine milkers. *J Agric Safety Health.* 2004;10:247–256.
19. Tsai TM, Syed SA. A transverse skin incision approach for decompression of pronator teres syndrome. *J Hand Surg Br.* 1994;19:40–42.
20. Werner CO, Rosen I, Thorngren KG. Clinical and neurophysiologic characteristics of the pronator syndrome. *Clin Orthop Relat Res.* 1985;197:231–236.

21. Zancolli ER III, Zancolli EP, Perrotto CJ. New mini-invasive decompression for pronator teres syndrome. *J Hand Surg Am*. 2012;37:1706–1710.
22. Miller-Breslow A, Terrono A, Millender LH. Nonoperative treatment of anterior interosseous nerve paralysis. *J Hand Surg Am*. 1990;15:493–496.
23. Sood MK, Burke FD. Anterior interosseous nerve palsy. A review of 16 cases. *J Hand Surg Br*. 1997;22:64–68.
24. Spinner M. *Injuries to the Major Branches of Peripheral Nerves of the Forearm*. Philadelphia, PA: Saunders; 1978.
25. Stern MB. The anterior interosseous nerve syndrome (the Kiloh-Nevin syndrome). Report and follow-up study of three cases. *Clin Orthop Relat Res*. 1984;187:223–227.
26. Ulrich D, Piatkowski A, Pallua N. Anterior interosseous nerve syndrome: retrospective analysis of 14 patients. *Arch Orthop Trauma Surg*. 2011;131:1561–1565.
27. Lee AK, Khorsandi M, Nurbhai N, Dang J, Fitzmaurice M, Herron KA. Endoscopically assisted decompression for pronator syndrome. *J Hand Surg Am*. 2012;37:1173–1179.
28. Haussmann P, Patel MR. Intraepineurial constriction of nerve fascicles in pronator syndrome and anterior interosseous nerve syndrome. *Orthop Clin North Am*. 1996;27:339–344.

Ulnar Neuropathy—Cubital Tunnel Syndrome

Ron Ron Cheng and Abhay K. Varma

4

Case Presentation

A 42-year-old, right-handed female presents with a 10-month history of numbness and tingling affecting the ring finger, little finger, and adjacent part of the palm of the left hand. Initially, the symptoms were intermittent but they have now progressed to become constant. For the last 4 months, the patient has also noticed impaired dexterity in her left hand. She works as an administrative assistant and is experiencing increasing difficulty with using her left hand in typing on a keyboard. Intermittently, she experiences pain over the medial aspect of her left elbow that radiates along the medial forearm to the hand. She denies any history of trauma. Examination of the left upper extremity demonstrates very slight wasting of the first dorsal interosseous muscle, weakness of the abductor digiti minimi and opponens digiti minimi, a positive Tinel sign at the elbow, a positive Froment sign, and a positive Wartenberg sign. Sensation is impaired over the ventral and dorsal aspect of the little finger, the medial half of the ring finger, and the ventral and dorsal aspect of the medial palm. There is no impairment of sensation proximal to the wrist. The remainder of the neurologic examination is normal. Palpation of the ulnar nerve at the medial epicondyle through range of motion does not reveal subluxation of the ulnar nerve.

Questions

1. What is the differential diagnosis?
2. What is the likely diagnosis?
3. What is the next step in the workup of this condition?
4. Is any imaging modality useful?

Assessment and Planning

The neurosurgeon suspects ulnar nerve entrapment at the elbow (cubital tunnel syndrome). The differential diagnosis includes thoracic outlet syndrome, C8-T1 radiculopathy, entrapment of the ulnar nerve at Guyon's canal, inflammatory neuropathy involving the ulnar nerve (e.g., Parsonage-Turner syndrome), or a tumor/mass involving the ulnar nerve. In this case, the clinical exam findings and clinical history are all consistent with entrapment of the ulnar nerve at the cubital tunnel. The patient has not provided any history suggestive of an inflammatory neuritis and the findings are isolated to the ulnar nerve. The muscles of the hand innervated by the median nerve are normal, which argues against thoracic outlet syndrome or C8-T1 radiculopathy. The patient also does not report any radiating pain originating in the neck. Furthermore, the clearly demarcated border of sensory loss is typical of a peripheral neuropathy, rather than a radiculopathy, where hazy borders of sensory loss are more typical. In this case, the sharply demarcated border fits the ulnar sensory distribution. Several findings localize the lesion/entrapment to the cubital tunnel rather than Guyon's canal. First, there is a positive Tinel sign at the elbow. Second, the distribution of sensory loss helps differentiate the two. The palmar cutaneous branch and dorsal cutaneous branch both arise proximal to Guyon's canal. As a result, compression at Guyon's canal does not affect these two branches. In this case, the sensory distribution includes the palm and dorsal surface of the hand, localizing the lesion to the cubital tunnel rather than Guyon's canal.

Electrodiagnostic study of the left upper extremity can help differentiate between radiculopathy and neuropathy and can localize the site of compression. Ultrasonographic evaluation and MR neurography evaluation of the ulnar nerve at the elbow are useful adjuncts, and they can help establish the diagnosis while excluding mass lesions affecting the ulnar nerve.

Ulnar nerve entrapment within the cubital tunnel is the second most common entrapment neuropathy, surpassed only by median nerve compression within the carpal tunnel.[1,2] The mainstays of diagnosis in cubital tunnel syndrome remain clinical history and examination supplemented by electrodiagnostic testing. While imaging is not the primary diagnostic modality employed in ulnar neuropathy, it may provide valuable information regarding the severity and causes of entrapment. In cases where trauma or fracture of the bones surrounding the cubital tunnel is in the history or is suspected, X-ray or CT evaluation may be helpful. Otherwise, the mainstays of evaluation are ultrasound and MR imaging. Ultrasound is a cost-effective and relatively quick means of evaluating ulnar nerve entrapment, presence of subluxation over the bony medial epicondyle, and the presence of compressive lesions.[3] Ultrasound has been shown to have superior sensitivity and equivalent specificity in comparison to MR imaging.[4] Additionally, an advantage of ultrasound over MR imaging is that ultrasound allows dynamic evaluation, which MR imaging does not. Regardless of the modality, imaging studies are extensions of the physical examination. They can help localize the site of entrapment and can exclude mass lesions, which is the primary purpose of obtaining imaging studies in these circumstances.

MR neurography findings suggestive of an entrapment neuropathy include T2 hyperintensity of the ulnar nerve, nerve enlargement proximal to the site of entrapment, fascicular abnormalities, perineural fat stranding, and, sometimes, distal muscle denervation changes. Abrupt signal change in the nerve in a bright–black–bright pattern indicates severe constriction.[5] In the present case, MR neurography was obtained and demonstrated T2 hyperintensity, enlargement proximal to the cubital tunnel, and disruption of the fascicular pattern of the ulnar nerve, as well as perineural fat stranding (Figure 4.1).

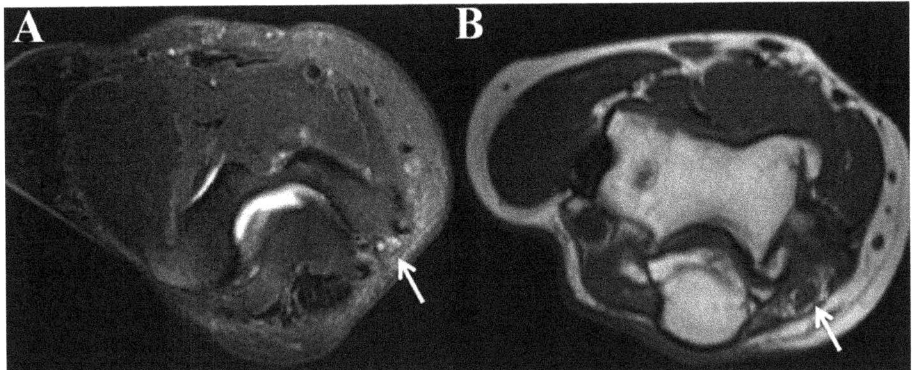

Figure 4.1. A, T2-weighted MR imaging of the elbow demonstrates enlargement, hyperintense signal, and fascicular abnormality of the ulnar nerve in the cubital tunnel (arrow). B, T1-weighted MR imaging of the elbow demonstrates perineural fat stranding of the ulnar nerve in the cubital tunnel (arrow).

Oral Boards Review—Diagnostic Pearls

1. Wartenberg sign: Fifth digit stays in a slightly abducted position because of weakness of the third palmar interosseous muscle. The unopposed action of the extensor digiti minimi and extensor digitorum communis cause the finger to rest in a slightly abducted position.
2. Muscle atrophy: In long-standing and severe ulnar nerve palsy, muscle wasting, including the dorsal interosseous muscle and hypothenar muscles, is noticeable.
3. Ulnar claw hand: Hyperextension at the metacarpophalangeal joints of the fourth and fifth digits, with partial flexion of both interphalangeal joints, occurs secondary to weakness of the third and fourth lumbricals, with unopposed action of the extensor digitorum communis and extensor digiti minimi.
4. Froment sign: Weakness of the adductor pollicis leads the patient to compensate by using the flexor pollicis longus (innervated by the anterior interosseous nerve) when attempting to hold a piece of paper between the volar surface of a straightened thumb and the radial surface of the index finger.
5. Sensory impairment affects the hypothenar eminence (innervated by the ulnar palmar cutaneous branch), the volar surface of the fifth digit and the ulnar half of the fourth digit (superficial sensory division innervation), and the dorsal medial third of the hand and fingers (innervated by the ulnar dorsal cutaneous nerve). If sensory loss extends up the medial border of the forearm (supplied by the medial antebrachial cutaneous nerve), proximal to the wrist crease, consider a more proximal pathology (involvement of the medial cord of the brachial plexus or C8/T1 nerve roots). Sparing of the ulnar dorsal cutaneous nerve and ulnar palmar cutaneous nerve distribution

should prompt consideration of compression at Guyon's canal rather than at the cubital tunnel.

6. If nonconformal deficits are identified, be mindful of the possibility of median and ulnar nerve communications in the forearm (Martin-Gruber anastomosis) or the hand (Riche-Cannieu anastomosis).
7. Electrodiagnostic studies can help identify compression in the cubital tunnel but can be nonlocalizing in chronic cases. MR neurography and ultrasound are increasingly being used to identify nerve compression in the cubital tunnel and can help exclude mass lesions affecting the ulnar nerve.

Questions

1. What are your options for management? Nonsurgical? Surgical?
2. What intervention would you offer this patient?
3. What prognosis would you give the patient?
4. How would the presence or absence of subluxation of the nerve over the medial epicondyle influence your surgical decision?

Decision-Making

Patients with intermittent symptoms and absence of motor involvement should be offered conservative management, including rest, elbow bracing, and/or activity modification. Failure of conservative management, severe or progressive neurologic deficits, and/or the presence of a mass lesion should prompt discussion of surgical intervention and surgical options. Surgical options include in situ decompression performed with an open approach or endoscopically and nerve transposition, including both subcutaneous and submuscular. The choice between open and endoscopy-assisted approaches largely depends on individual surgeon experience. In typical cases, in situ decompression is the initial operation of choice. In cases of severe ulnar neuropathy, in cases where there is subluxation of the nerve over the medial epicondyle, and in cases of recurrent or persistent ulnar neuropathy following initial decompression, the authors favor ulnar nerve transposition.

Questions

1. When would you offer surgical intervention to a patient with ulnar nerve entrapment at the elbow?
2. Which nerve should be actively identified and safeguarded during ulnar nerve exploration at the elbow?
3. If, intraoperatively, you decide to transpose the nerve, what anatomic structures would you look for to prevent proximal nerve compression after transposition?

Surgical Procedure

Anatomy

Originating as the terminal branch of the medial cord, the ulnar nerve pierces the intermuscular septum in the arm and passes through the arcade of Struthers, although there is controversy whether this structure actually exists.[6] The arcade of Struthers is formed by a combination of a variety of structures, including the brachial fascia, the internal brachial ligament, and the medial intermuscular septum.[6] The ulnar nerve continues through the arm between the medial intermuscular septum and the medial head of the triceps. Understanding the anatomy of the medial intermuscular septum is important, as it is particularly important to release this structure during transposition. The medial intermuscular septum attaches on the humerus between the lesser tubercle and medial epicondyle and separates the brachialis and triceps muscles.

To enter the forearm, the ulnar nerve passes posterior to the medial epicondyle in a groove between the medial epicondyle of the humerus and the olecranon process of the ulna. It is in this vicinity that the medial antebrachial cutaneous nerve crosses the ulnar nerve in the subcutaneous tissue. Just distal to the medial epicondyle, the nerve enters the cubital tunnel as it passes deep to Osborne's ligament, which is the thickened proximal aspect of Osborne's fascia between the ulnar and humeral heads of the flexor carpi ulnaris. The nerve courses distally between the two heads of the flexor carpi ulnaris beneath Osborne's fascia. The ulnar nerve exits the cubital tunnel as it passes beneath the muscular substance of the flexor carpi ulnaris and then continues in a plane between the flexor carpi ulnaris and flexor digitorum profundus.

Branches of the nerve that may be encountered during cubital tunnel decompression include an articular branch to the elbow arising near the cubital tunnel entrance and multiple motor branches to the flexor carpi ulnaris and flexor digitorum profundus that arise within the cubital tunnel. Typical points of compression along the course of the ulnar nerve include the arcade of Struthers, medial intermuscular septum, medial epicondyle, postcondylar groove, Osborne's ligament, and Osborne's fascia.

Open Decompression

Open decompression can be performed under general anesthesia or local anesthesia with conscious sedation. The patient is positioned supine with the arm abducted and externally rotated at the shoulder, resting on an arm board. The forearm is fully supinated and slightly flexed at the elbow. A curvilinear incision is made centered over the cubital tunnel between the medial epicondyle and olecranon, with the proximal aspect of the incision along the plane between the biceps and triceps and the distal aspect of the incision bisecting the heads of the flexor carpi ulnaris (Figure 4.2A). Once the incision is made, dissection of the subcutaneous tissue is performed in order to identify the ulnar nerve between the two heads of the flexor carpi ulnaris. Care should be taken to

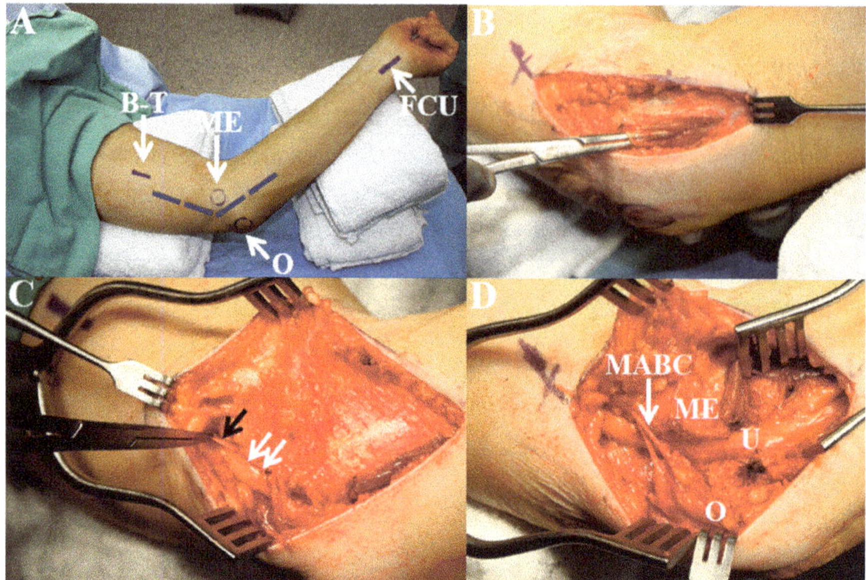

Figure 4.2. A, The arm is positioned with the shoulder abducted and externally rotated and with the elbow slightly flexed. The incision (dashed line) is planned to cross between the olecranon (O) and medial epicondyle (ME), heading proximally toward the cleft between the biceps and triceps (B-T) and distally toward the flexor carpi ulnaris tendon (FCU). B, Osborne's ligament, extending between the olecranon and medial epicondyle, is the usual site of compression of the ulnar nerve. C, The ulnar nerve (double white arrow) is located proximally, adjacent to the medial intermuscular septum (black arrow). This is a potential point of compression. Division of the medial intermuscular septum is particularly important in cases where transposition is performed. D, The ulnar nerve (U) has been fully decompressed. Branches of the medial antebrachial cutaneous nerve (MABC) have been preserved. O = olecranon; ME = medial epicondyle.

identify and safeguard the medial antebrachial cutaneous nerve during the subcutaneous dissection. Once the ulnar nerve is identified, Osborne's fascia and Osborne's ligament roofing the cubital tunnel are carefully incised (Figure 4.2B). Some surgeons favor circumferential decompression to ensure the nerve is free, while others perform an in situ decompression in order to preserve the vasa nervorum, to avoid potential nerve injury, and to avoid postoperative scarring. The medial epicondyle is then examined for any bony abnormalities that may be compressing the nerve as it enters the cubital tunnel. Neurolysis is carried proximally, dividing the arcade of Struthers and cutting a wedge in the medial intermuscular septum (Figure 4.2C). This step is particularly important if transposition is anticipated. At this point, the neurolysis is complete (Figure 4.2D). The nerve is then tested for evidence of subluxation throughout range of motion of the elbow. If no subluxation is present, the wound is copiously irrigated and is closed in layers. If subluxation is present, the procedure is converted to transposition.

Endoscopic Decompression

Endoscopic decompression aims to achieve in situ decompression of the nerve, with excellent visibility, via a small incision. The ideal candidate for endoscopic release is a patient with primary (idiopathic) cubital tunnel syndrome. Relative or absolute contraindications include surgeon's inexperience, subluxation of the ulnar nerve, space-occupying lesions, long-standing elbow contractures requiring release, prior trauma with extensive scar formation, and prior open decompression with transposition of the nerve. A 1.5- to 2-cm longitudinal skin incision is made between the medial epicondyle and the olecranon. Dissection is carried down through the subcutaneous tissue, toward the roof of the cubital tunnel. Osborne's ligament is divided over a short distance in its proximal aspect, exposing the ulnar nerve. In the next step (under endoscopic visualization), depending on the technique, dissecting instruments are placed either within the cubital tunnel or superficial to Osborne's fascia. In the former technique, the fascia overlying the ulnar nerve is divided from within, and in the latter technique, the superficial muscle fascia is first divided, followed by the release of the ulnar nerve from its investing connective tissues.

Subcutaneous Transposition

Transposition requires more dissection than in situ decompression, necessitating general anesthesia, but patient positioning and incision are the same as those described for open in situ decompression. As in open decompression, the incision is made over the cubital tunnel. Neurolysis is also carried out as for in situ decompression, with circumferential neurolysis being mandatory for transposition. Particular attention is paid to dividing the medial intermuscular septum and to releasing any points of tethering at the distal end of the neurolysis, as these can serve as iatrogenic points of compression or acute angulation when the nerve is transposed. Resection of a small portion of the flexor carpi ulnaris muscle is sometimes required to achieve an adequate transposition. The pocket for the nerve is prepared by sweeping all of the subcutaneous tissue off the fascia overlying the common flexor-pronator mass. The nerve is then transposed anterior to the medial epicondyle. The proximal and distal aspects of the nerve are then rechecked for points of tethering or acute angulation. The subcutaneous tissue overlying the now transposed nerve is then sutured to the fascia of the medial epicondyle to prevent the nerve from dislocating back into the cubital tunnel. Once the surgeon is satisfied with the transposition, the wound is copiously irrigated and is closed in layers.

Submuscular Transposition

As in subcutaneous transposition, the ulnar nerve is transposed anteriorly to the medial epicondyle after being liberated from the cubital tunnel. A Z-flap may be created from the pronator teres and flexor carpi ulnaris muscles and investing fascia, and the two musculofascial ends are then reapproximated over the transposed ulnar nerve for stabilization.

Oral Boards Review—Management Pearls

1. Surgical options include simple decompression (neurolysis), endoscopic neurolysis, anterior subcutaneous transposition, and anterior submuscular transposition.
2. Safeguard the medial antebrachial cutaneous nerve, particularly the dorsal branch, during surgical exposure of the ulnar nerve at the elbow.
3. Flex the elbow intraoperatively after decompression of the cubital tunnel to check for anterior dislocation of the nerve during flexion.
4. Look for and release the arcade of Struthers when transposing the nerve and pay careful attention to dividing the medial intermuscular septum.

Pivot Points

1. If sensory impairment involves the medial aspect of the forearm, think of a proximal lesion involving the lower brachial plexus, as in thoracic outlet syndrome.
2. If there is prior history of trauma to the elbow region or upper arm, consider alternatives to compression in the cubital tunnel. Order imaging accordingly.

Aftercare

An arm sling may be prescribed postoperatively for comfort. In most patients, it is not required for more than 5 to 7 days. Analgesics should be restricted to nonsteroidal anti-inflammatory drugs (NSAIDs) and acetaminophen. Opioids should be the exception rather than the rule. Because the incision crosses the joint line, some surgeons leave sutures in for 10 to 14 days. The decision to start postoperative occupational/physical therapy depends on the degree of preoperative motor deficit. It is advisable to initiate this treatment once the discomfort of surgery subsides.

Complications and Management

Complications specific to surgery include incomplete decompression, post decompression nerve subluxation, and injury to the medial antebrachial cutaneous nerve. Incomplete decompression can result in persistent symptoms. Re-exploration for recurrent or persistent symptoms requires transposition of the nerve. Potential sites of compression, such as the arcade of Struthers, medial intramuscular septum, the medial epicondyle, Osborne's ligament, and Osborne's fascia, should be assessed at surgery. If clinically indicated, imaging of the elbow should be performed prior to re-exploration, to exclude other pathology in that region. Subluxation can be avoided by intraoperative assessment of nerve dislocation during flexion and extension of the elbow. If subluxation is diagnosed postoperatively, transposition is required to alleviate the symptoms, if present. If the subluxation of the nerve is asymptomatic, further surgery is not required purely for subluxation. Injury to the medial antebrachial cutaneous nerve can result in a painful neuroma with disabling symptoms. Surgical management involves excision of the neuroma with intramuscular implantation of the proximal nerve end. If the injury is recognized intraoperatively, options for management include intramuscular implantation of the proximal nerve end or microsurgical primary repair of the nerve injury.

Patients who undergo a submuscular transposition run a slight risk of weakness in the muscle that was divided and reattached in the course of surgery.

Oral Boards Review—Complication Pearls

1. Flex and extend the elbow during surgery to identify subluxation of the nerve.
2. Be cognizant of the presence of the medial antebrachial cutaneous nerve during exposure to avoid injury to this nerve. If injury is recognized intraoperatively, options for management include intramuscular implantation of the proximal cut nerve end or microsurgical primary repair of the nerve.
3. Re-exploration for failed cubital tunnel decompression should include a longer exposure of the nerve, with assessment of each potential compression site. Transposition should be performed for persistent or recurrent symptoms.

Evidence and Outcomes

With open in situ decompression, approximately 85% of patients have complete resolution of symptoms or only mild residual symptoms.[7–10] In patients with severe muscle atrophy or severe electrodiagnostic findings, improvement can be expected but may not be to the same degree as in patients with only sensory impairment or mild weakness. Patients should be informed that recovery may continue to occur even beyond 2 years postoperatively.[11] Postoperatively, patients can expect improvement in a number of metrics, including key-pinch strength, two-point discrimination, activities of daily living, and pain, and, overall, patients report a high rate of satisfaction.[12]

There is a paucity of large randomized controlled trials (level I evidence) of the management of ulnar neuropathy at the elbow. A meta-analysis of randomized controlled studies and a Cochrane review found no difference in outcomes following in situ decompression and anterior transposition, although the rates of both deep and superficial infections with anterior transposition are higher.[13–15] Although the data are of moderate quality, the outcomes are the same in both groups, even when the ulnar neuropathy is severe.[13] Despite this, many surgeons, including the authors, continue to utilize anterior transposition for severe cases. Based on the available data, it is recommended that in situ decompression, either open or endoscopic, be offered in primary cases of cubital tunnel syndrome. In one randomized controlled trial comparing open and endoscopic neurolysis, outcomes were similar between the two groups, but the endoscopic group had more postoperative hematomas. No significant advantages were seen in the endoscopic group.[16] Anterior transposition should be considered in primary cases where preoperative or intraoperative subluxation of the nerve is identified. In revision cases, anterior subcutaneous transposition or submuscular transposition can be offered. The latter is more appropriate for revision cases with minimal subcutaneous tissue. Although the data are limited, the available data suggest that outcomes are similar for submuscular and subcutaneous transposition, with submuscular transposition having a higher rate of adverse events.[17,18]

References

1. Nellans K, Tang P. Evaluation and treatment of failed ulnar nerve release at the elbow. *Orthop Clin North Am*. 2012;43:487–494.
2. Shi Q, MacDermid JC, Santaguida PL, Kyu HH. Predictors of surgical outcomes following anterior transposition of ulnar nerve for cubital tunnel syndrome: a systematic review. *J Hand Surg Am*. 2011;36:1996–2001.
3. Ali ZS, Pisapia JM, Ma TS, Zager EL, Heuer GG, Khoury V. Ultrasonographic evaluation of peripheral nerves. *World Neurosurg*. 2016;85:333–339.
4. Zaidman CM, Seelig MJ, Baker JC, Mackinnon SE, Pestronk A. Detection of peripheral nerve pathology: comparison of ultrasound and MRI. *Neurology*. 2013;80:1634–1640.
5. Chalian M, Behzadi AH, Williams EH, Shores JT, Chhabra A. High-resolution magnetic resonance neurography in upper extremity neuropathy. *Neuroimaging Clin N Am*. 2014;24:109–125.
6. Tubbs RS, Deep A, Shoja MM, Mortazavi MM, Loukas M, Cohen-Gadol AA. The arcade of Struthers: an anatomical study with potential neurosurgical significance. *Surg Neurol Int*. 2011;2:184.
7. Bacle G, Marteau E, Freslon M, et al. Cubital tunnel syndrome: comparative results of a multicenter study of 4 surgical techniques with a mean follow-up of 92 months. *Orthop Traumatol Surg Res*. 2014;100:S205–208.
8. Goldfarb CA, Sutter MM, Martens EJ, Manske PR. Incidence of re-operation and subjective outcome following in situ decompression of the ulnar nerve at the cubital tunnel. *J Hand Surg Eur*. 2009;34:379–383.
9. Keiner D, Gaab MR, Schroeder HW, Oertel J. Comparison of the long-term results of anterior transposition of the ulnar nerve or simple decompression in the treatment of cubital tunnel syndrome—a prospective study. *Acta Neurochir (Wien)*. 2009;151:311–315; discussion 316.
10. Mitsionis GI, Manoudis GN, Paschos NK, Korompilias AV, Beris AE. Comparative study of surgical treatment of ulnar nerve compression at the elbow. *J Shoulder Elbow Surg*. 2010;19:513–519.
11. Matsuzaki H, Yoshizu T, Maki Y, Tsubokawa N, Yamamoto Y, Toishi S. Long-term clinical and neurologic recovery in the hand after surgery for severe cubital tunnel syndrome. *J Hand Surg Am*. 2004;29:373–378.
12. Song JW, Waljee JF, Burns PB, et al. An outcome study for ulnar neuropathy at the elbow: a multicenter study by the surgery for ulnar nerve (SUN) study group. *Neurosurgery*. 2013;72:971–981.
13. Caliandro P, La Torre G, Padua R, Giannini F, Padua L. Treatment for ulnar neuropathy at the elbow. *Cochrane Database Syst Rev*. 2016;11:CD006839.

14. Macadam SA, Gandhi R, Bezuhly M, Lefaivre KA. Simple decompression versus anterior subcutaneous and submuscular transposition of the ulnar nerve for cubital tunnel syndrome: a meta-analysis. *J Hand Surg Am*. 2008;33:1314 e1311–1312.
15. Zlowodzki M, Chan S, Bhandari M, Kalliainen L, Schubert W. Anterior transposition compared with simple decompression for treatment of cubital tunnel syndrome. A meta-analysis of randomized, controlled trials. *J Bone Joint Surg Am*. 2007;89:2591–2598.
16. Schmidt S, Kleist Welch-Guerra W, Matthes M, Baldauf J, Schminke U, Schroeder HW. Endoscopic vs open decompression of the ulnar nerve in cubital tunnel syndrome: a prospective randomized double-blind study. *Neurosurgery*. 2015;77:960–970; discussion 970–961.
17. Liu CH, Chen CX, Xu J, et al. Anterior subcutaneous versus submuscular transposition of the ulnar nerve for cubital tunnel syndrome: a systematic review and meta-analysis. *PLOS ONE*. 2015;10:e0130843.
18. Liu CH, Wu SQ, Ke XB, et al. Subcutaneous versus submuscular anterior transposition of the ulnar nerve for cubital tunnel syndrome: a systematic review and meta-analysis of randomized controlled trials and observational studies. *Medicine (Baltimore)*. 2015;94:e1207.

Ulnar Neuropathy—Guyon's Canal Syndrome

Abhay K. Varma and Ron Ron Cheng

5

Case Presentation

A 36-year-old, right-handed woman presents with a 4-year history of progressive numbness and weakness of the right hand. The numbness primarily affects her ring finger and little finger. For the last 2 years, she has noticed progressive deformity of the fourth and fifth digits. She is experiencing increasing difficulty in performing daily chores, including activities of daily living that involve use of both hands. She also reports intermittent pain over the volar aspect of her right wrist. Examination of the left upper extremity demonstrates significant wasting of the first dorsal interosseous muscle, weakness of the abductor digiti minimi and opponens digiti minimi, a positive Froment sign, and a positive Wartenberg sign. Tinel test at the elbow is negative. Sensation is impaired over the ventral aspect of the little finger and the medial half of the ring finger. The dorsal aspect of these fingers have preserved sensation and the ventral and dorsal aspects of the medial palm have preserved sensation. There is no impairment of sensation proximal to the wrist. Palpation of the ulnar nerve at the elbow through range of motion does not reveal subluxation of the ulnar nerve. An ill-defined fullness is noted upon palpation of the medial half of the volar aspect of the wrist. There is a positive Tinel sign at this location. The remainder of the neurologic examination is normal.

Questions

1. What is the likely site of ulnar nerve compression?
2. What are the boundaries of this anatomic site?
3. What are the variations in compression at this site?
4. What is the next step in the workup of this condition?
5. Is any imaging modality useful?

Assessment and Planning

Ulnar nerve entrapment at the wrist, possibly secondary to a mass lesion, is the likely diagnosis. The differential diagnosis includes idiopathic entrapment at Guyon's canal, cubital tunnel syndrome, thoracic outlet syndrome, C8-T1 radiculopathy, and inflammatory neuropathy involving the ulnar nerve (e.g., Parsonage-Turner syndrome). In this case, the findings are consistent with ulnar neuropathy. The sensory examination helps localize the lesion. Preservation of the ulnar dorsal cutaneous nerve and ulnar palmar cutaneous nerve sensory distributions suggests a lesion distal to the take-off of both of these branches, making Guyon's canal the most likely area of entrapment. Preservation of the median-innervated muscles of the hand argues against thoracic outlet syndrome. The patient provides no subjective history consistent with an inflammatory neuropathy, and the findings are isolated to the ulnar nerve, making Parsonage-Turner syndrome less likely. The ill-defined fullness in the area of Guyon's canal suggests the possible presence of a mass that warrants further evaluation.

Electrodiagnostic studies can be used as an extension of the neurologic examination to help confirm localization. Imaging, including ultrasonography, CT, and/or MR imaging, should be performed. CT can be particularly helpful when bony abnormalities are suspected or when there is a history of trauma. CT (of bony pathology) and MR imaging (of soft tissue masses, aberrant muscle, and vascular lesions) complement each other.[1] MR imaging often discloses T2 hyperintensity, particularly in the deep branch of the ulnar nerve, and is very sensitive and specific for the diagnosis of ulnar tunnel syndrome. The main trunk of the ulnar nerve more proximally seems to demonstrate less T2 hyperintensity. T2 hyperintensity in the deep branch has been shown to correlate with conduction velocity abnormalities on electrodiagnostic studies.[2] The role of ultrasound in the diagnosis of ulnar tunnel syndrome is not well established. Ultrasound can identify soft tissue mass lesions and differentiate cystic from solid lesions.

In this patient, electrodiagnostic studies establish the presence of nonlocalizing ulnar neuropathy, and MR imaging of the wrist demonstrates compression of the ulnar nerve by a solid mass in the ulnar tunnel.

Oral Boards Review—Diagnostic Pearls

1. Ulnar nerve entrapment within the ulnar tunnel (Guyon's canal) is much less common than cubital tunnel syndrome.
2. Ganglia and chronic repetitive trauma over the hypothenar eminence (for example, in occupational or long-distance cyclists) are the two leading causes of ulnar tunnel syndrome.[3] Benign lesions, hook of hamate fractures, ulnar artery pathology or aberrancy, anomalous hypothenar muscles, and crystal deposition disease are the other reported causes.[4–16]
3. Imaging of the wrist is essential in suspected cases of ulnar tunnel syndrome, as impingement by an organic lesion is common.
4. Ulnar claw hand is more profound in ulnar tunnel syndrome because the flexor digitorum profundus is spared and causes unopposed distal finger flexion due to weakness in the lumbricals.
5. Three zones of compression are recognized, based on the ulnar nerve branching pattern in the ulnar tunnel.
   a. Zone 1—Compression of the nerve prior to its division in the ulnar tunnel. Sensory loss involves the volar surfaces of the fifth digit and the medial half of the fourth digit, including the nail beds. The hypothenar eminence is commonly spared, because the palmar ulnar cutaneous branch

is not affected. Intrinsic hand muscles are affected, while the flexor carpi ulnaris and flexor digitorum profundus are spared.

b. Zone 2—Only the deep motor branch is affected as it exits the tunnel at the level of the hamate. Motor deficits are similar to those in zone 1, with no sensory loss. The palmaris brevis muscle is spared (tested by looking for corrugation of the medial border of the palm when the patient "tightens" the hypothenar eminence), because it is supplied by the proximal superficial sensory division.

c. Zone 3—Only the superficial sensory division is affected. This is the least common variant. There is primarily sensory impairment on the volar surface of the fourth and fifth digits. Palmaris brevis contraction is absent. Motor function is otherwise preserved.

Questions

1. Does conservative management have a role in the care of this patient?
2. Can electrodiagnostic study be nonlocalizing in a compressive neuropathy?
3. What other compressive neuropathy is common in these patients?

Decision-Making

Nonoperative treatment is offered to patients when an organic pathology is not identified and there is no motor weakness or muscle wasting. A neutral wrist splint and activity modification to avoid local pressure or repetitive trauma to the wrist are recommended.

Surgical intervention is indicated when a compressive pathology is identified, there is motor involvement, or conservative management has failed. The aim of surgery is to decompress the ulnar nerve and to remove any compressive pathology. In this case, a mass lesion was identified and profound motor weakness was present, both indications for surgery.

Questions

1. When would you offer surgical intervention to a patient with ulnar nerve compression at the wrist?
2. Which nerve(s) should be actively identified and safeguarded during ulnar nerve exploration at the wrist?
3. What specific compressive site would you look for in a patient with zone 2 compression?

Surgical Procedure

Anatomy

After exiting the cubital tunnel, the ulnar nerve courses distally in a plane between the flexor carpi ulnaris and flexor digitorum profundus. As the nerve heads toward Guyon's canal (i.e., the ulnar tunnel) prior to entering the canal, it gives off the dorsal cutaneous branch more proximally and then the palmar cutaneous branch more distally. Just proximal to the entrance into Guyon's canal, the ulnar artery and ulnar nerve can be located slightly posterior and lateral to the tendon of the flexor carpi ulnaris. The contents of Guyon's canal include the ulnar nerve, the ulnar artery, and a network of veins. Within the canal, the ulnar nerve is slightly deep and medial to the ulnar artery. The boundaries of Guyon's canal are the palmar carpal ligament, palmaris brevis muscle, and hypothenar connective tissue, forming the roof; the transverse carpal ligament, pisohamate ligament, pisometacarpal ligament, tendons of the flexor digitorum profundus, and tendon of the opponens digiti minimi, forming the floor; the transverse carpal ligament and hook of hamate, forming the lateral wall; and the pisiform bone, tendon of the flexor carpi ulnaris, and abductor digiti minimi muscle, forming the medial wall (Figure 5.1).

Within the confines of the distal canal, approximately 6 mm distal to the pisiform, the ulnar nerve bifurcates into a superficial and a deep branch.[17] The superficial

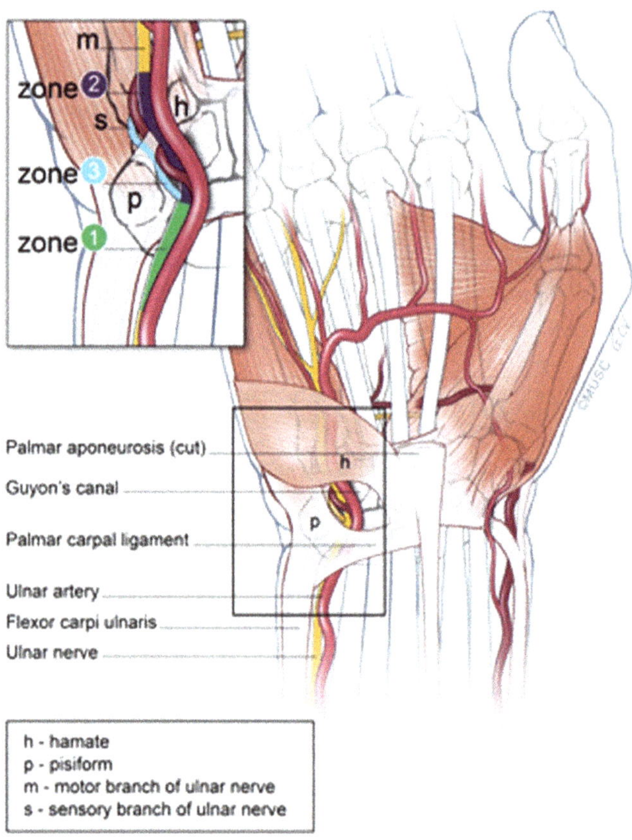

Figure 5.1. Surgical anatomy of Guyon's canal with zones of compression (inset).

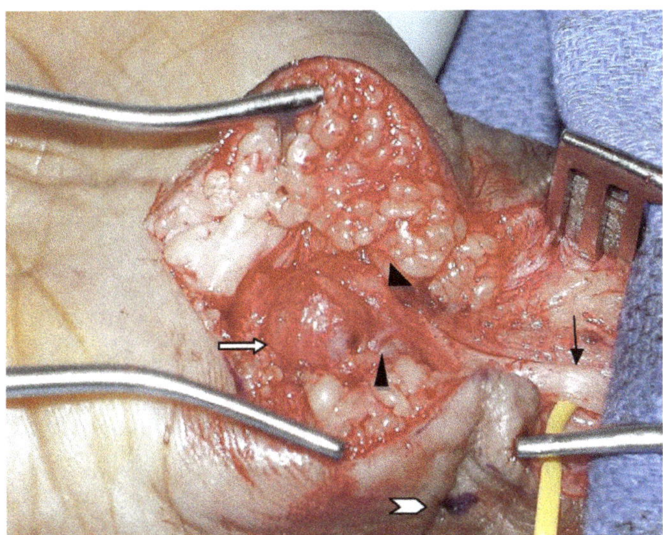

Figure 5.2. Giant cell tumor (white arrow) displacing the two branches (black arrowheads) of the ulnar nerve (black arrow). The pisiform is marked on the surface (white arrowhead).

branch is predominantly sensory but does supply motor innervation to the palmaris brevis. The deep branch is the main motor branch, providing innervation to the ulnar-innervated hand intrinsic muscles.

Technique

Surgery can be performed under general, regional, or local anesthesia, depending on patient and surgeon preference and comfort level. The patient is positioned with the shoulder abducted and externally rotated and the arm supinated on an arm board. A Z-shaped longitudinal incision is made between the hamate and pisiform bones, starting 4 cm proximal to the wrist crease and extending another 3 to 4 cm into the palm. During dissection of the subcutaneous tissue, care should be taken to avoid injury to the palmar cutaneous branches of the median and ulnar nerves. Once the skin is divided, the flexor carpi ulnaris tendon is identified proximal to the wrist. The ulnar nerve and artery run posterior and lateral to the tendon. The nerve is traced distally into the tunnel, and the palmar carpal ligament, palmaris brevis muscle, and the hypothenar fat and fascia are divided to unroof the tunnel and decompress the nerve. Any compressive lesion, if present, is excised (Figure 5.2). The nerve is traced distally beyond its bifurcation, and the tendinous origin of the hypothenar muscles from the hook of hamate should be inspected for compression of the deep motor branch. Once neurolysis is complete, the wound is copiously irrigated and is closed in layers.

Oral Boards Review—Management Pearls

1. Safeguard the palmer cutaneous branches of the ulnar and median nerves during ulnar tunnel decompression.

2. Be cognizant of vascular structures in the ulnar tunnel, including the ulnar artery.
3. Release the canal up to the hook of hamate.
4. Preserve the vasa nervorum during dissection.

Pivot Points

1. Rule out a proximal site of ulnar nerve compression or cervical spinal cord pathology.
2. Actively look for concurrent carpal tunnel syndrome.
3. Point tenderness over the hook of hamate should raise suspicion of bony pathology.

Aftercare

Sutures are removed 10 to 14 days after surgery. Postoperative splinting is offered to patients with severe pain. Postoperative hand therapy is offered to patients with reduced mobility of the hand from pain and edema.

Complications and Management

The most likely complications are incomplete decompression and misdiagnosis. If there is lack of improvement following surgical intervention, these two possibilities should be considered. Injury to the palmar cutaneous branches of the ulnar and median nerves and ulnar artery are other potential complications.

Oral Boards Review—Complication Pearls

1. Thorough work-up, including meticulous clinical evaluation, electrodiagnostic studies, and appropriate imaging studies, is imperative prior to offering surgical intervention.
2. Protect the ulnar artery and palmar cutaneous branches during surgery.

Evidence and Outcomes

Compression of the ulnar nerve in the ulnar tunnel is a much less frequently encountered entrapment neuropathy than cubital tunnel compression; consequently, there is paucity of large case series in the literature. In one series of 13 patients, significant improvements in clinical and electrodiagnostic parameters were observed postoperatively, and 90% of patients reported subjective improvement.[18] Surgical intervention is recommended when there is a clearly identified compressive pathology, motor weakness/muscle wasting, or lack of response to nonsurgical treatment. The recommended surgical approach is open neurolysis. At present, there is inadequate experience with endoscopic decompression of the ulnar tunnel to make recommendations regarding the safety or efficacy of this approach.

References

1. Shen L, Masih S, Patel DB, Matcuk GR Jr. MR anatomy and pathology of the ulnar nerve involving the cubital tunnel and Guyon's canal. *Clin Imaging*. 2016;40(2):263–274.
2. Kollmer J, Baumer P, Milford D, et al. T2-signal of ulnar nerve branches at the wrist in Guyon's canal syndrome. *PLOS ONE*. 2012;7(10):e47295.
3. Shea JD, McClain EJ. Ulnar-nerve compression syndromes at and below the wrist. *J Bone Joint Surg Am*. 1969;51(6):1095–1103.
4. Wang B, Zhang J, Li G, Zhang Z. Fibroma of a tendon sheath causing Guyon's canal syndrome: case report. *J Plast Surg Hand Surg*. 2016;50(4):246–248.
5. Wang B, Zhao Y, Lu A, Chen C. Ulnar nerve deep branch compression by a ganglion: a review of nine cases. *Injury*. 2014;45(7):1126–1130.
6. Michot A, Chaput B, Alet JM, Pelissier P. Arterial myopericytoma resulting in Guyon's canal syndrome. *Hand Surg Rehabil*. 2016;35(3):231–233.
7. Dobson PF, Purushothaman B, Michla Y, England S, Krishnan MK, Tourret L. Delayed ulnar nerve palsy secondary to ulnar artery pseudoaneurysm distal to Guyon's canal following penetrating trauma to the hand. *Ann R Coll Surg Engl*. 2013;95(5):e75–e76.
8. Paraskevas GK, Ioannidis O, Economou DS. Anomalous muscle causing ulnar nerve compression at Guyon's canal. *J Plast Surg Hand Surg*. 2012;46(3-4):288–290.
9. Ozdemir O, Calisaneller T, Gerilmez A, Gulsen S, Altinors N. Ulnar nerve entrapment in Guyon's canal due to a lipoma. *J Neurosurg Sci*. 2010;54(3):125–127.
10. Kwak KW, Kim MS, Chang CH, Kim SH. Ulnar nerve compression in Guyon's canal by ganglion cyst. *J Korean Neurosurg Soc*. 2011;49(2):139–141.
11. Jeong C, Kim HM, Park IJ. Compression of the ulnar nerve in Guyon's canal by an angioleiomyoma. *J Hand Surg Eur*. 2010;35(7):594–595.
12. Pai V, Harp A, Pai V. Guyon's canal syndrome: a rare case of venous malformation. *J Hand Microsurg*. 2009;1(2):113–115.
13. Francisco BS, Agarwal JP. Giant cell tumor of tendon sheath in Guyon's canal causing ulnar tunnel syndrome. A case report and review of the literature. *Eplasty*. 2009;9:e8.
14. Kim SS, Kim JH, Kang HI, Lee SJ. Ulnar nerve compression at Guyon's canal by an arteriovenous malformation. *J Korean Neurosurg Soc*. 2009;45(1):57–59.
15. Capitani D, Beer S. Handlebar palsy—a compression syndrome of the deep terminal (motor) branch of the ulnar nerve in biking. *J Neurol*. 2002;249(10):1441–1445.
16. Bachoura A, Jacoby SM. Ulnar tunnel syndrome. *Orthop Clin North Am*. 2012;43(4):467–474.
17. Ombaba J, Kuo M, Rayan G. Anatomy of the ulnar tunnel and the influence of wrist motion on its morphology. *J Hand Surg*. 2010;35(5):760–768.
18. Kaiser R, Houstava L, Brzezny R, Haninec P. The results of ulnar nerve decompression in Guyon's canal syndrome [in Czech]. *Acta Chir Orthop Traumatol Cech*. 2012;79(3):243–248.

Radial Neuropathy—Saturday Night Palsy and Posterior Interosseous Neuropathy

Sethesh Mansinghani, Xiaoming Qi, and Jason H. Huang

6

Case Presentation

A 69-year-old right-handed man presents with a chief complaint of weakness in the fingers of his left hand. The symptoms started 2 months earlier, after a fall in which he landed on his left arm. X-rays taken at that time were negative for any fractures. His past medical history is significant for hypertension and is negative for diabetes. Physical examination reveals full strength with elbow flexion and extension. The brachioradialis muscle shows full strength. Wrist extension is 4/5, with radial deviation. At the left metacarpophalangeal (MCP) joints, extension strength is 2/5. Thumb extension is 2/5. Sensation is intact in both the upper and the lower extremities. The patient's deep tendon reflexes are normal.

Questions

1. What is the most likely diagnosis?
2. What is the most appropriate diagnostic testing?
3. What are the next steps in managing this patient?

Assessment and Planning

In this patient, the presentation of finger drop without wrist drop is typical for posterior interosseous nerve (PIN) neuropathy. Electromyography (EMG) is the best diagnostic study to localize the lesion and to confirm the diagnosis. In this patient, EMG shows normal motor unit potentials with full recruitment from the left triceps, brachioradialis, and extensor carpi radialis longus (ECRL) and brevis (ECRB), and reduced recruitment with a variable degree of positive sharp waves and fibrillation potentials from the extensor digitorum communis (EDC), extensor carpi ulnaris (ECU), and extensor pollicis longus (EPL). The electrophysiologic findings confirmed a typical PIN injury.

The differential diagnosis for PIN palsy includes trauma, entrapment, mass lesions, and inflammatory neuropathies. PIN palsy should be differentiated from C7 radiculopathy, radial tunnel syndrome, and more proximal radial nerve injury (e.g., at the spiral groove). Any past trauma should be elicited during the history. EMG, thorough clinical examination, and imaging (including X-rays, ultrasound, and MR imaging) can all be used to work through the differential diagnoses and to localize the nerve injury.

Typical points of compression of the PIN include fibrous bands around the radiocapitellar joint, the leash of Henry, the ECRB, and the arcade of Frohse. The defining feature of PIN palsy is painless weakness with no sensory loss. Often, however, patients may present with poorly localizing pain. The PIN, a branch of the radial nerve, carries motor signals to the superficial layer of the posterior extensor compartment, with the notable exceptions of the ECRL and ECRB, which are innervated by the radial nerve proper proximal to the origin of the PIN. Thus, due to sparing of the ECRL and ECRB, patients will not present with wrist drop. Patients instead present with mildly decreased wrist extension and a radial drift of the hand due to weakness of the ECU, decreased finger extension at the MCP joints due to EDC weakness, and decreased thumb extension due to weakness of the EPB and EPL. Patients typically do not have noticeably weak thumb abduction despite abductor pollicis longus weakness, due to compensation from the median-innervated abductor pollicis brevis (APB).[1–8]

A variant of PIN palsy is radial tunnel syndrome. Compression of the PIN occurs in the typical locations. However, the presentation is markedly different than that of typical PIN palsy. Patients with radial tunnel syndrome present with pain only, without sensory loss or motor dysfunction. Anatomically, the radial tunnel runs from the radiocapitellar joint to the proximal edge of the supinator. Pain associated with radial tunnel syndrome is often aching in character and is located in the dorsum of the proximal forearm. Resisted finger extension or supination often reproduces the symptoms. While no true weakness is found, patients may complain of weakness that in reality is secondary to pain.

More proximal radial nerve injuries in the spiral groove are often associated with fractures of the humerus and with prolonged pressure while unconscious, secondary to either improper positioning during general anesthesia or intoxication (Saturday night palsy). An intoxicated, obtunded person is less likely to self-reposition in response to discomfort caused by improper positioning of the arm over a chair back or headrest compressing the lateral surface of the arm. The same pressure phenomenon can occur when the arm is improperly positioned while under general anesthesia. Regardless of the cause of the injury, patients with injury of the radial nerve in the spiral groove typically present with wrist and finger drop. The triceps strength is intact because the nerve branches to the triceps take off proximal to the spiral groove. They may also have diminished sensation in the distribution of the superficial sensory radial nerve, which can be tested in the dorsal first webspace.

Oral Boards Review—Diagnostic Pearls

1. Physical findings that are extremely important for accurate diagnosis of PIN neuropathy are:
   a. Finger drop (marked extensor weakness of thumb and fingers)
   b. No wrist drop (minimal or no wrist extensor weakness due to sparing of ECRB and ECRL)
   c. Radial deviation with wrist extension due to palsy of ECU
   d. No sensory loss

2. Injury of the radial nerve in the spiral groove is associated with humeral fractures and prolonged pressure when intoxicated (Saturday night palsy) or under general anesthesia.
    a. Physical examination reveals:
        i. Weakness of wrist extensors (wrist drop) and finger extensors (finger drop).
        ii. Normal triceps muscle.
        iii. Decreased sensation in superficial radial sensory distribution.
3. Differential diagnosis of isolated wrist and finger extensor weakness includes lead poisoning.

Decision-Making

Based on the likely mechanism of injury and the localization of the lesion via the physical examination, the neurosurgeon should determine the appropriate diagnostic tests to obtain. EMG should typically be ordered. To assess the PIN, latency potentials of the brachioradialis (a muscle innervated proximal to the PIN) and the extensor carpi ulnaris (a muscle innervated by the PIN) should be measured. In acute denervation, decreased recruitment, increased insertional activity, and fibrillation potentials and/or positive sharp waves are present. In chronic lesions seen after 3 to 6 months, decreased recruitment may still be seen, along with giant motor unit potentials and polyphasia due to peripheral axonal ingrowth. In the case presented here, EMG localizes the lesion to the PIN.

When a history of trauma is present, as in this case, plain X-rays can be useful to detect evidence of fracture or callus formation. Plain X-rays are negative for bony pathology in this case. If the neurosurgeon suspects a mass, MR imaging should be obtained. The space-occupying lesions that most commonly affect the PIN include benign nerve sheath tumors (neurofibromas and schwannomas), ganglion cysts, and lipomas. In cases of entrapment, the PIN may demonstrate T2 hyperintensity. In cases of trauma, a neuroma can occasionally be visualized. In the patient presented, no mass lesion is identified, but T2 hyperintensity is observed in the PIN near its origin. The neurosurgeon suspects a closed traumatic injury to the PIN.

The mechanism of injury is important in determining appropriate treatment. For closed traumatic injuries (for example, injuries related to compression or fractures), a period of 3 months of conservative management with or without physical therapy is reasonable to observe for, and to allow, spontaneous improvement. A wrist splint and hand therapy should be used in order to keep the fingers supple and to maintain range of motion. If, instead, the mechanism of injury involves a laceration or a tumor, surgical treatment is the definitive option. In this case, the patient fails to improve with 3 months of conservative management and surgery is recommended.

Surgical Procedure

In the authors' practice, general anesthesia is preferred for surgical exploration. On the other hand, with a cooperative patient who cannot tolerate general anesthesia, we have occasionally used conscious sedation with local anesthetics. The use of a sterile

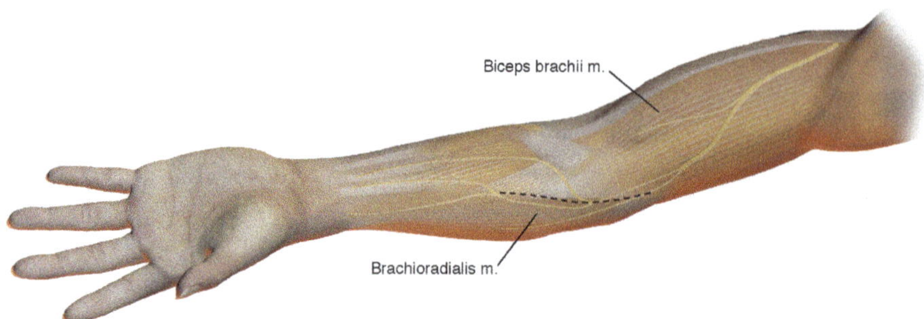

Figure 6.1. The typical incision (dotted line) for exposure of the lateral arm and forearm portion of the radial nerve.

tourniquet is optional but promotes a bloodless field to foster easy identification of the radial nerve and the numerous cutaneous nerves that require preservation. The patient is positioned supine with the affected arm abducted on an arm board. The PIN can be approached either anteriorly or posteriorly. For the anterior approach, which the authors favor, the incision typically begins on the anterolateral aspect of the arm, approximately 5 cm proximal to the elbow crease. The incision is continued distally, turning medially in the elbow crease for 2 to 3 cm before continuing down the midportion of the volar aspect of the arm for approximately 3 to 5 cm (Figure 6.1).

The operation begins with identification of the radial nerve in the interval between the brachioradialis and brachialis (Figure 6.2). Use of intraoperative monitoring and stimulation can facilitate accurate identification. If the radial nerve, rather the PIN, is compressed, proximal dissection to the lateral intermuscular septum is then undertaken. The incision may need to be extended proximally to ensure adequate exposure of the septum, which can run for 8 cm and is most often the primary source of compression and entrapment. The borders of the lateral intermuscular septum (below the cutaneous nerves) are then carefully developed. Decompression is carried out longitudinally along the course of the radial nerve distally and proximally through the entirety of the septum. The surgeon can also use transverse cuts across the septum to ensure decompression in two directions. Then a finger can be used to inspect the

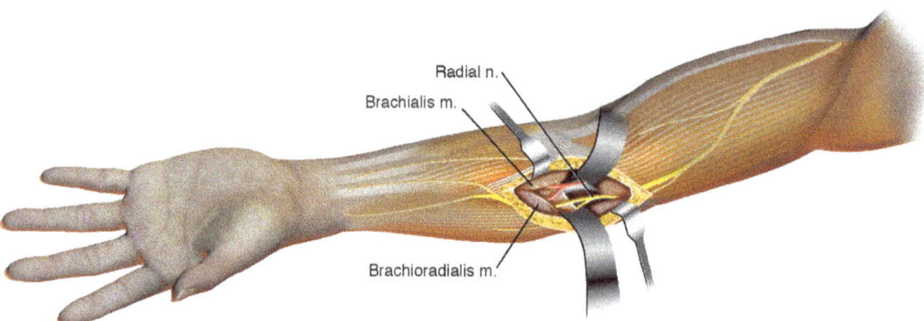

Figure 6.2. Retraction of the brachialis medially and the brachioradialis laterally exposes the radial nerve between the two muscles.

radial nerve circumferentially to ensure no further fibrous bands or points of compression exist along its course.

To decompress the PIN, the first step remains identification of the radial nerve in the interval between the brachioradialis and brachialis. All potential points of compression of the PIN should be inspected and addressed, including fibrous bands around the radial head, the border of the ECRB, the leash of Henry, and the arcade of Frohse. The radial nerve is traced distally in order to identify the branch point of the superficial sensory radial nerve and the PIN, which will be located in the interval between the brachioradialis and ECRL. The posterior cutaneous nerve of the forearm defines this space and should be identified prior to deep dissection. Identification of the superficial sensory radial nerve allows the surgeon to track back proximally to find the PIN with the overlying ECRB. Once all four nerves are exposed (posterior cutaneous nerve of the forearm, radial nerve, superficial sensory radial nerve, and PIN), nerve stimulation can confirm accurate identification of the PIN. Decompression of the PIN begins with cuts laterally and longitudinally along the nerve's course through the ECRB. This will expose the supinator and arcade of Frohse lying inferiorly. The PIN dives deep to the supinator (it is sometimes identified as the deep branch of the radial nerve). A longitudinal decompression is then carried out through the supinator distally, taking care to avoid injuring the two veins that run parallel to the PIN. Any fibrous bands crossing the PIN are divided.

If a neuroma-in-continuity has been identified, at this point, intraoperative nerve action potentials can be recorded across the lesion. If nerve action potentials are present across the lesion, neurolysis alone is sufficient and will allow for a high rate of recovery. If nerve action potentials are absent across the lesion, the surgeon must decide whether to resect the neuroma. If nerve action potentials are absent across the lesion, the authors favor resection of the neuroma followed by primary repair, if feasible, or by graft repair if the gap length would place a primary repair under tension. Harvest sites for the nerve graft should be sterilely prepped at the start of the procedure, and the possible need for nerve graft harvest should be discussed with the patient preoperatively. In the case presented here, with weakness but not absent motor function in the PIN-innervated musculature, one would expect nerve action potentials to be present and neurolysis alone to be sufficient.[2,5–7,9]

Oral Boards Review—Management Pearls

1. Conservative treatment starts with physical therapy for 2 to 3 months.
2. Most injuries where the nerve remains in continuity can be managed nonoperatively because the chance of spontaneous recovery is high.
3. In the presence of a mass lesion, surgery is recommended to be performed earlier.
4. Along the distal half of the humerus, the radial nerve is relatively superficial and is subject to compression (such as by a low-placed, tight blood pressure cuff), iatrogenic injury from injections, penetrating injuries (e.g., bullet wounds or knife wounds), and even blunt trauma.

5. If no improvement is observed after a period of conservative treatment, then surgical exploration should to be considered.
6. The PIN may be approached using an anterior incision, a posterior incision, or a combination of both.
7. The operative treatment options are external neurolysis and release of entrapment, internal neurolysis, and resection of neuroma-in-continuity with primary or graft repair.
8. We recommend the use of general anesthesia without paralytic agents and the use of intraoperative nerve conduction studies.
9. Have the patient's consent for, and be prepared for, nerve grafting.
10. Prep and drape graft harvest sites (e.g., lower extremity for sural nerve harvest) when suspicion for neuroma-in-continuity is high.

Pivot Points

1. Radial nerve injuries are more common in the spiral groove, at the intermuscular septum or just distal to it, and are less common more proximally in the axillary area.
2. Posterior interosseous neuropathy patients have significant extensor weakness of both thumb and fingers (finger drop) but much less wrist extensor weakness (no wrist drop) due to sparing of the ECRB and ECRL.
3. In PIN neuropathy, there will be some radial deviation with wrist extension due to palsy of the ECU.
4. In PIN neuropathy, there is no sensory loss.
5. Patients who have failed 2 to 3 months of conservative treatment, such as physical therapy, need to be considered for surgical exploration, since PIN entrapment may lead to permanent nerve injury.

Aftercare

Generally, patients are allowed early, active range of motion as tolerated to prevent adhesion formation, although some advocate for a course of splinting. Elevation of the arm above the heart level is helpful for relief of throbbing pain. Narcotics may be used as well before transitioning to nonsteroidal anti-inflammatory medications when tolerated. Perioperative antibiotics are continued for 24 hours postoperatively.

Data are lacking on the role of physical therapy in recovery after decompression of either the radial nerve at the spiral groove or the PIN. Nonetheless, a physical therapy rehabilitation program is recommended to promote a faster recovery and a rapid return to work and/or daily activities. Gentle massage of the operative area is encouraged to reduce scar hypertrophy.

Complications and Management

Care should be taken to avoid injury to arteries or cutaneous nerves. However, bleeding and subsequent use of monopolar electrocautery can cause local injury, which may produce sensory disturbance in the distribution of the injured cutaneous nerve, or it may cause the patient to develop a new pain syndrome of neuropathic origin. We use bipolar coagulation set on low current for hemostasis.

Oral Boards Review—Complications Pearls

1. For all radial nerve exploration surgeries, use fine-tipped bipolar coagulation set on low current and avoid the use of monopolar cautery to minimize the risk of damage to the nerves.
2. Have the patient's consent for, and be prepared for, nerve grafting.
3. Use headlight and loupe magnification for dissection. Use an operative microscope for nerve repair.

Evidence and Outcomes

Outcomes of PIN neurolysis are generally good.[3,4] In the largest reported series of PIN palsy, outcomes were graded using the Louisiana State University Health Sciences Center (LSU) grading system, and 20 of 21 patients with PIN entrapment regained LSU Grade 3 or better function. Overall, 43 of 45 patients with a PIN lesion regained LSU Grade 3 or better function.[4] There is increasing clinical evidence for the effectiveness of initial conservative treatment and for good outcomes with surgical decompression of either the radial nerve at the spiral groove or the PIN in patients who fail initial conservative treatment.[3] However, no randomized controlled clinical trials have been performed regarding the effectiveness of treatment for either radial nerve entrapment at the spiral groove or PIN entrapment, perhaps due to the relatively infrequent occurrence of the condition.

References

1. Dang AC, Rodner CM. Unusual compression neuropathies of the forearm, part I: radial nerve. *J Hand Surg Am*. 2009;34:1906–1914.
2. Fessler RG, Sekhar LN. *Atlas of Neurosurgical Techniques: Spine and Peripheral Nerves*. New York, NY: Thieme; 2016.
3. Huisstede BM, Miedema HS, van Opstal T, et al. Interventions for treating the posterior interosseous nerve syndrome: a systematic review of observational studies. *J Peripher Nerv Syst*. 2006;11:101–110.
4. Kim DH, Murovic JA, Kim YY, Kline DG. Surgical treatment and outcomes in 45 cases of posterior interosseous nerve entrapments and injuries. *J Neurosurg*. 2006;104:766–777.
5. Kline D, Hudson AR, Kim DH. *Atlas of Peripheral Nerve Surgery*. Philadelphia, PA: W. B. Saunders; 2001.
6. Mackinnon S. *Nerve Surgery*. New York, NY: Thieme; 2015.
7. Midha R, Zager EL. *Surgery of Peripheral Nerves: A Case-Based Approach*. New York, NY: Thieme; 2008.
8. Spinner RJ. Outcomes for peripheral nerve entrapment syndromes. *Clin Neurosurg*. 2006;53:285–294.
9. Trescot AM. *Peripheral Nerve Entrapments: Clinical Diagnosis and Management*. Cham, Switzerland: Springer; 2016.

Suprascapular Neuropathy

Andrés A. Maldonado and Robert J. Spinner

7

Case Presentation

A 42-year-old man presents to his primary care physician complaining of right posterior shoulder pain and weakness in shoulder abduction and external rotation. He reports that his symptoms began approximately 9 months prior to presentation. He denies any history of trauma. The patient is otherwise healthy. Referral is made to a neurologist.

The neurologist observes atrophy of the shoulder musculature affecting the spinati muscles (Figure 7.1). Muscle testing reveals right trapezius 5/5, deltoid 5/5, rhomboids 5/5, supraspinatus 2/5, infraspinatus 2/5, and latissimus dorsi 5/5; muscles innervated by the median, radial, and ulnar nerves are all 5/5. Left-sided motor testing is all normal. Sensation is normal in the limb. Abduction over the initial 30° of motion is significantly weak. There is no Tinel sign in the neck or in the upper limb. The remainder of the neurologic examination by the neurologist is unremarkable.

Questions

1. What is the likely diagnosis?
2. What is the most appropriate imaging modality?
3. What additional complementary tests would be necessary to confirm the diagnosis?

Assessment and Planning

The neurologist suspects entrapment of the suprascapular nerve (SSN). The diagnosis of suprascapular neuropathy is a challenging one to make from the history and physical examination alone, especially since suprascapular neuropathy can often coexist with other shoulder pathology. The differential diagnosis of SSN entrapment includes C5 radiculopathy, rotator cuff injury, and Parsonage-Turner syndrome. Patients involved in overhead athletic activities, particularly volleyball, baseball, tennis, basketball, and swimming, are at risk for developing suprascapular neuropathy.

The SSN arises in the supraclavicular fossa at the trifurcation of the upper trunk. The SSN is most lateral and arises from the posterior division of the upper trunk; the anterior division of the upper trunk is the most medial of these neural structures. The SSN follows the course of the omohyoid on its deep surface, heading toward the suprascapular notch. It then passes through the suprascapular notch, under the

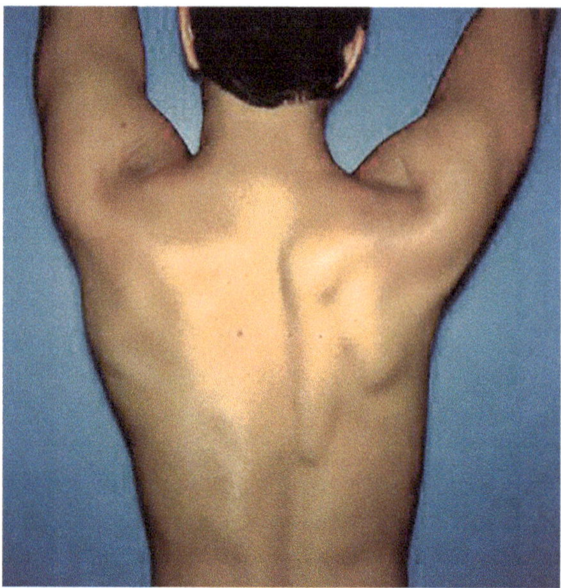

Figure 7.1. This patient presented with posterior shoulder pain and weakness in shoulder abduction and external rotation and was found to have atrophy of the right supra- and infraspinatus muscles.

suprascapular ligament (the suprascapular artery and vein typically pass above the ligament). Beneath the ligament, the SSN may be vulnerable (by sling effect) to entrapment or tethering (Figure 7.2). The SSN innervates the supraspinatus muscle (which effects shoulder abduction, primarily in the first 30°) and the infraspinatus muscle (shoulder external rotation) and also provides sensation to the shoulder joint.[1] The shoulder is a complex joint and many muscles are involved in active motion. Suprascapular neuropathy frequently leads to loss of shoulder active range of motion. Contrary to what's stated in many textbooks, weakness or paralysis of either the supraspinatus or deltoid alone may still allow a full arc of motion due to the other functioning muscle, especially if the patient is young and muscular. In these cases, weakness is still often noted

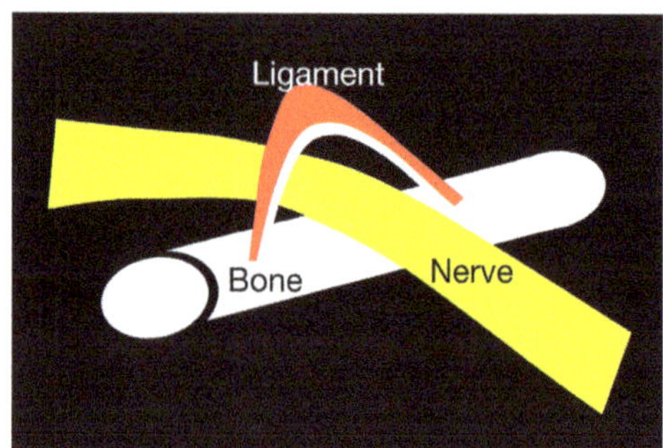

Figure 7.2. Schematic showing nerve compression by a ligament. For example, the suprascapular nerve may be tethered by the transverse scapular ligament, as has been well described by Rengachary et al.[1,7] The suprascapular artery and vein typically run above the ligament.

in resisted abduction, and fatiguing often occurs with overhead activities. Lesions affecting the SSN rarely result in any cutaneous disturbance.

The differential diagnosis of SSN entrapment includes C5 radiculopathy, Parsonage-Turner syndrome, and rotator cuff pathology. C5 radiculopathy in the younger population is usually the result of a disc herniation or an acute injury. In older patients, cervical radiculopathy is often a result of foraminal narrowing from a combination of osteophyte formation, decreased disc height, and degenerative changes of the uncovertebral joints anteriorly and the facet joints posteriorly. Unlike suprascapular neuropathy, C5 radiculopathy also affects the deltoid, rhomboid, and midcervical paraspinal muscles clinically and electrophysiologically. Parsonage-Turner syndrome is a neuritis with a predilection for involvement of certain nerves, including the anterior and posterior interosseous nerves and SSN, in combination or in isolation. The fact that an isolated SSN lesion may occur from an inflammatory etiology can be confusing; when the clinician is considering an entrapment, the presence of subtle features on history or on workup may sway the clinician toward diagnosis of an inflammatory etiology rather than entrapment. Parsonage-Turner syndrome is thought to be an immune-mediated disorder, and triggers, such as viral infection, immunization, or previous surgery, have been associated with the syndrome. The classical clinical history may be present, consisting of sudden-onset pain (often scapular pain), followed by resolution of the pain and then the development of weakness. When present, this history may suggest Parsonage-Turner syndrome. Furthermore, in Parsonage-Turner syndrome, unlike in isolated suprascapular entrapment, electromyography (EMG) may reveal subclinical changes in other muscles, and MR imaging may show subtle changes of denervation in other muscles. Finally, rotator cuff pathology should be considered. Rotator cuff pathology is the most common cause of shoulder pain. The two main causes of rotator cuff tears are injury and degeneration. Previous high-load shoulder injury followed by intensive pain is typical in rotator cuff injuries. Degenerative tears are more frequent in patients over 40 years old who engage in repetitive shoulder activity. MR imaging can be helpful in assessing for rotator cuff injury.

Imaging is helpful in assessing all disorders of the shoulder, including suprascapular neuropathy. Imaging should include plain radiographs (anteroposterior, Grashey AP oblique, scapular outlet, and axillary views) in order to rule out fracture, tumors, and arthropathy. MR imaging is useful to evaluate for soft tissue lesions contributing to nerve injury, such as cysts, retracted rotator cuff tears, or space-occupying lesions. As mentioned previously, MR imaging is also helpful in assessing the rotator cuff for pathology and in assessing muscles not innervated by the SSN for subtle denervation changes. MR imaging of the cervical spine is also helpful in assessing for pathology contributing to a radiculopathy.

Electrodiagnostic studies are another important component of the evaluation of potential SSN entrapment. EMG and nerve conduction studies (NCS) remain the most clinically useful ancillary tests to establish the diagnosis and to eliminate other possibilities in the differential diagnosis. Moreover, these studies are important to monitor nerve function before, during (occasionally), and after the treatment of any of the causes of suprascapular neuropathy. The sensitivity and specificity of EMG and NCS vary from 74% to 91% for various pathologies, but they have not been extensively studied specifically for suprascapular neuropathy.[2–4] Abnormal findings can localize the area of compression or nerve injury or both.[3]

In the present case, shoulder radiographs, MR imaging of the brachial plexus and shoulder, and electrodiagnostic studies are obtained. The X-rays and MR imaging are normal. The electrodiagnostic studies show a severe suprascapular neuropathy with fibrillation potentials in the supra- and infraspinatus muscles. EMG of the deltoid, rhomboids, and cervical paraspinal muscles is normal.

Oral Boards Review—Diagnostic Pearls

1. For diagnosis of suprascapular neuropathy, physical examination must correlate with electrodiagnostic studies.
2. The differential diagnosis of SSN entrapment includes C5 radiculopathy, Parsonage-Turner syndrome, and rotator cuff pathology.
3. MR imaging should be considered to rule out an underlying mass lesion and evidence of denervation beyond the spinati (i.e., findings suggestive of Parsonage-Turner syndrome).

Questions

1. What are the treatment options for suprascapular neuropathy?
2. How do the clinical and radiologic findings influence surgical planning?
3. What are the most common zones of compression of the SSN?

Decision-Making

The etiology of suprascapular neuropathy is the most important factor in choosing the appropriate treatment. The exact timing of surgical intervention is somewhat controversial. When deciding between nonoperative and operative management, one must balance the competing facts that earlier intervention could prevent irreversible nerve damage and muscle atrophy and that a favorable natural history may eliminate the need for surgical intervention. Many cases of Parsonage-Turner syndrome recover late or recovery maximally over 2½ years.

In the absence of a space-occupying lesion, nonoperative measures are considered the initial treatment of choice. These measures consist of nonsteroidal anti-inflammatory drugs (NSAIDs), activity modification, and physical therapy as part of a rehabilitation program.

The indications for a surgical procedure are the failure of nonoperative management with lack of clinical or electrical improvement in 6 to 9 months, and the presence of a space-occupying lesion causing compression of the SSN. Direct nerve decompression is typically recommended in cases of symptomatic isolated suprascapular neuropathy. Because of the wider appreciation of overlap with Parsonage-Turner syndrome, there has been a paradigm shift in the treatment and timing of surgery. Some surgeons have favored observing longer to see if spontaneous recovery occurs. In fact, good results after surgery may, in fact, be due to a favorable natural history of suprascapular neuropathy or Parsonage-Turner syndrome, rather than the nerve decompression.[5] Suprascapular neuropathy due to a mass lesion is still best addressed by mass resection.[6,7]

In the absence of a mass lesion, when surgery is undertaken, the most common locations of compression must be addressed. The two most common locations and etiologies of compression are the suprascapular notch, with or without a rotator cuff tear, and the spinoglenoid notch, with or without a concomitant paralabral cyst.[3] Approaches to the SSN are designed to allow access to these specific locations.

Surgical Procedure

Multiple techniques have been described to decompress the nerve at the suprascapular notch.[8] In the standard open approach, the operation is performed under general anesthesia without the use of long-acting paralytics in order to allow intraoperative nerve stimulation. The SSN is typically exposed through a posterior approach. The authors prefer to place the patient in the prone position using pinions and to approach the nerve in an anatomic position (Figure 7.3). A 6- to 8-cm incision is made centered at the level of the coracoid process and 1 cm superior to the scapular spine. Trapezius fibers are split. Alternatively, the trapezius may be detached from the scapular spine and subsequently repaired at the end of the procedure. The dissection is deep. The atrophied supraspinatus is reflected inferiorly (which eases the dissection to some degree). The operative microscope can be helpful in this part of the operation. The SSN passes obliquely beneath the scapular ligament and appears pearly white. The ligament is released and neurolysis is performed (Figure 7.4). Occasionally, the ligament may be ossified.

Other surgeons have described a superior or anterior approach to the suprascapular notch. Other approaches can be employed depending on the site of pathology (mass lesion) or entrapment (Figure 7.5). An arthroscopic approach can also address joint-related intraneural or extraneural ganglion cysts or decompress the nerve at the suprascapular notch.

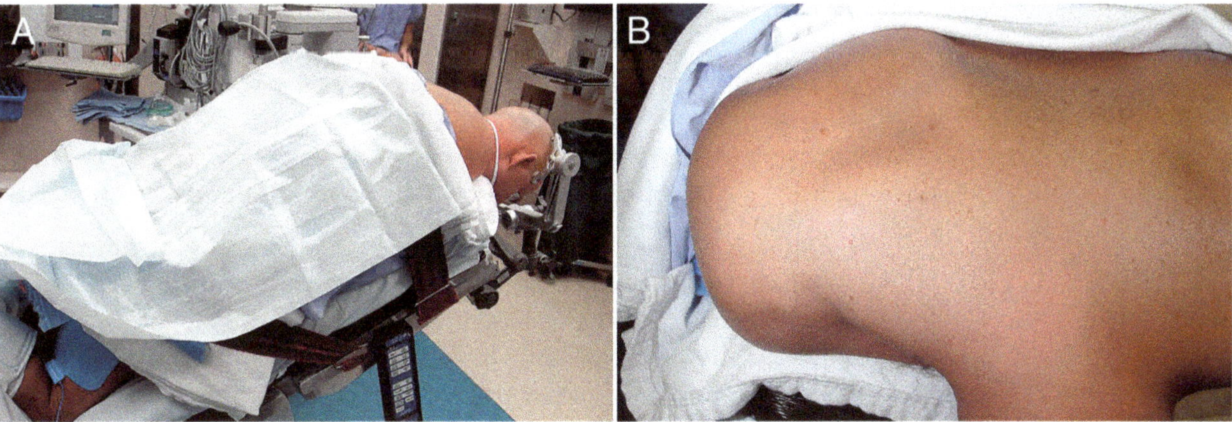

Figure 7.3. Positioning for the posterior approach in suprascapular nerve decompression. A, The patient is positioned prone in pinions, allowing anatomic exposure of the suprascapular nerve. B, The position allows good surgical access to the scapula from either a cephalad or a caudad approach. The microscope can be utilized easily in this position.

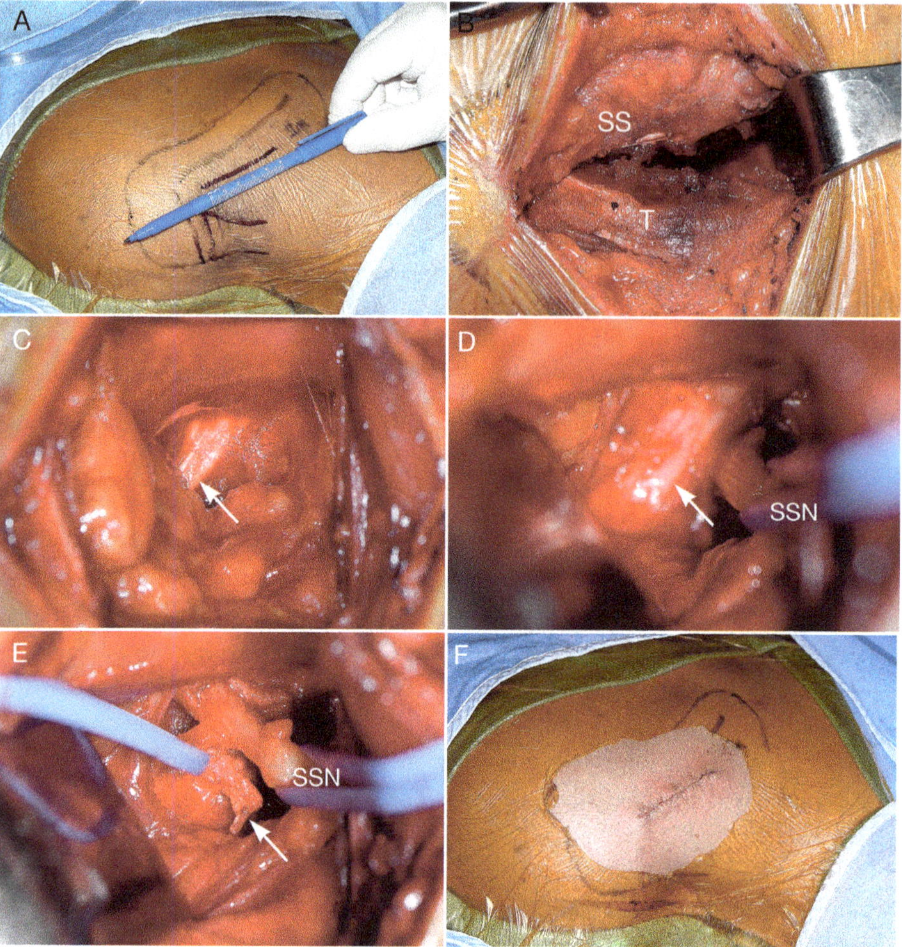

Figure 7.4. Posterior approach to the suprascapular nerve at the transverse scapular ligament. A, A 6- to 8-cm incision is planned posteriorly. B, The trapezius (T) muscle-splitting approach is used. SS = scapular spine. C, The transverse scapular ligament (arrow) is seen. D, The suprascapular nerve (SSN) is identified proximal to the ligament and is protected in a vessel loop. E, The ligament is released. A muscular branch to the supraspinatus is seen (in a vessel loop). F, Skin closure.

Oral Boards Review—Management Pearls

1. EMG is important to confirm the diagnosis, to localize the site of the lesion, to determine the severity of the neuropathy, and to rule out coexisting lesions or more widespread disease.
2. MR imaging of the shoulder is useful to identify rotator cuff pathology, a mass lesion, or denervation atrophy beyond the SSN territory.
3. Indications for surgery are lack of clinical or electrical improvement in 6 to 9 months or the presence of a mass lesion.
4. Release of the transverse scapular ligament for SSN decompression is commonly performed through an open, posterior approach.

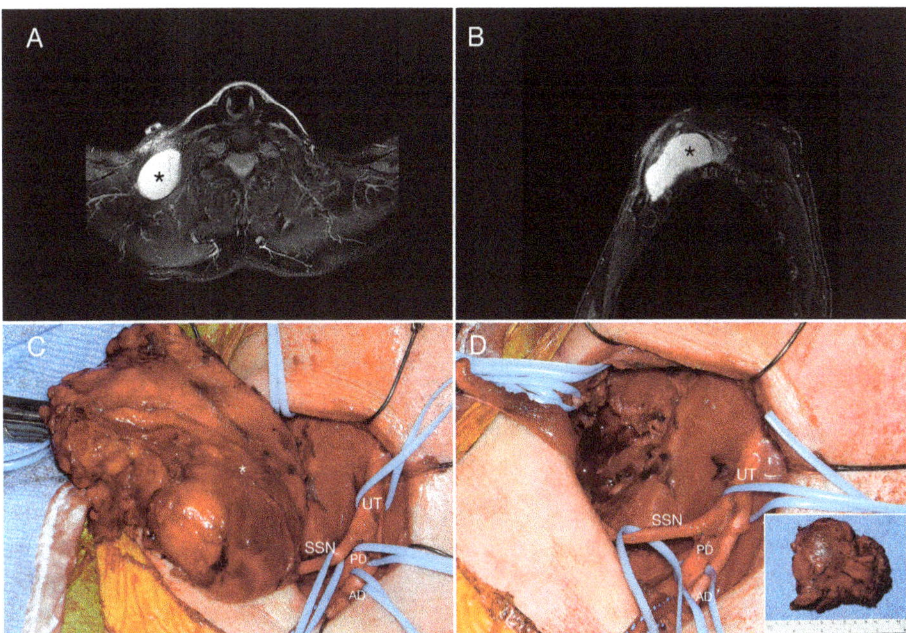

Figure 7.5. Suprascapular nerve compression by a cystic hygroma. Axial (A) and sagittal (B) T2-weighted MR images of the cystic lesion (asterisk). C, A supraclavicular approach allows good access to the mass and the underlying brachial plexus. The upper trunk (UT) at its trifurcation is seen. SSN = suprascapular nerve; PD = posterior division of the upper trunk; AD = anterior division of the upper trunk. D, The mass has been resected (inset) and the nerves have been decompressed.

Pivot Points

1. If a mass lesion (such as a ganglion cyst) is found compressing the nerve, there is no consensus regarding whether the scapular ligament should be released.
2. Massive rotator cuff tears can cause traction injury on the SSN at the suprascapular notch. If a rotator cuff tear and suprascapular neuropathy are found, controversy exists about whether the rotator cuff repair should be accompanied by a concomitant nerve decompression.

Aftercare

Surgery can be done as an outpatient procedure or with an overnight observation. There are no special considerations for immediate postoperative care. Routine perioperative antibiotics are generally given, but they are not continued more than 24 hours postoperatively. Perioperative pain management is provided for the first 10 days. Narcotic pain medicine may be supplemented with NSAIDs. Steroids are generally not necessary or indicated. Progressive shoulder range of motion should be started from postoperative day 1.

In patients with a mass lesion, we recommend MR imaging 3 months after surgery to assess resection and to serve as a baseline. Electrodiagnostic studies can be performed 3 to 9 months after surgery to confirm muscle recovery.

Complications and Management

The most common complication is lack of recovery postoperatively. No recovery or worsening supra- and infraspinatus muscle atrophy can result in a permanent deficit in shoulder abduction and external rotation. If there is no clinical recovery 1 to 2 years after surgery, tendon transfers should be considered as a secondary reconstructive option. Lower trapezius tendon transfer to the infraspinatus tendon has been popularized recently, with good results for external rotation.[8–12]

Nerve pain is another potential complication after any nerve surgery. Patients will describe a deep, dull, and chronic pain, localizing it to the superior, posterior, and lateral aspects of their shoulder, with occasional radiation to the neck or lateral arm. Neuropathic pain medications (e.g., gabapentin, pregabalin, duloxetine) should be considered if the pain does not resolve after surgery. Nerve stimulation can also be considered for refractory cases.

Oral Boards Review—Complications Pearls

1. If there is no motor improvement, tendon transfers should be considered as a secondary reconstructive option to improve shoulder external rotation and abduction.
2. Neuropathic pain medications and nerve stimulation are the two options to treat nerve pain that has not improved with surgical decompression.

Evidence and Outcomes

No prospective studies exist because suprascapular neuropathy is rare, and only a few isolated series are available to guide management. Case series have documented experience with various approaches to surgical management of the pathology, generally with excellent results for pain relief, good results for the improvement in supraspinatus muscle function, and fair results for the improvement in infraspinatus muscle function.[6,13] Significant improvement in pain is seen in approximately 80% to 90% of patients postoperatively.[14–16] Motor improvement is seen in the majority of patients, with better improvement in supraspinatus function than in infraspinatus function.[14,15]

While surgical treatment is generally associated with good to excellent results, nonoperative management has also been associated with good outcomes. In one series of 15 patients managed nonoperatively with physical therapy as part of a rehabilitation program, the result was good or excellent for 12 of 15 patients. Due to persistent symptoms, the remaining three patients underwent operative decompression.[5] Data like these have led many to think that, in the absence of a space-occupying lesion, isolated cases of suprascapular neuropathy may frequently have an inflammatory etiology rather than being caused by an entrapment. Regardless, in the absence of a space-occupying lesion, the data support a trial of nonoperative management.

References

1. Rengachary SS, Burr D, Lucas S, Hassanein KM, Mohn MP, Matzke H. Suprascapular entrapment neuropathy: a clinical, anatomical, and comparative study. Part 2: anatomical study. *Neurosurgery.* 1979;5:447–451.
2. Kraft GH. Axillary, musculocutaneous and suprascapular nerve latency studies. *Arch Phys Med Rehabil.* 1972;53:383–387.
3. Moen TC, Babatunde OM, Hsu SH, Ahmad CS, Levine WN. Suprascapular neuropathy: what does the literature show? *J Shoulder Elbow Surg.* 2012;21:835–846.
4. Nardin RA, Rutkove SB, Raynor EM. Diagnostic accuracy of electrodiagnostic testing in the evaluation of weakness. *Muscle Nerve.* 2002;26:201–205.
5. Martin SD, Warren RF, Martin TL, Kennedy K, O'Brien SJ, Wickiewicz TL. Suprascapular neuropathy. Results of non-operative treatment. *J Bone Joint Surg Am.* 1997;79:1159–1165.
6. Antoniadis G, Richter HP, Rath S, Braun V, Moese G. Suprascapular nerve entrapment: experience with 28 cases. *J Neurosurg.* 1996;85:1020–1025.
7. Rengachary SS, Neff JP, Singer PA, Brackett CE. Suprascapular entrapment neuropathy: a clinical, anatomical, and comparative study. Part 1: clinical study. *Neurosurgery.* 1979;5:441–446.
8. Elhassan BT, Wagner ER, Werthel JD. Outcome of lower trapezius transfer to reconstruct massive irreparable posterior-superior rotator cuff tear. *J Shoulder Elbow Surg.* 2016;25:1346–1353.
9. Elhassan B, Bishop A, Shin A, Spinner R. Shoulder tendon transfer options for adult patients with brachial plexus injury. *J Hand Surg Am.* 2010;35:1211–1219.
10. Elhassan BT, Wagner ER, Spinner RJ, Bishop AT, Shin AY. Contralateral trapezius transfer to restore shoulder external rotation following adult brachial plexus injury. *J Hand Surg Am.* 2016;41:e45–51.
11. Gracitelli ME, Assuncao JH, Malavolta EA, et al. Trapezius muscle transfer for external shoulder rotation: anatomical study. *Acta Ortop Bras.* 2014;22:304–307.
12. Hartzler RU, Barlow JD, An KN, Elhassan BT. Biomechanical effectiveness of different types of tendon transfers to the shoulder for external rotation. *J Shoulder Elbow Surg.* 2012;21:1370–1376.
13. Vastamaki M, Goransson H. Suprascapular nerve entrapment. *Clin Orthop Relat Res.* 1993;297:135–143.
14. Gosk J, Rutowski R, Wiacek R, Reichert P. Experience with surgery for entrapment syndrome of the suprascapular nerve. *Orthop Traumatol Rehabil.* 2007;9:128–133.
15. Kim DH, Murovic JA, Tiel RL, Kline DG. Management and outcomes of 42 surgical suprascapular nerve injuries and entrapments. *Neurosurgery.* 2005;57:120–127.
16. Shah AA, Butler RB, Sung SY, Wells JH, Higgins LD, Warner JJ. Clinical outcomes of suprascapular nerve decompression. *J Shoulder Elbow Surg.* 2011;20:975–982.

Neurogenic Thoracic Outlet Syndrome

Pascal Lavergne and Hélène T. Khuong

8

Case Presentation

A 27-year-old female is referred to a neurosurgeon by her primary care physician with a 3-year history of progressive left hand weakness and numbness over the medial aspect of her left forearm and hand. The patient is otherwise healthy. She works as a secretary and has noticed impairment in typing over the past year. She reports an occasional feeling of heaviness in her left upper extremity. When further questioned, she mentions increased numbness when using her left arm overhead. Examination of her left hand shows moderate atrophy of the thenar eminence, hypothenar eminence, and first dorsal webspace, with intrinsic muscle weakness (Figure 8.1). Sensation to light touch and pinprick is decreased over the medial aspect of left hand and forearm. Horner's sign is present. The remainder of her neurologic exam is within normal limits. Her vascular examination is normal, including provocative maneuvers.

Questions

1. What is the most likely diagnosis?
2. What is the differential diagnosis?
3. What is the appropriate workup?

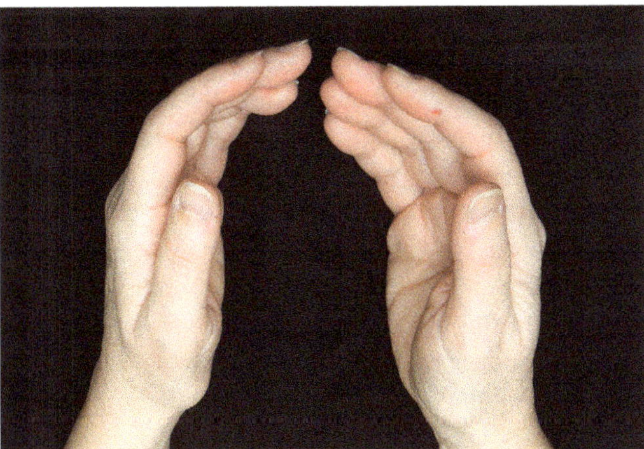

Figure 8.1. When compared to the right hand, the left hand shows atrophy in the thenar eminence and first dorsal webspace.

Assessment and Planning

Neurogenic thoracic outlet syndrome (nTOS) is suspected. The differential diagnosis includes cervical radiculopathy or myelopathy, carpal tunnel syndrome, and ulnar neuropathy, as well as Pancoast tumor. The respective incidences and prevalences of these entities are variable, carpal tunnel syndrome being quite common and nTOS rare in comparison. The reported incidence and prevalence of nTOS vary due to lack of established diagnostic criteria. Moreover, two distinct entities are often considered to be part of the nTOS spectrum: true nTOS and disputed TOS. The difference between the true and disputed forms lies in the neurologic examination. Disputed TOS is an upper extremity pain syndrome in which the neurologic examination is normal.[1]

nTOS is an entrapment neuropathy, and accurately identifying the site of compression through clinical, radiologic, and electrophysiologic examination influences further management. Three anatomic passageways have been described as being possible sites of compression along the trajectory of the brachial plexus from the cervical spine to the axilla: the interscalene triangle, the costoclavicular space, and the subcoracoid space. The interscalene triangle is bordered by the anterior scalene anteriorly, the middle scalene posteriorly, and the first rib inferiorly. The lower trunk is usually involved, with compression from hypertrophic or anomalous muscle. The costoclavicular space is defined by the clavicle anteriorly, the first rib posteromedially, and the scapula posterolaterally. Compression of the lower trunk in this space may relate to an elongated C7 transverse process, a cervical rib, or fibrous bands that extend between an anomalous bony structure and the first thoracic rib. The subcoracoid space lies just beneath the coracoid process and deep to the pectoralis minor tendon. Pectoralis minor syndrome occurs at this site, triggered by rotation of the brachial plexus around the tendon.[2–5]

nTOS usually has an insidious presentation. Whiplash injury or repeated trauma is sometimes reported. Numbness, with or without tingling, is usually present. Hand weakness and muscle atrophy are slow to evolve. Examination of the neck, shoulder, and upper extremity aims to confirm the presence of TOS and to exclude other causes. General evaluation looks for muscle imbalance, particularly forward flexion of the neck and drooping shoulders, while active and passive shoulder range of motion are evaluated for possible rotator cuff pathology, and Spurling's test is assessed for the presence of cervical disc disease. A Tinel sign may be present over the supraclavicular area. Many diagnostic maneuvers for TOS have been described. Although useful, their specificity is not very high. In addition to specific maneuvers, a detailed neurologic exam is essential, looking for specific hand atrophy (Gilliat-Sumner hand), weakness, and sensory changes in a C8-T1 distribution. Horner's sign, when present, comes from involvement of the sympathetic fibers as they exit the spinal cord along the T1 nerve root.

Initial radiologic investigation begins with plain cervical X-rays to identify a cervical rib or elongated transverse process. In case of such abnormality, a cervical CT scan will help to adequately visualize the bony anatomy. Cervical spine MR imaging helps to rule out more commonly found cervical radiculopathy or myelopathy. MR imaging allows visualization of the path of the brachial plexus. In addition to MR neurography, MR tractography now permits better imaging of nerve fascicles and may help to define the type of injury and regeneration potential.[1,6,7]

Nerve conduction studies (NCS) and electromyography (EMG) are very helpful in demonstrating nerve or muscle impairment and in confirming localization of the

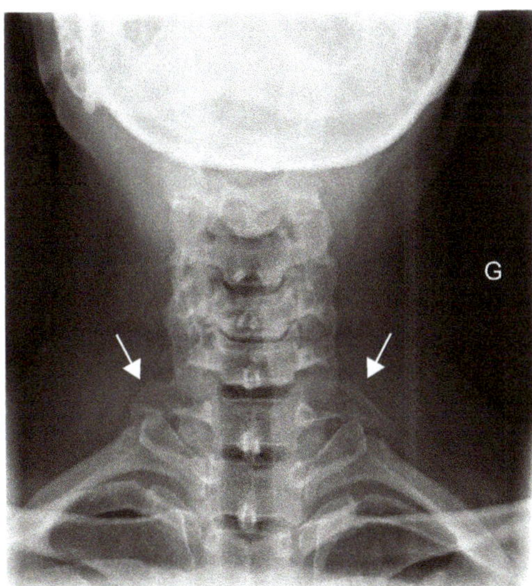

Figure 8.2. Cervical spine X-ray (anteroposterior view) showing bilateral elongated C7 transverse processes (arrows).

lesion. Typical findings of nTOS include low-amplitude median motor responses and ulnar sensory responses, low or normal ulnar motor responses, and normal median sensory responses. Altered sensory conduction is present in the medial antebrachial cutaneous nerve. EMG may show acute or chronic neurogenic changes, with fibrillations or decreased recruitment, particularly in the abductor pollicis brevis (APB) and first dorsal interosseous (FDI) muscles.

In the case described here, plain X-ray and CT scan show bilateral elongated C7 transverse processes (Figures 8.2 and 8.3). MR imaging excludes coexistent

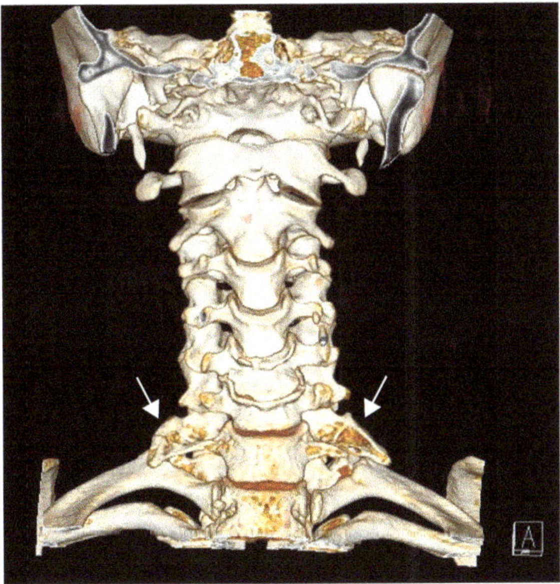

Figure 8.3. CT scan with 3-dimensional reconstruction showing bilateral elongated C7 transverse processes (arrows).

cervical disease but fails to demonstrate a clear site of compression or a fibrous band extending to the first rib. NCS/EMG shows classic denervation signs in a C8-T1 distribution.

Questions

1. Is conservative management appropriate for this patient?
2. What are the nonsurgical treatment options?
3. How would the management change in a case of disputed TOS?

Oral Board Review—Diagnostic Pearls

1. Physical examination is helpful in diagnosis of nTOS.
   a. Reproducing symptoms with shoulder hyperabduction and neck rotation (Wright's test, also called hyperabduction maneuver), with ipsilateral head rotation and inspiration (Adson's test), or by opening and closing the hand while the shoulder is abducted and externally rotated (Roos test or elevated arm stress test [EAST]) points to a diagnosis of TOS.
   b. Muscle atrophy and weakness involve both ulnar- and median-innervated intrinsic hand muscles, predominantly the abductor pollicis brevis muscle (Gilliat-Sumner hand).
   c. Sensory loss is found in the ulnar and medial antebrachial cutaneous nerve territories.
2. Plain X-ray can reveal cervical ribs or elongated transverse processes.
3. CT scan is optional but helps with understanding abnormal bony anatomy.
4. Cervical spine MR imaging is essential to rule out cervical radiculopathy or myelopathy, as well as the more rarely found spinal cord neoplasm or syringomyelia.
5. NCS and EMG help to demonstrate neural compression and to localize the lesion.
6. Vascular imaging, either CT angiography or digital subtraction angiography, is useful to rule out vascular TOS.
7. Disputed TOS is predominantly a pain syndrome with few neurologic or radiological findings.

Decision-Making

Ideal timing for surgical decompression has yet to be described in the literature and recommendations vary between authors. Some suggest that any type of TOS, either true nTOS or disputed TOS, should undergo a trial of conservative management. Conservative management in a patient with nTOS includes reduction of activities that exacerbate symptoms, especially overhead work. Physical therapy works on correcting poor posture and strengthening shoulder girdle musculature. Other nonpharmacologic measures, such as customized bracing or transcutaneous electrical nerve stimulation (TENS), may be tried, but their effect is often limited and evidence for their efficacy is low.[8,9]

Pharmacologic measures help to reduce pain in nTOS. Nonsteroidal anti-inflammatory agents, narcotics, antidepressants, antiepileptic drugs, and muscle relaxants are among the most commonly used. Stellate ganglion, cervical root, cervical epidural, and interscalene nerve blocks have been tried.[8,10] Botulinum toxin injection targeted toward the anterior scalene or pectoralis minor muscle can improve symptoms, although research has failed to demonstrate its definitive efficacy.[11]

Even with the myriad conservative management modalities available, patients often respond poorly, and surgical treatment is elected. In this context, some advocate that, for patients with true nTOS, with an identified site of compression and NCS/EMG neurogenic changes, early surgery could prevent irreversible denervation and lead to better functional outcomes.

The surgical approach should target the site of compression identified through clinical and ancillary studies. The supraclavicular approach is often preferred in nTOS cases because it offers the easiest access to brachial plexus structures and allows for lower trunk neurolysis.[12] Recognized compression points, such as the scalene muscles, a cervical rib, the first thoracic rib, an elongated transverse process, or various fibrous bands, may be released. If the identified compression point is the pectoralis minor tendon, an infraclavicular approach is used. Although it is more commonly used to treat vascular TOS, a transaxillary approach has been described and may be used for first rib resection.

When the surgeon is planning a supraclavicular approach, patients should be counseled about potential complications, including brachial plexus injury, vascular structure injury, infection, surgical site hematoma, phrenic or long thoracic nerve injury, persistence of symptoms, symptom recurrence, incisional pain, intercostobrachial neuralgia, and pneumothorax.

Questions

1. Which surgical approaches can be used for nTOS?
2. Which neural structures should be neurolysed during surgical decompression?
3. How should bony abnormalities be approached surgically?
4. Which potential complications should be explained while obtaining consent?

Surgical Procedure

The surgical procedure is performed under general anesthesia. Either intraoperative EMG monitoring of the involved upper extremity or nerve stimulation may be used. Headlight illumination with loupe magnification and/or use of the surgical microscope is critical to diminish procedural risks.

The patient is positioned supine with a bolster between the shoulders for neck extension. The head is rotated to the contralateral side (Figure 8.4). The arms should be mobile enough to allow easy abduction or adduction of the shoulder. Before final positioning and draping, important anatomic landmarks, such as the midline, the posterior border of the sternocleidomastoid (SCM) muscle, the angle of the mandible,

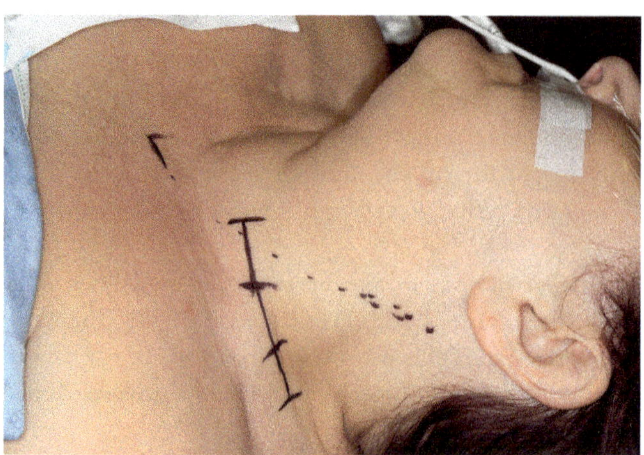

Figure 8.4. The typical incision for the supraclavicular approach begins at the posterior border of the sternocleidomastoid muscle and proceeds parallel to the clavicle.

the clavicle, and the deltopectoral groove, are identified and marked. The neck, upper torso, and proximal arm are prepped and draped, for a possible infraclavicular approach, if needed.

The classic incision is made approximately one to two fingerbreadths above and paralleling the clavicle, starting at the posterior border of the SCM muscle and extending toward the lateral third of the clavicle. The skin incision exposes the platysma muscle, which is divided with monopolar cautery or scissors and then is retracted with self-retaining retractors, exposing the SCM. The avascular plane beneath the platysma is dissected. The external jugular vein is then identified, ligated, and divided. Next, the clavicular head of the SCM is detached with monopolar cautery and retracted medially. Dissecting in the fat layer beneath the SCM exposes muscle bellies of the omohyoid and its intervening tendon. The omohyoid muscle is either retracted inferiorly or tagged and divided at its tendon. The transverse cervical vessels are then ligated and divided. At this point, the scalene fat pad is fully visualized.

The scalene fat pad is elevated and retracted laterally, and it must be preserved to fill the supraclavicular fossa during closure. The anterior scalene muscle is then exposed, with the phrenic nerve running on its anterior surface. This important nerve is identified and protected, and then it is followed superiorly until its junction with the C5 nerve root. The combination of the C5 and C6 nerve roots forms the upper trunk. Inferior to the upper trunk lies the middle trunk, formed by the C7 nerve root. Deeper and inferior dissection allows identification of the lower trunk, formed by the junction of the C8 and T1 nerve roots. Being the deepest, the lower trunk is more difficult to expose. To aid in exposure, anterior scalenectomy is performed and can be therapeutic if the compression originates in the interscalene triangle. During scalenectomy, care is taken to protect the phrenic nerve as well as to look out for the subclavian artery, which can arc rostrally and obscure the lower trunk. The entire compressed trunk, most typically the lower trunk, must then be circumferentially neurolysed, taking care not to injure the long thoracic

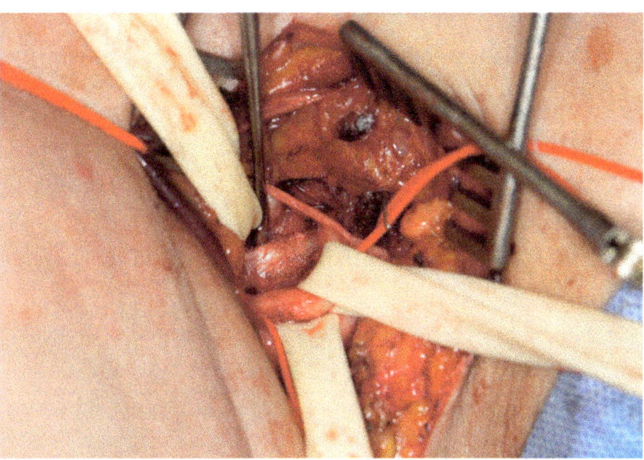

Figure 8.5. Operative photograph showing a rigid fibrous band attached to a prominent C7 transverse process, between the C7 and C8 nerve roots. The phrenic nerve is seen crossing the surgical field after anterior scalenectomy.

nerve. While performing neurolysis, the surgeon should look out for compressive structures, such as a hypertrophied scalene muscle, a cervical rib, or fibrous bands that extend from an elongated transverse process often connected to the first rib (Figure 8.5). Anomalous bony structures are then resected with a Kerrison or Leksell rongeur, and any compressive fibrous bands are resected, if possible (Figure 8.6). At the end of surgery, all neural elements should be free of any possible residual compression or irritation. When decompression is complete, the field is copiously irrigated, hemostasis is achieved, and a multilayered closure is performed. The scalene fat pad and omohyoid muscle are returned to their native anatomic location, the platysma muscle is closed with resorbable suture, and the skin is closed according to the surgeon's preference.

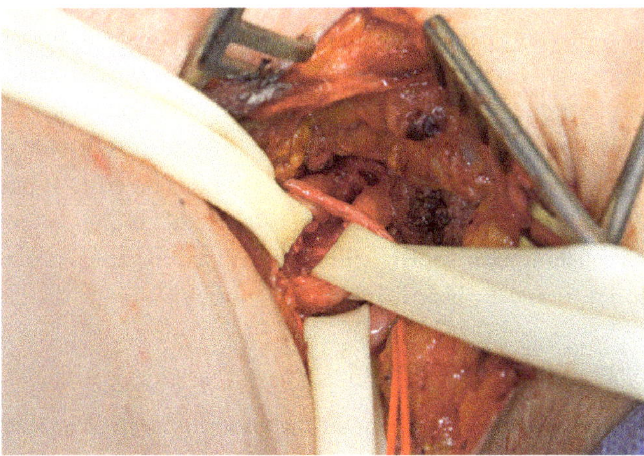

Figure 8.6. Operative photograph after resection of the fibrous band and the lateral part of the C7 transverse process.

Oral Board Review—Management Pearls

1. A trial of conservative management, including pharmacologic treatment and physical therapy, may help resolve subjective symptoms.
2. The goal of surgery in the presence of muscle atrophy is to stop further neurologic deterioration.
3. Compressive fibrous bands are often not visualized on imaging studies, including MR imaging.
4. Classic surgical approaches include supraclavicular and transaxillary exposures. The transaxillary approach offers good visualization of the first rib, while the supraclavicular approach targets compressed brachial plexus elements.

Pivot Points

1. If muscle atrophy is present, surgical decompression is preferable to conservative management.
2. In the presence of anatomic variations, surgery may yield a better outcome than conservative management.
3. A positive muscle block in the pectoralis minor or anterior scalene muscle localizes the compression point and should direct surgical management toward the targeted muscle.

Aftercare

Patients are typically kept overnight in the hospital for pain management. The follow-up interval is at the discretion of the surgeon, but usually a follow-up appointment at 2 weeks is recommended to ensure proper wound healing. The next follow-up is typically at 3 or 6 months and can include NCS/EMG to look for signs of reinnervation, especially in the case of true nTOS. Disputed TOS is followed clinically, except if electrophysiologic signs were present preoperatively. Postoperative imaging studies are usually not required, except in cases with persistent or recurring symptoms.

Physical therapy is an important part of the healing process. It should begin 2 to 3 weeks postoperatively, once the operative pain is gone. The goals of physical therapy are to restore muscle balance by stretching and strengthening upper extremity musculature. Hand rehabilitation, ideally with a specialized therapist, is essential in cases of nTOS with significant intrinsic hand muscle atrophy.

Complications and Management

The supraclavicular approach is a methodical approach that has low risk of complication if performed adequately, but it exposes many critical neurovascular structures that must be preserved at all cost. Nerve injury to the brachial plexus or vascular injury to the subclavian vessels can be catastrophic. In the case of a brachial plexus injury not identified intraoperatively, early reoperation and coaptation with or without grafting must be performed. Vascular injury must be managed immediately and the assistance of a vascular surgeon is required. Phrenic nerve injury leads to hemidiaphragm palsy, while winged scapula results from a long thoracic nerve injury. Pneumothorax is a rare but possible complication. It occurs more frequently during a first rib resection and is usually easily dealt with by placement of a chest tube for a few days. A rare but disappointing complication is complex regional pain syndrome, which can lead to significant disability. Early pharmacologic management and physical therapy may help to prevent long-term consequences.

Oral Boards Review—Complication Pearls

1. Intraoperative electrophysiologic monitoring, with avoidance of systemic paralytic agents, is essential to avoid iatrogenic nerve injury.
2. Care must be taken to identify and to protect the phrenic and long thoracic nerves. Postoperative chest X-ray will help to rule out phrenic nerve injury and hemidiaphragm paresis.
3. Other nonneural surrounding structures that may be injured intraoperatively include the stellate ganglion, thoracic duct, and lymphatic vessels, as well as the subclavian artery and vein.
4. Persistence or recurrence of symptoms may be due to incomplete decompression, excessive scarring at the surgical site, or improper identification of the site of compression. Appropriately selected patients may benefit from revision surgery.

Evidence and Outcome

Very few high-quality studies exist that focus on treatment and outcomes of nTOS. This is due to a combination of factors: variability in diagnostic criteria among different studies, few well-designed prospective studies, and diversity in surgical approaches. Recently, a review of treatment of TOS found very few randomized controlled trials with 6-month follow-up.[13] With variability in diagnostic criteria and surgical approach, reported rates of postoperative good outcome also vary significantly, ranging from 40% to over 90%.[14–17] The key to good outcomes is principally good patient selection for surgical treatment when clinical, radiologic, and electrophysiologic studies are concordant. Recent advances in neuroimaging can aid in patient selection by better demonstration of the point of compression and may eventually lead to improved surgical outcomes.

References

1. Magill ST, Brus-Ramer M, Weinstein PR, Chin CT, Jacques L. Neurogenic thoracic outlet syndrome: current diagnostic criteria and advances in MRI diagnostics. *Neurosurg Focus*. 2015;39:E7.
2. Ferrante MA. The thoracic outlet syndromes. *Muscle Nerve*. 2012;45:780–795.
3. Freischlag J, Orion K. Understanding thoracic outlet syndrome. *Scientifica (Cairo)*. 2014;2014:248163.

4. Hooper TL, Denton J, McGalliard MK, Brismee JM, Sizer PS Jr. Thoracic outlet syndrome: a controversial clinical condition. Part 1: anatomy, and clinical examination/diagnosis. *J Man Manip Ther.* 2010;18:74–83.
5. Huang JH, Zager EL. Thoracic outlet syndrome. *Neurosurgery.* 2004;55:897–902; discussion 902–893.
6. Baumer P, Kele H, Kretschmer T, et al. Thoracic outlet syndrome in 3T MR neurography—fibrous bands causing discernible lesions of the lower brachial plexus. *Eur Radiol.* 2014;24:756–761.
7. Filler A. Magnetic resonance neurography and diffusion tensor imaging: origins, history, and clinical impact of the first 50,000 cases with an assessment of efficacy and utility in a prospective 5000-patient study group. *Neurosurgery.* 2009;65:A29–A43.
8. Hooper TL, Denton J, McGalliard MK, Brismee JM, Sizer PS Jr. Thoracic outlet syndrome: a controversial clinical condition. Part 2: non-surgical and surgical management. *J Man Manip Ther.* 2010;18:132–138.
9. Watson LA, Pizzari T, Balster S. Thoracic outlet syndrome part 2: conservative management of thoracic outlet. *Man Ther.* 2010;15:305–314.
10. Lum YW, Brooke BS, Likes K, et al. Impact of anterior scalene lidocaine blocks on predicting surgical success in older patients with neurogenic thoracic outlet syndrome. *J Vasc Surg.* 2012;55:1370–1375.
11. Finlayson HC, O'Connor RJ, Brasher PM, Travlos A. Botulinum toxin injection for management of thoracic outlet syndrome: a double-blind, randomized, controlled trial. *Pain.* 2011;152:2023–202.
12. Terzis JK, Kokkalis ZT. Supraclavicular approach for thoracic outlet syndrome. *Hand (N Y).* 2010;5:326–337.
13. Povlsen B, Hansson T, Povlsen SD. Treatment for thoracic outlet syndrome. *Cochrane Database Syst Rev.* 2014;11:CD007218.
14. Landry GJ, Moneta GL, Taylor LM Jr, Edwards JM, Porter JM. Long-term functional outcome of neurogenic thoracic outlet syndrome in surgically and conservatively treated patients. *J Vasc Surg.* 2001;33:312–317; discussion 317–319.
15. Martens V, Bugden C. Thoracic outlet syndrome: a review of 67 cases. *Can J Surg.* 1980;23:357–358.
16. Mingoli A, Feldhaus RJ, Farina C, et al. Long-term outcome after transaxillary approach for thoracic outlet syndrome. *Surgery.* 1995;118:840–844.
17. Sheth RN, Campbell JN. Surgical treatment of thoracic outlet syndrome: a randomized trial comparing two operations. *J Neurosurg Spine.* 2005;3:355–363.

Peroneal Neuropathy—Fibular Tunnel Syndrome

Thomas J. Wilson and Robert J. Spinner

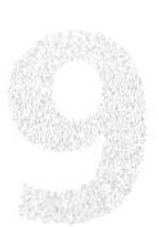

Case Presentation

A 43-year-old woman presents with the chief complaint of left foot drop. Approximately 6 weeks earlier, she had been at an amusement park and the following day began noticing foot drop. Over the ensuing 3 days, she noted progression of the foot drop. She also began to note paresthesias and pain over the lateral aspect of her leg and the dorsum of her foot. She described the pain as beginning around her knee and radiating down her leg. She was initially evaluated by her primary care physician, who ordered MR imaging of her lumbar spine. The study revealed mild, multi-level degenerative disease without any significant central canal or neuroforaminal stenosis. She was prescribed an ankle–foot orthosis (AFO), which she continues to wear. Since that time, she has not noted any improvement in her strength and continues to have pain and paresthesias in the same distribution. On physical examination, she has normal strength in her upper and lower extremities, with the exception of 1/5 dorsiflexion, 1/5 toe extension, 1/5 extensor hallucis longus, and 1/5 eversion on the left. Plantar flexion and inversion are both full strength bilaterally. She has decreased sensation to fine touch and pinprick along the lateral aspect of the left leg and over the dorsum of the left foot. Patellar and Achilles reflexes are 2+ bilaterally, and no pathologic reflexes are present. Straight leg raise (SLR) test is negative. Percussion about the fibular neck on the left yields pain and paresthesias in the same distribution as her baseline pain and paresthesias.

Questions

1. What is the most likely diagnosis?
2. What are the next steps in the diagnostic evaluation?
3. When, in relation to the time of injury, should the next diagnostic steps be performed?
4. What is the most likely site of injury/compression?

Assessment and Planning

A diagnosis of common peroneal neuropathy is suspected. The other major diagnosis to be considered when a patient presents with foot drop is an L5 radiculopathy. Distinguishing between common peroneal neuropathy and L5 radiculopathy can be accomplished by clinical history and physical examination. The history of pain starting around the knee and radiating distally, as opposed to originating in the back and radiating down the entire leg, is a helpful finding. Testing of inversion and eversion can be particularly helpful in differentiating between common peroneal neuropathy and L5 radiculopathy. Dorsiflexion weakness with eversion weakness is typical of peroneal neuropathy, while dorsiflexion weakness with inversion weakness is typical of L5 radiculopathy. Also, the finding of percussion tenderness at the fibular neck and a negative SLR test can help diagnose a common peroneal neuropathy. The diagnosis can then be confirmed by electrodiagnostic studies and imaging.

Oral Boards Review—Diagnostic Pearls

1. Inversion and eversion testing can help differentiate foot drop secondary to peroneal neuropathy from foot drop secondary to L5 radiculopathy.
   a. L5 radiculopathy is characterized by dorsiflexion weakness plus weakness of inversion.
   b. Common peroneal neuropathy is characterized by dorsiflexion weakness plus weakness of eversion.
2. Results of provocative maneuvers, including a negative SLR test and positive Tinel test at the fibular neck, suggest common peroneal neuropathy.
3. Presentation with predominant weakness of muscles innervated by the deep peroneal nerve suggests the possibility of an intraneural ganglion cyst.
4. High-resolution imaging (MR imaging or ultrasound) should be utilized in the evaluation of patients presenting with unusual neuropathies, including peroneal neuropathy, which has a high association with mass lesions, the most common of which is an intraneural ganglion cyst.

Common peroneal neuropathy is the most common compressive neuropathy of the lower extremity.[1] It often presents with acute, progressive foot drop. The most common site of compression of the peroneal nerve is as it courses around the neck of the fibula beneath the fascia of the peroneus longus.[2] The most common points of compression are a fibrous band deep to the superficial head of the peroneus longus, a fibrous band on the surface of the deep head of the peroneus longus, and at the confluence of the origins of the soleus muscle and the peroneus longus.[3] A number of factors have been shown to predispose an individual to peroneal neuropathy, including weight loss, diabetes mellitus, and prolonged pressure, such as can occur with habitual leg crossing or prolonged squatting.[2,4–6] Iatrogenic causes should also be considered, such as compression from positioning with prolonged pressure during surgery, knee surgery with compression, stretch, or direct injury to the nerve, pneumatic sequential compression devices, casting/bracing, or pressure from an AFO.[2,4,6–9] The peroneal division of the sciatic nerve is also more susceptible to stretch injury when stretch occurs at the hip. The peroneal division is positioned more laterally than the tibial division of the nerve, and the relative distance between the points of fixation—the piriformis muscle and the fibular neck for the peroneal nerve versus the piriformis muscle and the tarsal tunnel for the tibial nerve—is shorter for the peroneal nerve. Thus, stretch injury, such as can occur during hip surgery or traumatic hip dislocation, is more likely to injure the peroneal nerve than the tibial nerve.[10,11] Mass lesions should also be considered as the cause of peroneal neuropathy, particularly when the onset is insidious. The most common mass lesion of the peroneal nerve is an intraneural ganglion cyst. Less commonly, schwannomas, neurofibromas, and osteochondromas can involve or compress the peroneal nerve. In one series, mass lesions accounted for 13% of patients presenting with peroneal neuropathy.[12] In another series, in 41 patients presenting with foot drop, 18% of patients with an isolated peroneal neuropathy (5 of 28) had an intraneural ganglion cyst on ultrasound examination.[13] Patients with an intraneural ganglion cyst often present with weakness predominantly in the muscles innervated by the deep peroneal nerve.

Electrodiagnostic studies can be helpful in both confirming the diagnosis and localizing the pathology. It is important to note, however, that results of electrodiagnostic studies may not be revealing until 4 to 6 weeks after the initial injury or initial onset of symptoms. Both electromyography (EMG) and nerve conduction studies (NCS) should be performed. NCS of the extensor digitorum brevis and tibialis anterior should be included, and stimulation should be applied both above and below the fibular neck and the values compared. Slowing of conduction across the fibular neck is seen in patients with peroneal neuropathy. Needle EMG can be particularly helpful in both localizing the pathology and determining the severity of the lesion. Typical needle EMG includes the tibialis anterior, peroneus longus, short head of the biceps femoris, and a tibial-innervated muscle. In addition, the tibialis posterior is included because it is L5 innervated via the tibial nerve rather than the peroneal nerve. Involvement of the short head of the biceps femoris suggests a lesion more proximal than at the fibular neck. Gluteal muscles and lumbosacral paraspinal muscles are also tested to help localize the lesion and to rule out a proximal lesion (e.g., lumbosacral plexopathy or radiculopathy).[1,14]

High-resolution ultrasound can be a useful diagnostic adjunct in the diagnosis of peroneal neuropathy, both in confirming the diagnosis and in ruling out secondary causes. Visualizing the peroneal nerve proximal to the fibular head is difficult, but the nerve can be readily identified at the fibular head. Ultrasound has been shown to have higher sensitivity and specificity for peroneal neuropathy than electrodiagnostic studies have. Useful measurements include the area of the nerve, its transverse breadth, and its transverse length. The area of the nerve and its transverse length seem to be particularly useful because they have been shown to have a negative correlation with peroneal motor amplitude.[15] Ultrasound can also be used to identify mass lesions that may be causing the peroneal neuropathy.

While high-resolution ultrasound is being increasingly used, the imaging modality of choice for evaluation of the peroneal nerve is MR imaging, and it is particularly useful in evaluating for an underlying mass lesion, such as an intraneural ganglion cyst, the most common mass lesion causing peroneal neuropathy. In addition to standard MR imaging, MR neurography is being increasingly utilized. MR imaging is particularly helpful because the presence of a mass lesion changes the surgical plan. The most sensitive marker for peroneal neuropathy is T2 hyperintensity in the peroneal nerve. Other imaging characteristics that show high specificity but lower sensitivity include nerve size, fascicular morphology, and atrophy of muscle supplied by the nerve.[16]

While MR imaging can be useful in confirming the diagnosis, its main use and the reason that it should be utilized when evaluating patients with peroneal neuropathy is the identification of mass lesions causing the peroneal neuropathy. Identification of such lesions significantly alters the management plan and thus is imperative. Peroneal intraneural ganglion cysts have been shown to have an articular origin.[17] The joint origin may be difficult to visualize but it can be easiest to establish on axial or sagittal images. For example, standard bony landmarks can be incorporated into a clock face in order to make an accurate diagnosis of an intraneural ganglion on axial MR images. For the right peroneal nerve (mirror image for the left), the common peroneal nerve can be seen in the 7 or 8 o'clock position at the midportion of the fibular head. When an intraneural ganglion cyst is present on axial, T2-weighted imaging, the cyst and nerve can both be seen at the 7 or 8 o'clock position at the midportion of the fibular head, a finding that is referred to as the signet ring sign (Figure 9.1A). On the same image, the cyst within the articular branch can also be seen at the superior tibiofibular joint (STFJ) connection at the 12 or 1 o'clock position, which is referred to as the tail sign (Figure 9.1A). Similarly, a few axial images lower, at the midportion of the fibular neck, the cyst can be observed in the 10 to 12 o'clock position in the transverse limb of the articular branch, a finding called the transverse limb sign (Figure 9.1B).[18] These findings can be used to differentiate between intraneural and extraneural cysts, with important treatment ramifications.

Questions

1. Where is the most common site of compression of the peroneal nerve?
2. What factors predispose to peroneal neuropathy?
3. What is the imaging modality of choice in the evaluation of peroneal neuropathy?
4. How do the imaging findings influence surgical approach?

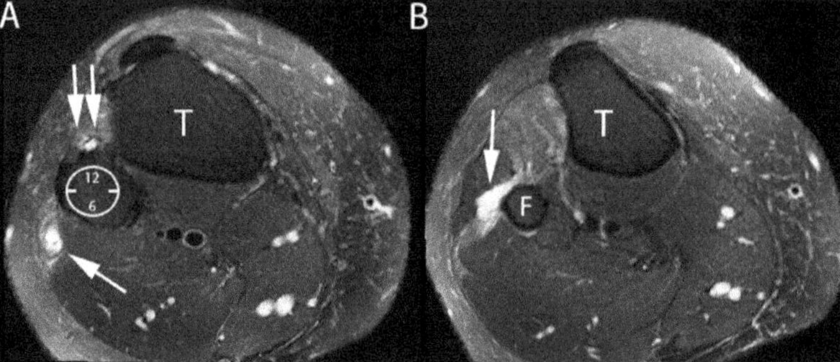

Figure 9.1. Axial, T2-weighted, fat-saturated MR images of the right lower extremity of a patient with a peroneal intraneural ganglion cyst. A, At the midportion of the fibular head, a clock face can be superimposed on the fibula. The signet ring sign (arrow) can be seen at the 7 o'clock position, while the tail sign (double arrow) can be seen at the 12 o'clock position. B, At the midportion of the fibular neck, using the same clock face, the transverse limb sign (arrow) can be seen between the 10 and 11 o'clock positions. F = fibula; T = tibia.

Decision-Making

No firm guidelines are available to guide decision-making. The authors typically consider the origin of the symptoms (idiopathic/entrapment versus mass lesion versus traumatic), the findings on electrodiagnostic studies, and the time course of symptoms. Nonoperative management is usually recommended when mass lesions are absent, the findings on electrodiagnostic studies are not severe, and there has not been rapid progression of motor symptoms. Conservative management typically consists of behavior modification aimed at reducing repetitive trauma or pressure on the nerve at the fibular head. Behaviors like repetitive leg crossing should be avoided, and padding the area around the fibular head can be considered, particularly during sleep. If the patient has weakness, a daily stretching regimen is important to avoid the development of contractures. As motor recovery occurs, strengthening exercises should be initiated. While awaiting motor recovery and throughout the initial phases of recovery, an AFO can be used to improve foot clearance during ambulation and to improve overall gait mechanics. Trial of conservative management is typically recommended for a period of 3 months.

The authors recommend surgical decompression when mass lesions are present, when motor symptoms are rapidly progressive, when electrodiagnostic studies show severe neuropathy, or when a trial of conservative management fails to show improvement.

Surgical Procedure

Anatomy

The common peroneal nerve is a terminal branch of the lumbosacral plexus. L4, L5, S1, and S2 contribute to the common peroneal nerve via the sciatic nerve. The peroneal component of the sciatic nerve lies lateral and posterior to the tibial component. The sciatic nerve exits the greater sciatic foramen and typically runs inferior to the piriformis muscle down the posterior aspect of the thigh. Before dividing into the common peroneal nerve and the tibial nerve, the peroneal component of the sciatic nerve supplies the short head of the biceps femoris. Just proximal to the popliteal fossa, the sciatic nerve divides into the tibial nerve and the common peroneal nerve. The common peroneal nerve courses across the lateral head of the gastrocnemius between the tendon of the biceps femoris and the gastrocnemius muscle and runs in the subcutaneous tissue as it wraps around the head of the fibula. As the common peroneal nerve passes beneath the peroneus longus muscle at the fibular neck, it trifurcates into the articular branch to the STFJ and the deep and superficial peroneal nerves. The deep peroneal nerve lies directly on the fibula, coursing distally, while the superficial peroneal nerve travels distally in the lateral compartment of the leg between the peroneus longus and peroneus brevis muscles. The deep peroneal nerve innervates the tibialis anterior, extensor hallucis longus, extensor digitorum longus, peroneus tertius, extensor digitorum brevis, and extensor hallucis brevis. The superficial peroneal nerve innervates the peroneus longus and peroneus brevis. The peroneal division of the sciatic nerve typically innervates the short head of the biceps femoris.

Technique

The patient is positioned in a semilateral position with a bump under the ipsilateral hip. The knee is slightly flexed and the entire lower limb is prepped and draped. If a tourniquet is utilized, the limb is exsanguinated. A short oblique incision is made overlying the fibular tunnel (Figure 9.2A). In the proximal portion of the incision, the common peroneal nerve lies medial to the tendon of the biceps femoris, which is readily palpable. The incision is carried deeper until the aponeurosis of the biceps femoris is identified, and the aponeurosis is traced distally until it meets the fascia of the peroneus longus. The aponeurosis of the biceps femoris contracts to form a tendon that attaches at the fibular head. The aponeurosis of the biceps femoris is then opened, revealing the common peroneal nerve beneath it. The opening is carried distally until the nerve travels deep to the peroneus longus. Here, the superficial fascia of the peroneus longus is opened in a cruciate fashion (Figure 9.2B), revealing the muscle fibers of the peroneus longus. The fibers of the peroneus longus are then retracted to reveal the deep fascia of the peroneus longus (Figure 9.2C). The deep component of the peroneus longus fascia is then divided. Neurolysis is carried distally until the trifurcation into the deep peroneal nerve, superficial peroneal nerve, and articular branch to the STFJ occurs. Identification of the trifurcation ensures adequate neurolysis. If a tourniquet has been utilized, it is released. Hemostasis is achieved. The incision is then irrigated and is closed in layers.

In cases of intraneural ganglion cysts, additional steps must be taken to improve clinical function and to reduce the risk of cyst recurrence. The source of intraneural ganglion cysts is thought to be transmission of synovial fluid into the articular branch of the peroneal nerve from a degenerative STFJ.[19–22] In surgical management, to allow more exposure, the skin incision is U-shaped and is directed toward the STFJ. The dissection is performed by dividing the fascia and peroneus longus muscle to expose the articular trunk along the fibular neck to the anterior aspect of the STFJ. The articular branch is then disconnected near the joint (Figure 9.3). The cyst is decompressed, but resection of the cyst and cyst wall are not necessary. To further reduce the risk of recurrence, complete synovectomy and removal of the articular cartilage from the proximal tibia and fibula are also performed. A drain is typically placed in the joint space and the anterior joint capsule and overlying fascia are reapproximated.

Oral Boards Review—Surgical Pearls

1. The common peroneal nerve can be identified medial to the tendon of the biceps femoris and deep to the bicipital aponeurosis (popliteal fascia).
2. The peroneus longus fascia is a C-shaped structure with a superficial and deep component, both of which must be divided to ensure adequate neurolysis.
3. Neurolysis is adequate when it is carried to the point of trifurcation of the common peroneal nerve into the articular branch, deep peroneal nerve, and superficial peroneal nerve.

4. Intraneural ganglion cysts are thought to occur via transmission of synovial fluid from a degenerative STFJ via the articular branch. In surgical management and to prevent recurrence, in addition to cyst decompression, the articular branch should be disconnected and the STFJ should be resected.
   a. The cyst and cyst wall do not need to be resected. Avoiding resection of the cyst and cyst wall lessens the risk of iatrogenic nerve injury.

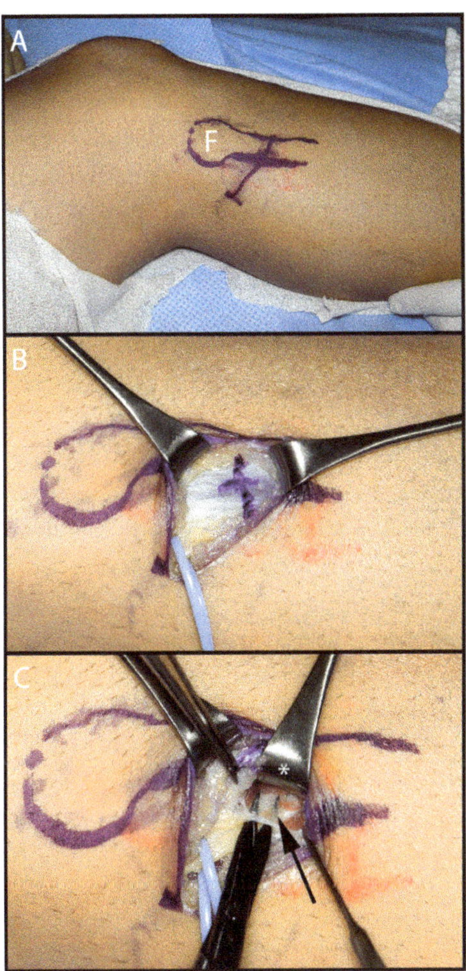

Figure 9.2. Intraoperative photographs of a right peroneal decompression. A, A short oblique incision is planned overlying the fibular tunnel just distal to the fibular head (F). B, The common peroneal nerve (blue vessel loop) is traced until it dives beneath the fascia of the peroneus longus. A cruciate opening (purple cruciate marking) is then made in the superficial fascia of the peroneus longus, exposing the muscle fibers. C, The peroneus longus is retracted (retractor marked *), revealing the compressive band and deep fascia of the peroneus longus (arrow). The compressive band and deep fascia are divided and the common peroneal nerve (blue vessel loop) is traced distally until it trifurcates into the superficial peroneal nerve (most lateral), deep peroneal nerve, and articular trunk (most medial).

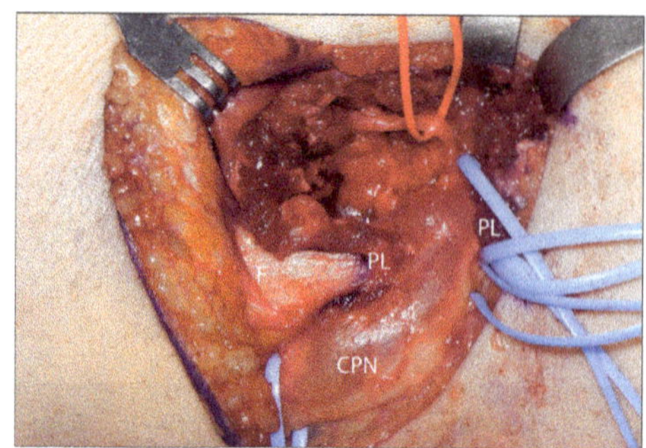

Figure 9.3. Intraoperative photograph of anatomy around the fibular head (F) during surgery for a right peroneal intraneural ganglion cyst. The peroneus longus has been divided (PL to PL) and the common peroneal nerve (CPN) has been traced until its trifurcation into the superficial peroneal nerve, deep peroneal nerve, and articular trunk. The common peroneal nerve contains a large intraneural ganglion cyst. The articular trunk is then followed toward the superior tibiofibular joint (STFJ). The articular branch (red vessel loop) will then be disconnected from the STFJ.

Aftercare

In cases of peroneal neurolysis, a compressive dressing is applied. The compressive dressing is typically removed after 48 hours. While ambulation can begin immediately postoperatively, the patient is encouraged to elevate the leg as much as possible for the first week.

When weakness is present, the patient is encouraged to perform daily stretches to avoid the development of a contracture. A strengthening regimen should also be undertaken, but the muscles should not be exercised to the point of fatigue. A gradual increase should occur as motor function recovers.

If recovery does not occur, additional options can be entertained, including nerve reconstruction (graft or transfer) or tendon transfer. Tendon transfer (typically using the posterior tibialis) can be performed late (with no time window), as long as the heel cord is supple, and it can restore reliable ankle dorsiflexion and eliminate the need for an AFO in the majority of cases.

Complications and Management

The main complication following peroneal nerve decompression is persistence of symptoms secondary to incorrect diagnosis or inadequate decompression. When patients are referred with persistent symptoms, electrodiagnostic studies should be performed to ensure the correct localization, and imaging studies should be performed to ensure that a structural cause of peroneal neuropathy has not been overlooked. If no structural cause is present, re-exploration can be considered; if re-exploration is undertaken, the surgeon should explore the nerve from the popliteal fossa to the trifurcation into the articular branch and the deep and superficial peroneal nerves.

Intraneural ganglion cysts can recur. Recurrence is typically the result of an inadequate operation that did not address the pathophysiology of peroneal intraneural ganglion cysts. In a series of 24 patients with intraneural ganglion cysts, when the cyst was drained and the articular branch was disconnected, no patient had intraneural recurrence.[21] When patients are referred with cyst recurrence, operative intervention should be undertaken to drain the cyst and to disconnect the articular branch. If extraneural recurrence of the cyst occurs and the STFJ was not resected, consideration should be given to resecting the STFJ.

Finally, recovery of peroneal nerve function may not occur despite adequate decompression. In these cases, other reconstructive options can be considered, including nerve transfer and tendon transfer. Gait should be normalized as much as possible through use of an AFO, and stretching should be continued to avoid the development of contractures.

Evidence and Outcomes

The prognosis after operative decompression for common peroneal neuropathy is quite good. Mont and colleagues previously reported that 97% of patients reported functional improvement postoperatively, to the point that the patients were able to discontinue use of an AFO. In contrast, only 33% of patients managed nonoperatively in the series had the same degree of improvement.[23] Mackinnon and colleagues also reported optimistic results. They found, however, after operative decompression, motor dysfunction and pain were more likely to improve than sensory disturbance. In their series, 83% of patients had motor improvement, 84% had improvement in pain, and 49% had improvement in sensory disturbance.[24] Thus, surgical decompression of the common peroneal nerve for pain or weakness should be considered useful and to have good outcomes.

References

1. Poage C, Roth C, Scott B. Peroneal nerve palsy: evaluation and management. *J Am Acad Orthop Surg*. 2016;24:1–10.
2. Katirji B. Peroneal neuropathy. *Neurol Clin*. 1999;17:567–591, vii.
3. Dellon AL, Ebmer J, Swier P. Anatomic variations related to decompression of the common peroneal nerve at the fibular head. *Ann Plast Surg*. 2002;48:30–34.
4. Elias WJ, Pouratian N, Oskouian RJ, Schirmer B, Burns T. Peroneal neuropathy following successful bariatric surgery. Case report and review of the literature. *J Neurosurg*. 2006;105:631–635.
5. Masakado Y, Kawakami M, Suzuki K, Abe L, Ota T, Kimura A. Clinical neurophysiology in the diagnosis of peroneal nerve palsy. *Keio J Med*. 2008;57:84–89.
6. Tacconi P, Manca D, Tamburini G, Cannas A, Giagheddu M. Bed footboard peroneal and tibial neuropathy. A further unusual type of Saturday night palsy. *J Peripher Nerv Syst*. 2004;9:54–56.
7. Asp JP, Rand JA. Peroneal nerve palsy after total knee arthroplasty. *Clin Orthop Relat Res*. 1990;261:233–237.
8. McGrory BJ, Burke DW. Peroneal nerve palsy following intermittent sequential pneumatic compression. *Orthopedics*. 2000;23:1103–1105.
9. Ryan MM, Darras BT, Soul JS. Peroneal neuropathy from ankle-foot orthoses. *Pediatr Neurol*. 2003;29:72–74.

10. Edwards BN, Tullos HS, Noble PC. Contributory factors and etiology of sciatic nerve palsy in total hip arthroplasty. *Clin Orthop Relat Res.* 1987;218:136–141.
11. King JC. Peroneal neuropathy. In: Frontera WR, Silver JK, Rizzo TD, eds. *Essentials of Physical Medicine and Rehabilitation.* Philadelphia, PA: W. B. Saunders; 2008;pp. 389–393.
12. Kim DH, Murovic JA, Tiel RL, Kline DG. Management and outcomes in 318 operative common peroneal nerve lesions at the Louisiana State University Health Sciences Center. *Neurosurgery.* 2004;54:1421–1428; discussion 1428–1429.
13. Visser LH. High-resolution sonography of the common peroneal nerve: detection of intraneural ganglia. *Neurology.* 2006;67:1473–1475.
14. Marciniak C. Fibular (peroneal) neuropathy: electrodiagnostic features and clinical correlates. *Phys Med Rehabil Clin N Am.* 2013;24:121–137.
15. Lo YL, Fook-Chong S, Leoh TH, et al. High-resolution ultrasound as a diagnostic adjunct in common peroneal neuropathy. *Arch Neurol.* 2007;64:1798–1800.
16. Lee PP, Chalian M, Bizzell C, et al. Magnetic resonance neurography of common peroneal (fibular) neuropathy. *J Comput Assist Tomogr.* 2012;36:455–461.
17. Spinner RJ, Desy NM, Rock MG, Amrami KK. Peroneal intraneural ganglia. Part I. Techniques for successful diagnosis and treatment. *Neurosurg Focus.* 2007;22:E16.
18. Spinner RJ, Luthra G, Desy NM, Anderson ML, Amrami KK. The clock face guide to peroneal intraneural ganglia: critical "times" and sites for accurate diagnosis. *Skeletal Radiol.* 2008;37:1091–1099.
19. Lipinski LJ, Rock MG, Spinner RJ. Peroneal intraneural ganglion cysts at the fibular neck: the layered "U" surgical approach to the articular branch and superior tibiofibular joint. *Acta Neurochir (Wien).* 2015;157:837–840.
20. Spinner RJ, Amrami KK, Angius D, Wang H, Carmichael SW. Peroneal and tibial intraneural ganglia: correlation between intraepineurial compartments observed on magnetic resonance images and the potential importance of these compartments. *Neurosurg Focus.* 2007;22:E17.
21. Spinner RJ, Atkinson JL, Tiel RL. Peroneal intraneural ganglia: the importance of the articular branch. A unifying theory. *J Neurosurg.* 2003;99:330–343.
22. Spinner RJ, Desy NM, Rock MG, Amrami KK. Peroneal intraneural ganglia. Part II. Lessons learned and pitfalls to avoid for successful diagnosis and treatment. *Neurosurg Focus.* 2007;22:E27.
23. Mont MA, Dellon AL, Chen F, Hungerford MW, Krackow KA, Hungerford DS. The operative treatment of peroneal nerve palsy. *J Bone Joint Surg Am.* 1996;78:863–869.
24. Humphreys DB, Novak CB, Mackinnon SE. Patient outcome after common peroneal nerve decompression. *J Neurosurg.* 2007;107:314–318.

Tibial Neuropathy—Tarsal Tunnel Syndrome

Daniel A. Lyons and David L. Brown

10

Case Presentation

A 36-year-old female presents to her primary care physician complaining of a several-month history of pain along the medial aspect of her right ankle, with numbness and intermittent shooting pain extending down the plantar surface of her foot to her fourth and fifth toes. She is otherwise healthy, jogs several times per week, and denies prior trauma to her right lower extremity. She notes that her symptoms are often worse at night and are partially relieved with rest and elevation. Examination reveals tenderness to palpation posterior to the medial malleolus. Her physician recommends a conservative course of activity modification, nonsteroidal anti-inflammatory drugs (NSAIDs), and physical therapy—for a presumptive diagnosis of tarsal tunnel syndrome (TTS). On follow-up 3 months later, her symptoms have not improved, and therefore a referral is made to a peripheral nerve surgeon. Detailed neurologic examination reveals a positive Tinel sign posterior to the medial malleolus, with shooting pain extending distally to the heel and the fourth and fifth toes. Semmes-Weinstein monofilament testing reveals decreased sensation along the lateral half of the plantar surface of the foot. No evidence of wasting of the abductor hallucis or the abductor digiti quinti is appreciated.

Questions

1. What is the likely diagnosis?
2. What is the proper timing of the diagnostic workup?
3. What are the most appropriate modalities to consider in confirming the diagnosis?

Assessment and Planning

TTS is suspected as the cause of the patient's symptoms. TTS is caused by compression of the tibial nerve and its branches within the tarsal tunnel at the ankle. The anatomic boundaries of the main (proximal) tarsal tunnel include the flexor retinaculum (laciniate ligament) superficially, the abductor hallucis muscle inferiorly, and the medial talus, sustentaculum tali, and medial calcaneus along the deep surface. The tibial nerve, flexor hallucis longus (FHL) tendon, flexor digitorum longus (FDL) tendon, tibialis posterior (TP) tendon, the posterior tibial artery, and the venae comitantes are contained within the main tarsal tunnel. The site of compression is rarely the tarsal tunnel itself; instead, compression occurs in one of the three well-defined fibrous tunnels of the branches of the tibial nerve, namely the medial and lateral plantar nerves and the calcaneal branch. The anatomy of the calcaneal branch is highly variable. It typically arises from the tibial nerve and pierces the flexor retinaculum. Alternatively, it may arise proximal to the flexor retinaculum and run on its superficial surface, or it may be a branch arising from the lateral plantar nerve.[1,2] The bifurcation of the tibial nerve into the medial and lateral plantar nerves typically occurs near the distal edge of the flexor retinaculum, only rarely occurring proximal to the flexor retinaculum.[1] The medial plantar nerve passes deep to the abductor hallucis, while the lateral plantar nerve pierces the abductor hallucis muscle.

The differential diagnosis of TTS is broad and includes plantar fasciitis, constrictive footwear, polyneuropathy (often diabetes-related), L3-S1 radiculopathy, tumor/neuroma/ganglion, ischemia, calcaneal stress fracture, osteophyte, proximal tibial nerve injury, tenosynovitis, and local fascial and/or ligamentous injuries.[3–5] The misdiagnosis of TTS in cases of plantar fasciitis is not uncommon (particularly in athletes). However, plantar fasciitis does not typically present with paresthesias. Although the true incidence of TTS is not known, there is a higher prevalence in female athletes and in the middle-aged and elderly.[4–6] The most common causes of TTS (in descending order of frequency) are idiopathic causes, trauma, varicosities, heel varus, fibrosis, and ganglion cysts.[6]

The diagnosis of TTS is often made clinically, based on a detailed history and physical exam. Antoniadis and Scheglmann[7] reported that over 50% of patients with compressive neuropathy of the tarsal tunnel will have a positive Tinel sign, while Kinoshita et al. found that simultaneous dorsiflexion and eversion of the affected ankle reproduced or aggravated symptoms in 82% of patients with TTS.[8] Additional signs and symptoms of TTS include unilateral lower extremity involvement, poorly localized paresthesias and burning along the plantar foot and heel, wasting of the intrinsic foot musculature, decreased two-point discrimination, worsening progression of symptoms throughout the day, and symptomatic improvement with rest and elevation.[5] Imaging and electrodiagnostic studies should be considered when the diagnosis of TTS cannot be ascertained from clinical history and examination.

First-line diagnostic studies of the foot and ankle include conventional radiography to rule out local trauma (e.g., calcaneal fracture), osteophytes, or other bony deformities. MR imaging remains the gold standard for identifying space-occupying lesions within the tarsal tunnel that may lead to compression of the tibial nerve (e.g., ganglion cysts, lipomas, schwannomas, varicosities, or tenosynovitis).[5] In patients with suspected TTS, Frey et al. found that MR imaging had a sensitivity of 88% in detecting a pathologic condition.[9] Both MR imaging and diagnostic ultrasound may be useful in identifying pathology at the tarsal tunnel, including increased thickness of the flexor retinaculum and increased cross-sectional area of the tibial nerve.[5] Ultrasound can also identify variant branching anatomy of the tibial nerve, a finding that can be useful for operative planning.

Electrodiagnostic studies, such as nerve conduction studies (NCS) and electromyography (EMG), assess sensory conduction velocities as well as the amplitude and duration of motor-evoked potentials at the tibial nerve.[5,6,10] Increased duration of motor conduction and reduced amplitudes within the tibial nerve at the ankle are indicative of nerve compression.[10] However, the validity of electrodiagnostic testing remains controversial, as there is limited evidence in the literature demonstrating adequate sensitivity and specificity for TTS.[3] Additionally, electrodiagnostic studies have been shown to have a high rate of false-negative results.[3,5,6] Conversely, EMG of intrinsic foot muscles may have a high false-positive rate, leading to overdiagnosis of TTS. In up to 40% of normal, asymptomatic individuals, the foot intrinsics may show EMG abnormalities.[11–13] Neurosensory testing with the Pressure-Specified Sensory Device has shown promise for detecting subtler changes in sensory conduction and is useful for following progress postoperatively.[14]

In the current case, standard radiographs of the foot and ankle do not reveal any bony abnormalities. Ultrasound of the ankle identifies an increased cross-sectional area of the tibial nerve at the flexor retinaculum, without evidence of a local tumor. Electrodiagnostic studies reveal increased motor and sensory latencies of the tibial nerve, with decreased motor amplitude distal to the ankle. Using a combination of the clinical history, physical examination, and the supportive tests (ultrasound and electrodiagnostics), a diagnosis of tarsal tunnel syndrome is made.

Oral Boards Review—Diagnostic Pearls

1. Patients with TTS may have "normal" nerve conduction studies despite a high clinical suspicion (beware of false-negative results).
2. The role of electrodiagnostic studies in diagnosing TTS remains controversial, and electrodiagnostics have not been shown to predict which patients will respond to surgical decompression.
3. Lack of symptomatic relief following decompression may be due to prolonged nerve compression and irreversible fibrosis or, more likely, incomplete release of all four tunnels.

Questions

1. How do the clinical and radiologic findings influence conservative versus surgical planning?
2. What is the most appropriate timing for intervention in this patient?
3. What are the anatomic boundaries of the tarsal tunnels, and what structures are found in the tunnels?

Decision-Making

In the absence of a space-occupying lesion or a definitive point of tibial nerve compression, nonoperative measures should be pursued as initial treatment.[3,6] Conservative modalities include activity modification, NSAID therapy, steroid injection, custom orthotics, and referral to physical therapy for muscle strengthening and stretching exercises.[3,5,6] Limited data exist regarding the length of time that conservative measures should be tried prior to considering surgical intervention. Takakura et al. reported poor nerve recovery if surgical decompression was delayed more than 10 months after the onset of symptoms.[15]

Surgical decompression of the tarsal tunnels should be pursued only after conservative measures have failed or when a space-occupying lesion or point of tibial nerve compression has been identified.[3] Surgical intervention requires complete release of the flexor retinaculum at the medial ankle, as well as release of the three distinct tunnels enveloping the medial and lateral plantar nerves and the calcaneal branch. The roofs of the three fibrous canals should be excised to prevent recurrence.[14] Release of only the main proximal tunnel by incising the flexor retinaculum (without a more complete release/excision of the three additional, distal tunnels) is usually insufficient to relieve the symptoms associated with TTS and is probably the reason for mixed results of this procedure in the literature.[3,4] The most common complication of tarsal tunnel release is incomplete relief of symptoms. Preoperative discussion with the patient regarding potential complications should also include recurrence, infection, iatrogenic nerve injury, and chronic pain.[5,6]

Questions

1. Where does tibial nerve fibrosis most commonly occur in patients with TTS?
2. How should the central fibrous septa between the medial and lateral plantar nerve sheaths be managed intraoperatively, and why?

Surgical Procedure

Tarsal tunnel decompression requires meticulous dissection of the tibial nerve and its distal branches and therefore should be performed under general anesthesia and loupe magnification. The patient is positioned supine, and a tourniquet is applied to the lower leg. It is important to prepare the skin up to the knee circumferentially and to drape widely to allow for repositioning and manipulation of the lower leg and foot as needed during the operation.

Because the site of compression is rarely within the main tarsal tunnel, the goal of decompression surgery is complete release of the tibial nerve, the medial and lateral plantar nerves, and the calcaneal branch. It is therefore important, after release of the flexor retinaculum, to follow the tibial nerve branches distally and to perform complete tunnel release for each.

The operation is begun by making a 6- to 8-cm longitudinal, curvilinear, L-shaped, or hockey-stick incision posterior to the medial malleolus, halfway between the bone and the medial edge of the Achilles tendon (Figure 10.1). This allows access to the four components of the tarsal tunnel.

Next, blunt dissection is carried down to the level of the flexor retinaculum. To prevent iatrogenic injury to the underlying tibial nerve, the flexor retinaculum should be lifted and a small stab incision should be made centrally within the retinaculum, followed by complete proximal and distal release of all retinacular fibers (Figure 10.2).

Care should be taken to identify the posterior tibial artery and vein in order to avoid injury to them in the main tarsal tunnel. The division of the tibial nerve into the medial and lateral plantar nerves should be identified. Any space-occupying lesion should be removed in its entirety. Extension of the incision distally, following the course of the lateral plantar nerve, proceeds around the medial malleolus and toward the medial aspect of the foot.

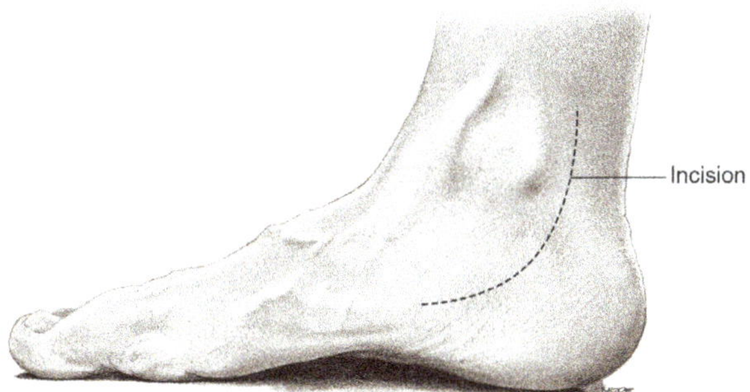

Figure 10.1. Access to the four components of the tarsal tunnel is achieved via a 6- to 8-cm longitudinal, curvilinear incision posterior to the medial malleolus, halfway between the bone and the medial edge of the Achilles tendon.

Decompression continues distally with release of the superficial fascia overlying the abductor hallucis muscle belly. Retraction of the muscle belly in a plantar direction will expose the medial and lateral plantar nerves, housed in separate, parallel fibrous tunnels. Both tunnels must be thoroughly released along their entire lengths, with finger palpation confirming no further points of constriction extending into the plantar aspect of the foot (Figure 10.3).

The central fibrous septa between the two tunnels should be excised to prevent subsequent fibrosis and recurrence of compression. Bipolar cauterization of the edges helps to ensure this result. The calcaneal branch can be visualized taking off from the main tibial nerve or from the lateral plantar nerve, often from the underneath surface. The calcaneal branch takes an inferior, vertical course toward the plantar heel and is contained in its own separate fibrous tunnel. Complete resection of the roof of this tunnel is also paramount.

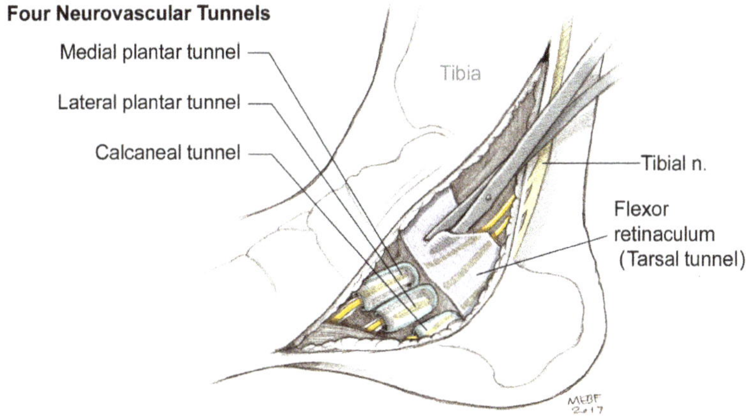

Figure 10.2. Decompression of the flexor retinaculum is carried out beginning proximally, ensuring complete release of all retinacular fibers. The division of the tibial nerve into the medial and lateral plantar nerves is identified, and they are traced distally. The calcaneal branch arises from the main tibial nerve or from the lateral plantar nerve.

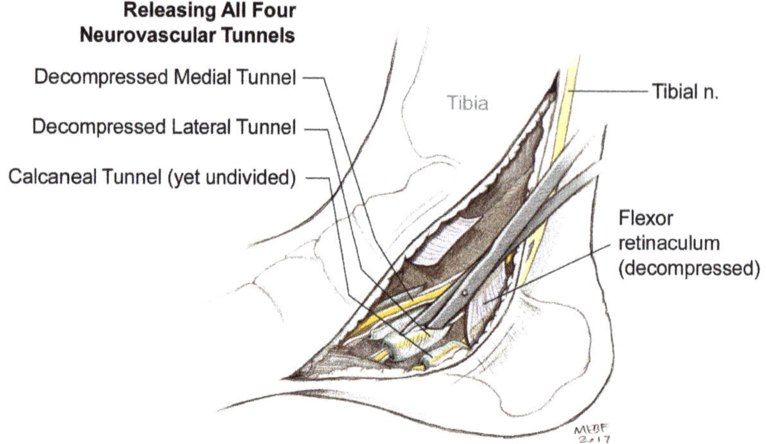

Figure 10.3. The roofs of the medial and lateral plantar tunnels must be released along their entire lengths, with finger palpation distally into the plantar aspect of the foot for confirmation. The fibrous septum between the two tunnels should also be excised to prevent subsequent fibrosis and recurrence of compression. Finally, release of the separate calcaneal tunnel completes the decompression.

Following decompression of the tibial nerve and all three of its distal branches, the nerves should be inspected for fibrosis. If fibrosis is found, an epineurial and/or interfascicular release should be considered. The most distal aspect of the tibial nerve (as it divides into the medial and lateral plantar nerves) is the region where fibrosis most commonly occurs.[3]

Oral Boards Review—Management Pearls

1. Only after conservative management has failed should a referral for nerve conduction studies and surgical evaluation be made, unless the patient has motor involvement or obvious atrophy of intrinsic foot muscles.
2. In select patients with TTS, early decompression should be considered in order to prevent permanent nerve fibrosis.
3. Complete release of the tibial, medial plantar, lateral plantar, and calcaneal nerves is required for adequate decompression in TTS.
4. A positive Tinel sign is one of the most predictable indicators of a favorable outcome after decompression.[3]

Pivot Points

1. Nerve recovery after tarsal tunnel decompression is limited in patients who have a sensory deficit without a positive Tinel sign.[3]
2. The endoscopic approach for tarsal tunnel decompression remains controversial. Endoscopic decompression may provide limited soft tissue injury

and a shorter recovery time, but the procedure may also increase the likelihood of iatrogenic injury and may fail to allow for complete decompression of the three distal tunnels.

Aftercare

Following decompression of the tibial nerve, a period of relative immobilization is generally prescribed. Some surgeons prefer to apply a short posterior leg splint for 2 weeks, with instructions for non-weight-bearing activity. Others apply a soft, bulky gauze dressing and allow the patient to walk slowly with a marching gait, raising and lowering the operated foot vertically. The goal is a balanced approach to early postoperative movement, to encourage nerve gliding while preventing wound-healing complications. Postoperative antibiotics are not prescribed. Narcotic pain medicine may be supplemented with NSAIDs. At 2 to 3 weeks, activity is increased to normal activities of daily living, while vigorous activities (e.g., sports) are delayed for 3 months.[6] Once the incision has healed and the sutures have been removed (generally by 3 weeks), some surgeons advocate water-walking, which may decrease the risk of allodynia.

Complications and Management

The most common complication of tarsal tunnel decompression is incomplete symptom relief. Other complications include minor wound-healing delay (estimated to occur in approximately 8% to 12% of patients), infection, permanent motor or sensory deficits, recurrence, and complex regional pain syndrome.[4,5] Patients must be counseled that nerve regeneration and axonal recovery may take up to a year after decompression.[3]

Oral Boards Review—Complication Pearls

1. The most common cause of operative failure is incomplete release of all four fibrous tunnels.
2. Lack of symptomatic improvement after tarsal tunnel decompression may be due to long-standing compression and nerve fibrosis.
3. Full nerve regeneration and symptom improvement may take a year.

Evidence and Outcomes

Success rates for tibial nerve decompression vary widely in the literature, ranging from 44% to 96%.[10,16] Cases with an identifiable lesion likely have better surgical outcomes than those without an identifiable lesion. Recurrence is rare, occurring in only 2% of patients.[16] Use of electrodiagnostic testing for diagnosis of TTS remains controversial, as does timing of operative intervention after failed conservative management. Outcomes may be better when operative intervention is not delayed beyond 10 to 12 months after the onset of symptoms.[15,17] As with most conditions, patient selection is important in yielding a high surgical success rate. Alternative diagnoses should be excluded, the clinical history and physical examination (including a positive Tinel sign at the tarsal tunnel) should support the diagnosis of TTS, and, ideally, a specific point of entrapment or space-occupying lesion should be identified.

References

1. Havel PE, Ebraheim NA, Clark SE, Jackson WT, DiDio L. Tibial nerve branching in the tarsal tunnel. *Foot Ankle.* 1988;9:117–119.
2. Park TA, Del Toro DR. The medial calcaneal nerve: anatomy and nerve conduction technique. *Muscle Nerve.* 1995;18:32–38.
3. Ahmad M, Tsang K, Mackenney PJ, Adedapo AO. Tarsal tunnel syndrome: A literature review. *Foot Ankle Surg.* 2012;18:149–152.
4. Dellon AL. The four medial ankle tunnels: a critical review of perceptions of tarsal tunnel syndrome and neuropathy. *Neurosurg Clin N Am.* 2008;19:629–648, vii.
5. McSweeney SC, Cichero M. Tarsal tunnel syndrome—A narrative literature review. *Foot (Edinb).* 2015;25:244–250.
6. Miller M, Thompson S. *DeLee & Drez's Orthopaedic Sports Medicine.* 4th ed. Philadelphia, PA: W. B. Saunders; 2014.
7. Antoniadis G, Scheglmann K. Posterior tarsal tunnel syndrome: diagnosis and treatment. *Dtsch Arztebl Int.* 2008;105:776–781.
8. Kinoshita M, Okuda R, Morikawa J, Jotoku T, Abe M. The dorsiflexion-eversion test for diagnosis of tarsal tunnel syndrome. *J Bone Joint Surg Am.* 2001;83-A:1835–1839.
9. Frey C, Kerr R. Magnetic resonance imaging and the evaluation of tarsal tunnel syndrome. *Foot Ankle.* 1993;14:159–164.
10. Kaplan PE, Kernahan WT Jr. Tarsal tunnel syndrome: an electrodiagnostic and surgical correlation. *J Bone Joint Surg Am.* 1981;63:96–99.
11. Boon AJ, Harper CM. Needle EMG of abductor hallucis and peroneus tertius in normal subjects. *Muscle Nerve.* 2003;27:752–756.
12. Falck B, Alaranta H. Fibrillation potentials, positive sharp waves and fasciculation in the intrinsic muscles of the foot in healthy subjects. *J Neurol Neurosurg Psychiatry.* 1983;46:681–683.
13. Gatens PF, Saeed MA. Electromyographic findings in the intrinsic muscles of normal feet. *Arch Phys Med Rehabil.* 1982;63:317–318.
14. Dellon AL. The Dellon approach to neurolysis in the neuropathy patient with chronic nerve compression. *Handchir Mikrochir Plast Chir.* 2008;40:351–360.
15. Takakura Y, Kitada C, Sugimoto K, Tanaka Y, Tamai S. Tarsal tunnel syndrome. Causes and results of operative treatment. *J Bone Joint Surg Br.* 1991;73:125–128.
16. Cimino WR. Tarsal tunnel syndrome: review of the literature. *Foot Ankle.* 1990;11:47–52.
17. Sammarco GJ, Chang L. Outcome of surgical treatment of tarsal tunnel syndrome. *Foot Ankle Int.* 2003;24:125–131.

Piriformis Syndrome and Other Nerve Entrapments of the Posterior Pelvis

Aaron G. Filler

11

Case Presentation

A 28-year-old female pedestrian was hit by a vehicle, causing her to fall in a sitting position as she struck the pavement. Subsequently, she experienced persistent bilateral buttock pain that was aggravated significantly by sitting and relieved in part by standing or lying down. On the right side, she experienced pain in the posterior thigh and anterolateral aspect of the lower leg, extending into the ankle, but not reaching the toes. On the left, she had upper buttock and low back pain, as well as lateral thigh pain extending to the knee. Additionally, she had a disturbing dysesthesia involving the perineum and genital area, along with distracting sexual arousal symptoms, as well as erythema and some edema in the genital region. She also experienced urinary frequency and decreased anorectal sensation, with occasional fecal incontinence.

Questions

1. Aside from cauda equina syndrome, what else belongs in the neurologic differential diagnosis in a patient with bowel and bladder dysfunction and low back symptoms?
2. Is MR imaging helpful for diagnosis of nerve entrapments?
3. If lumbar MR imaging is negative in this setting, what body region should be imaged next?
4. Do nerve entrapments generally require urgent diagnosis and treatment?

Assessment and Planning

Many neurosurgeons complete their entire training without learning the basics for approaching complex nerve entrapments in the posterior pelvis. Physical exam, history, MR neurography, and image-guided injections all play an important role in the diagnosis and management of entrapments in this location. Electrodiagnostic tests are less helpful than they are for spinal and extremity neural impingements because of the complex array of overlapping nerve courses and their depth from the skin surface. The main differential diagnosis includes lumbosacral spine pathology, which should be differentiated by physical examination, imaging, and electrodiagnostics.

History and physical examination maneuvers most classically associated with piriformis syndrome include buttock pain, tenderness to palpation over the greater sciatic notch, sitting pain, and exacerbation of pain with any examination maneuver that increases tension in the piriformis muscle, including the FAIR test (hip flexion, adduction, and internal rotation).[1,2] In the case presented, physical exam revealed an absence of lumbar tenderness and no lumbar aggravation with forward flexion, extension, lateral bending, or twisting at the waist. However, there was marked sciatic notch tenderness bilaterally and tenderness to palpation of the medial aspect of the ischial tuberosities bilaterally. On the left, there was upper buttock tenderness as high the superior margin of the iliac crest and over the greater trochanter laterally. The coccyx and sacrococcygeal joint were extremely painful to palpation, with mild tenderness to the right of the coccyx. History and physical examination were certainly consistent with piriformis syndrome and nerve entrapment in the posterior pelvis. Note that, while not perfectly uniformly, lumbar spine pathology is often exacerbated by standing and relieved by sitting, while piriformis syndrome is the opposite, often exacerbated by sitting and relieved by standing.

Passing through the small volume of the sciatic notch are the piriformis muscle (extending from the deep surface of the sacrum to an insertion on the greater trochanter), the sciatic nerve (L4 to S2), the nerve to the obturator internus (L5 to S2), the superior gluteal nerve (L4 to S1), and the pudendal nerve (S2 to S5). Thus, because L4, L5, S1, S2, S3, S4, and S5 components pass close together and may all be affected by spasm in the piriformis muscle, the analytic approach that is so useful for spinal disorders is often inapplicable in piriformis syndrome because of the overlap and apparent intermingling of the nerve elements supplying seven different myotomes and dermatomes. This is comparable to, but even more complex than, the situation with the brachial plexus, where the five elements of C5 through T1 are closely intermingled.

In addition, the sympathetic nerve chain is prominently represented by the impar ganglion (inferior hypogastric ganglion). The impar ganglion is an anomaly of the nervous system: a single midline structure equally controlling the right and left sides. Its location, at the deep surface of the sacrococcygeal joint, makes it different from most sympathetic ganglia because it is frequently subjected to compression and irritation, with positional aggravating and relieving factors. Impar ganglion dysfunction can affect urinary and rectal sphincter function and all aspects of sexual function. Furthermore, it is involved in sexual sensation. In an aggravated, irritable state, it may cause a persistent, intense, distracting sexual sensation. In a compressed, hypoactive state, it may cause the patient to experience normal somatic sensation in sexual structures, with a loss of normal sexual sensation. Irritative syndromes of the impar ganglion can produce swelling and erythema of the genitals and perineum and have also been associated with complex regional pain syndrome (CRPS).

In this case, further evaluation was performed with MR neurography, which revealed an anatomic variant on the right side in which both the piriformis muscle and the sciatic nerve were split, with part of the sciatic nerve passing through the piriformis muscle. This variant is present in approximately 13% of the population.[3–5] Both sides demonstrated dilation of the veins on the medial aspect of the obturator internus muscle, which can be indicative of obturator internus muscle spasm. The left superior gluteal nerve was enlarged and demonstrated T2 hyperintensity. MR neurography aids in the diagnosis, helps identify the anatomic origin of the entrapment, and, importantly, excludes tumors in the region of the sciatic notch.

Given the patient's history of trauma, a CT scan was also obtained to evaluate the bony anatomy. CT demonstrated an anteriorly displaced fracture of the first coccygeal segment and disruption of the sacrococcygeal joint.

On the basis of the history, physical examination, and imaging, piriformis syndrome and impar ganglion dysfunction were suspected. The patient was then referred for injection of the piriformis muscle for both diagnostic and therapeutic purposes. Open MRI-guided injection of the piriformis muscle with bupivacaine on the right side provided relief of the leg symptoms, and piriformis injection of the left side relieved the left upper buttock and lateral thigh symptoms. It is worth noting that, unlike virtually every other nerve in the body, the superior gluteal nerve has an upward course: it turns upward after exiting the sciatic notch. It exits below the fifth sacral segment, but due to its upward course, it affects muscles innervated as high as the L3 vertebra (upper portion of the gluteus medius), while also affecting the lateral thigh through its tensor fasciae latae branch. Impar ganglion block on the deep surface of the sacrococcygeal joint relieved the patient's pelvic genital dysesthesias and sphincter dysfunction for several weeks, but they subsequently recurred. Somatic pain and numbness in the genital area were relieved somewhat by pudendal blocks along the medial aspect of the obturator internus muscle when the blocks were done together with piriformis muscle anesthetic injection. Targeted injections provide very useful information in diagnosing the anatomic pain generators and also provide prognostic information, because relief of symptoms is highly correlated with surgical success.[6]

Oral Boards Review—Diagnostic Pearls

1. Physical exam of the posterior pelvis starts with three principal areas: the sacrococcygeal joint, the sciatic notch, and the medial aspect of the ischial tuberosity. Muscle spasm in the piriformis muscle can affect one or more of the nerves that either pass through or around the piriformis muscle.
   a. The S2, S3, and S4 spinal nerves typically pass through the proximal piriformis muscle attachment on the deep surface of the sacrum before giving rise to the pudendal nerve and the nerve to the obturator internus.
   b. Spasm of the obturator internus muscle can affect the obturator nerve (L2-4) where it passes through or just above the obturator internus muscle before passing through the obturator canal to reach the thigh adductors. Obturator internus spasm can cause inguinal area pain. Palpation of the medial aspect of the ischial tuberosity often elicits pain.
   c. The superior gluteal nerve (L4-S1) exits the sciatic notch, where its gluteus medius branch turns superiorly, potentially causing symptoms as high as the superior margin of the iliac crest at the L4-5 level. Its tensor

fasciae latae branch can cause symptoms as far down the leg as the tensor fasciae latae attachment on the lateral aspect of the knee.

d. Impingement of the sciatic nerve as it exits the sciatic notch can cause sciatica that mimics a lumbar radiculopathy.

2. Due to the insertion of the piriformis on the greater trochanter, piriformis spasm can cause greater trochanter pain similar to trochanteric bursitis.
3. MR neurography can be helpful for identifying nerve elements in the posterior pelvis that are irritated at common entrapment locations.
4. Injections can be helpful in identifying anatomic pain generators, and pain relief with injections correlates strongly with surgical success.

Decision-Making

Nonsurgical management options consist of medications, including muscle relaxants, nonsteroidal anti-inflammatory drugs (NSAIDs), and neuropathic pain medications, physical therapy, corticosteroid injections, and botulinum toxin injections. There is no consensus regarding initial nonsurgical management or duration of nonsurgical management. However, when symptoms persist despite conservative management and injections, surgery can be considered. In the case presented, two components of the syndrome formed an overwhelmingly distracting symptom complex: the severe impairment of the patient's ability to sit prevented attentive work and the recurrent episodes of incontinence over many months were embarrassing. Because the patient had no lasting benefit from injections, despite their diagnostic utility, surgical treatment came into consideration.

Questions

1. How can image-guided injections at the sites of the entrapments, such as open MRI-guided injection, affect decision-making?
2. What role does a history of positional aggravation play in diagnosis (e.g., severe symptoms while sitting, but relief of pain when standing or lying down)?

Surgical Procedure

The procedure is performed under general anesthesia, without the use of long-acting neuromuscular blockade in order to facilitate intraoperative nerve stimulation. The patient is positioned prone. Electromyography electrodes cover several different sciatic-innervated muscles (medial and lateral foot, gastrocnemius, tibialis anterior, hamstrings) and superior gluteal-innervated muscles (gluteus medius, tensor fasciae latae), and anal sphincter and obturator internus electrodes are placed as well. The ipsilateral low back, buttock, and upper thigh crossing the midline are sterilely prepped and draped. The surgical field should allow access to the ipsilateral buttock and to the midline proximal coccyx. In the modern era, surgery is performed through small, minimal access incisions in the mid-buttock, using a nondestructive surgical corridor between leaves of the gluteal musculature in order to reach the virtual space just outside the sciatic notch (which is generally fat-filled). Self-retaining retractors, such as those typically used for anterior cervical spine surgery, are very useful, and their usefulness can be augmented if they are attached to a table-fixed retractor system. An intraoperative nerve stimulation probe can be used to locate nerve elements before they can be seen and to confirm nerve identities.

Initially, the sciatic nerve (or nerve components in the case of the split sciatic/split piriformis variant) must be identified, as well as the superior and inferior gluteal nerves. The piriformis muscle is reliably identified by its insertion at the greater trochanter and its passage into the sciatic notch immediately superior to, and in contact with, the sciatic nerve. The superior gluteal nerve exits the sciatic notch along the dorsal aspect of the piriformis muscle. Once the nerve elements are all identified and mobilized, the superior segment of the piriformis muscle can be identified, encircled with 0-silk tie, injected with bupivacaine, and then fully transected and removed. The transection is performed by first incising the muscle at the sciatic notch, carefully protecting the superior gluteal nerve but cutting/coagulating the motor nerve to the piriformis muscle. A second incision in the muscle is then made at its insertion point. It is best to cut through very gradually, using bipolar cautery and scissors, so that the risk of inadvertent nerve injury is minimized. In the split configuration, the interneural segment of the piriformis muscle must be handled very carefully. It is slowly mobilized from the components of the sciatic nerve on its inferior and superior surfaces. The distal tendon is cut first in these circumstances. In some cases, the proximal portion of the muscle is not accessible, so it must be drawn gently downward and cut between the sciatic components. When the proximal part is accessible, it is carefully cut, taking care not to injure the pudendal nerve, which may be on its posterior and inferior surface.

Next, a retrosciatic dissection is performed, during which the full length of the nerve to the obturator internus is released by mobilizing it from adhesions. The pudendal nerve is identified medially on the deep surface of the sacroiliac ligament that forms the posterolateral margin of the sciatic notch, and then it is traced distally to where it crosses the inferior margin of the sacrospinous ligament to re-enter the pelvis through the lesser sciatic notch. In addition to mobilizing the nerve, it may be necessary to use a Kerrison punch or No. 11 blade to notch the inferior margin of the sacrospinous ligament if the pudendal nerve is found to be drawn tight across it as it turns into the pelvis. Access is limited, but in order to notch the sacrospinous ligament, the pudendal nerve must be fully mobilized and drawn posteriorly. Finally, if there is significant obturator internus muscle spasm (indicated by marked tenderness to palpation on the medial aspect of the obturator internus muscle), then well-identified branches of the nerve to the obturator internus are subjected to mild injury with heat and pressure from the bipolar forceps so that a 30% to 40% reduction in transmission in the nerve is accomplished in order to treat the muscle spasm. The nerve branches must be carefully distinguished from the inferior gluteal nerve and pudendal nerve in order to avoid unintended injury to the nerves. The wound is then copiously irrigated with antibiotic-impregnated irrigation. An adhesive barrier (for example, Seprafilm or Interceed) is applied (one sheet cut into approximately 1-cm squares). Lidocaine is injected into the muscle. After hemostasis is achieved, the gluteal fascia is closed. The skin and subcutaneous tissue are then closed in layers.

Next, to decompress the impar ganglion, a partial modified coccygectomy is performed. A separate 2-cm incision is made over the first coccygeal segment. Blunt dissection, bipolar cautery, and Metzenbaum scissors are then used to reach the periosteum of the coccyx. Mobility and the absence of dorsal element structures will generally differentiate the first coccygeal segment from the last sacral segment. The periosteum of the first coccygeal segment is opened sharply with a scalpel, in a cut parallel to midline. The first segment is carefully removed using the drill, Kerrison punches, and curets. Often, the superior portion of the second coccygeal segment is removed as well. After hemostasis is established, the periosteum is formally closed. This helps ensure maintenance of the integrity of the attachment of various pelvic floor structures to the distal coccygeal periosteum. The fascial layers are carefully closed in layers to help reduce the risk of sacral or coccygeal osteomyelitis in case of a surgical-site infection. Because of the substantial lateral tension applied to the incision line during sitting, the closure with subcutaneous and subcuticular sutures must be supplemented with interrupted horizontal mattress stitches (removed in 14 days). Skin glue can be applied over the closure line and nylon sutures.

Oral Board Review—Management Pearls

1. If resection of the piriformis muscle is indicated, all nerves in the region must be carefully identified and mobilized. The muscle must be cut proximally at the sciatic notch margin and distally near its point of tendinous insertion to fully remove it and minimize the risk of entrapment recurrence.
2. Use of an adhesive barrier will help prevent postoperative adhesions, which can otherwise cause symptom recurrence.

Aftercare

Patients who require only the transgluteal approach for piriformis resection generally have a very rapid recovery, with only a few days of significant incisional tenderness. Patients are encouraged to ambulate immediately, but for 2 weeks after surgery, patients are directed not to sit for longer than 30 minutes without getting up for a few minutes. No physical therapy is indicated, because therapists often apply vigorous piriformis stretches and massages, which are harmful after surgery. The patient is allowed to gradually resume full activities over a 3-month period, after which activity is unrestricted.

When the partial modified coccygectomy for impar ganglion decompression is included, there is more pain with sitting for 2 to 3 weeks postoperatively, but the pain generally resolves completely over that time period.

Postoperative antibiotic prophylaxis is continued for 7 to 10 days.

Complications and Management

One concerning complication is foot drop due to injury of the peroneal division of the sciatic nerve, that is most likely to happen in patients with the anatomic variant of a split piriformis muscle and split sciatic nerve. No specific data are available regarding the likelihood of this injury, although it has been reported.[7] Careful monitoring during the surgery and gentle manipulation of the interneural muscle segment can reliably prevent this complication.

Recurrent piriformis pain can occur if the muscle is cut only, rather than being removed, particularly if only the tendon is cut and the nerve to the piriformis muscle remains intact. In this situation, the piriformis remnant may remain in spasm and continue to be painful. Postoperative adhesions in the surgical area can also cause persistent pain. Adhesions can be reduced by the placement of an adhesive barrier at the end of the dissection and by the administration of tapering courses of methylprednisolone once or twice during the first 2 months postoperatively.

Any sign of wound infection must be treated early and aggressively. A wound infection can lead to recurrent adhesions in the piriformis area and can lead to a difficult sacral osteomyelitis if the coccygeal incision becomes infected. At the first sign of erythema suspicious for infection, the prophylactic antibiotic regimen should be discontinued and two new antibiotics should be started (e.g., erythromycin and rifampin) and continued for 10 days.

Oral Board Review—Complications Pearls

1. Avoidance of postoperative infection and rapid substitution of antibiotics when an infection emerges are crucial for avoiding postoperative adhesions and recurrent symptoms. Any concern from patients regarding potential surgical-site infection should be assessed immediately.
2. Steroid tapers can be helpful in preventing postoperative adhesions and in treating setbacks in pain resolution in the postoperative period.

Evidence and Outcomes

Approximately 50% of patients have been shown to respond to a combination of physiotherapy and medications (muscle relaxants and Level 1 or 2 pain medications). Among the patients not responding, an additional approximately 75% have a good or very good response to botulinum toxin injection. Finally, among patients failing both therapies, approximately 60% will respond to surgery.[8] Additional case reports and case series support the 60% surgical success rate.[6] A study that the author and colleagues performed had a surgical success rate of 80% with good or excellent results.[6] Overall, the surgical success rate in appropriately selected patients is likely to be 60% to 80%.

In another study, patients with a positive FAIR test had a good response to the combination of physical therapy and injection of lidocaine and triamcinolone. In fact, among patients with a positive FAIR test, nearly 80% had at least a 50% improvement with this combination therapy.[1] The injection of local anesthetic and the injection of local anesthetic plus steroids have been compared in a randomized, controlled trial and have been shown to have equivalent outcomes. Both were found to be highly effective in reducing the symptoms of piriformis syndrome,[9] but, while both were effective, the recurrence rate was high, with few patients having sustained relief of symptoms.[6]

Botulinum toxin injection also has demonstrated efficacy in piriformis syndrome. One study found fair to excellent results in 90% of patients, but the duration of efficacy was unclear because the study evaluated results only out to 16 weeks after injection.[10] An additional study corroborated the findings, supporting the efficacy of botulinum toxin in piriformis syndrome.[11]

References

1. Fishman LM, Dombi GW, Michaelsen C, et al. Piriformis syndrome: diagnosis, treatment, and outcome—a 10-year study. *Arch Phys Med Rehabil.* 2002;83:295–301.
2. Hopayian K, Song F, Riera R, Sambandan S. The clinical features of the piriformis syndrome: a systematic review. *Eur Spine J.* 2010;19:2095–2109.
3. Beaton LE, Anson BJ. The relation of the sciatic nerve and its subdivisions to the piriformis muscle. *Anat Rec.* 1937;70:1–5.
4. Natsis K, Totlis T, Konstantinidis GA, Paraskevas G, Piagkou M, Koebke J. Anatomical variations between the sciatic nerve and the piriformis muscle: a contribution to surgical anatomy in piriformis syndrome. *Surg Radiol Anat.* 2014;36:273–280.
5. Smoll NR. Variations of the piriformis and sciatic nerve with clinical consequence: a review. *Clin Anat.* 2010;23:8–17.
6. Filler AG, Haynes J, Jordan SE, et al. Sciatica of nondisc origin and piriformis syndrome: diagnosis by magnetic resonance neurography and interventional magnetic resonance imaging with outcome study of resulting treatment. *J Neurosurg Spine.* 2005;2:99–115.
7. Justice PE, Katirji B, Preston DC, Grossman GE. Piriformis syndrome surgery causing severe sciatic nerve injury. *J Clin Neuromuscul Dis.* 2012;14:45–47.
8. Michel F, Decavel P, Toussirot E, et al. Piriformis muscle syndrome: diagnostic criteria and treatment of a monocentric series of 250 patients. *Ann Phys Rehabil Med.* 2013;56:371–383.
9. Misirlioglu TO, Akgun K, Palamar D, Erden MG, Erbilir T. Piriformis syndrome: comparison of the effectiveness of local anesthetic and corticosteroid injections: a double-blinded, randomized controlled study. *Pain Physician.* 2015;18:163–171.
10. Lang AM. Botulinum toxin type B in piriformis syndrome. *Am J Phys Med Rehabil.* 2004;83:198–202.
11. Yoon SJ, Ho J, Kang HY, et al. Low-dose botulinum toxin type A for the treatment of refractory piriformis syndrome. *Pharmacotherapy.* 2007;27:657–665.

Brachial Plexitis—Parsonage-Turner Syndrome

Sandra Hearn

12

Case Presentation

A 44-year-old office worker presents with bilateral upper extremity complaints. Two months earlier, he fell from a tree, landing on his right side. He sustained multiple rib fractures and a liver laceration. He denied arm symptoms at the time of injury. Three weeks later, he noticed onset of right periscapular pain, accompanied by numbness radiating from the antecubital fossa to the hand. No weakness was noted at that time. Ten days later, he began experiencing periscapular pain on the left side. He did not experience paresthesias, but he developed weakness of the left external rotators of the shoulder. On both sides, the periscapular pain has been worse at night and has interfered with his sleep.

At the time of his presentation to clinic, his right upper extremity pain and paresthesias have almost fully resolved. The left periscapular pain is beginning to improve, but he is most troubled by persistent left shoulder weakness. He denies neck pain, bowel or bladder symptoms, lower extremity symptoms, shortness of breath, or skin vasomotor changes. He has no history of diabetes mellitus or alcohol abuse.

Physical examination reveals decreased bulk over the left infraspinous fossa and decreased strength of left external rotation of the shoulder. There is no scapular winging at rest, with flexion, or with abduction of the shoulders. Sensation is intact to light touch and reflexes are normal in the bilateral upper extremities. Provocative tests to assess for shoulder impingement are negative.

Questions

1. What is the likely diagnosis?
2. What features of the history and physical exam support this diagnosis?

Assessment and Planning

The patient's presentation suggests Parsonage-Turner syndrome, also known as neuralgic amyotrophy and idiopathic brachial plexitis. In this disorder, symptoms occur secondary to immune-mediated inflammation of portions of the brachial plexus and peripheral nerves of the upper extremity. Classic features in this case include the sudden onset of severe shoulder and upper arm pain, the sequence of pain followed by weakness, prominent night pain, the nonmechanical nature of the pain, presence of paresthesias, and sensory and motor complaints that do not share a radicular or peripheral nerve pattern. A history of preceding regional trauma and progression to a bilateral process also frequently occur in Parsonage-Turner syndrome. The differential diagnosis includes cervical radiculopathy, direct trauma or compression of the brachial plexus, entrapment neuropathy, focal motor neuron disease, and musculoskeletal causes of shoulder pain, such as rotator cuff impingement, rotator cuff tear, and arthritis.[1] A detailed neurologic examination and advanced imaging of the cervical spine with attention to concordant myotomes can help localize the pathology and exclude structural lesions. Distinguishing hallmarks of Parsonage-Turner syndrome include the prominent component of weakness in the absence of a concordant mechanism of injury and pain unrelated to physical activity. Of note, positive impingement signs or mechanical pain should not exclude Parsonage-Turner syndrome, especially in the subacute or chronic phase, as the neurologic weakness and shoulder girdle dysfunction of Parsonage-Turner syndrome can secondarily cause musculoskeletal pain.

The incidence of Parsonage-Turner syndrome is approximately 1 in 1,000 individuals, with the classic form occurring approximately 70% of the time.[2,3] While both idiopathic and hereditary forms exist, the idiopathic form accounts for the majority of cases.[3] The classic presentation of Parsonage-Turner syndrome is characterized by an acute pain episode lasting 1 day to 2 months, followed by weakness, usually of the shoulder girdle muscles and/or the scapular stabilizers. There is often a second pain phase, typified by shooting or radiating pain that travels to the arms or trunk. This phase can take weeks to months to resolve. There is often, although not universally, a history of recent trauma, ranging from trivial to significant. When a history of trauma is present, it is important to elicit a detailed timeline from the patient. Traumatic nerve injury should be maximal at the time of the injury.

While any portion of the brachial plexus and any nerve of the upper extremity can be affected, there is a predilection for the long thoracic, suprascapular, axillary, posterior interosseous, musculocutaneous, and anterior interosseous nerves (Table 12.1). Neural involvement is often patchy and multifocal, affecting select fascicles within a larger nerve. About two thirds of patients present with scapular instability; this

Table 12.1.
Common Deficits in Parsonage-Turner Syndrome

Commonly Affected Nerve	Major Muscles Affected	Clinical Deficit
Long thoracic	Serratus anterior	Medial scapular winging
Suprascapular	Supraspinatus	Shoulder abduction
	Infraspinatus	Shoulder external rotation
Axillary	Deltoid	Shoulder abduction
Musculocutaneous	Brachialis	Elbow flexion
	Biceps	Elbow flexion, supination
Posterior interosseous	Finger and thumb extensors	Finger drop
Anterior interosseous	Flexor digitorum profundus Flexor pollicis longus	Inability to make "OK" sign

physical exam finding, in the absence of a mechanical inciting event, should raise suspicion for Parsonage-Turner syndrome.[4] The presentation is bilateral and asymmetric in about a third of cases.[4] Recurrent episodes occur frequently, with approximately 25% of idiopathic cases recurring.[4]

Departing from the description above, about a third of cases present with atypical features. These presentations may be painless, sensory only, involve regions beyond the upper extremity (typically the lumbosacral plexus or the phrenic, recurrent laryngeal, facial, or hypoglossal nerves), or involve the autonomic nervous system (usually presenting with distal vasomotor changes in the upper extremity).[4] In addition, a single nerve can sometimes be affected rather than multiple nerves or a portion of the plexus. One particular nerve that often seems to be affected in isolation is the spinal accessory nerve, and its involvement leads to a unilateral trapezius palsy. In the absence of a mechanical cause or trauma, unilateral trapezius palsy should raise suspicion for Parsonage-Turner syndrome.[5] In cases where the presentation is consistent with a mononeuropathy, detailed neurologic examination and electrodiagnostic testing often reveal subclinical involvement of additional nerves.

The exact pathogenesis of Parsonage-Turner syndrome remains unclear. A familial form has been identified that is associated with a mutation in septin-9 (*SEPT9*); however, the majority of cases arise sporadically. The role of a preceding event that primes the immune system prior to an attack has been postulated. Over 50% of Parsonage-Turner syndrome patients report such a preceding event. The nature of such events is highly varied, including infection, vaccination, surgery, pregnancy, childbirth, and immunotherapy. Cases of Parsonage-Turner syndrome have also been retrospectively correlated with recent local injury or overuse of the shoulder girdle region. The notion that biomechanical wear on the mobile elements of the plexus may loosen the blood–nerve barrier, allowing for development of autoantibodies to the nerve components during a heightened immune state, represents a unifying hypothesis.[3]

Parsonage-Turner syndrome in the postsurgical context deserves particular attention. Cases of Parsonage-Turner syndrome arising after surgery can be mistaken for iatrogenic perioperative nerve injury. Presence of multifocal and/or bilateral symptoms or a gap in time between surgery and symptom onset (although not always present with Parsonage-Turner syndrome) should heighten the suspicion for an inflammatory etiology. Moreover, as surgery is a risk factor for recurrence of Parsonage-Turner syndrome, further neurosurgical interventions when the diagnosis is uncertain should be approached with caution.

Oral Boards Review—Diagnostic Pearls

1. Parsonage-Turner syndrome is a clinical diagnosis. Imaging and electrodiagnostic studies can be helpful in excluding other diagnoses but cannot establish a diagnosis of Parsonage-Turner syndrome.
2. Characteristic features of the history and physical exam that should raise consideration of Parsonage-Turner syndrome diagnosis include:
   a. Sudden-onset upper extremity or shoulder-region pain without proximate mechanical cause

   b. Nonmechanical pain (not affected by activity or position) that is worse at night
   c. Pain preceding upper extremity weakness
   d. Scapular winging
   e. Patchy, nonradicular sensory and/or motor deficits
3. A history of recent shoulder trauma or overuse, an antecedent immunologic trigger (e.g., illness, surgery, pregnancy), or a prior similar episode should increase suspicion for Parsonage-Turner syndrome.
   a. Consider this etiology in patients with a new peripheral neurologic deficit in the postoperative setting.
4. Atypical or unremitting symptoms should prompt consideration of alternative diagnoses, such as cervical radiculopathy or a compressive brachial plexus lesion. Consider spinal and/or brachial plexus MR imaging.
5. Diagnosis of Parsonage-Turner syndrome is important in avoiding unnecessary and inappropriate surgical intervention when symptoms are erroneously ascribed to another cause (for example, cervical spinal surgery for mild or discordant abnormalities seen on imaging).

Questions

1. How does the diagnostic impression affect surgical decision-making?
2. What diagnostic tests can support the clinical impression?

Decision-Making

Arriving at an accurate diagnosis is paramount in order to avoid unnecessary surgery that can potentially worsen the condition. The management of Parsonage-Turner syndrome is nonsurgical and centers on rehabilitation. The diffuse, patchy nature of the inflammatory pathophysiology and the lack of a structural cause of injury limit the effectiveness of a focal neurosurgical intervention. Furthermore, many cases of Parsonage-Turner syndrome represent self-limited episodes, and good long-term outcomes are observed with conservative management.

Parsonage-Turner syndrome is a clinical diagnosis. However, when features of the history and physical examination preclude a clear diagnostic impression, other testing, including electrodiagnostic studies and imaging, can be helpful in ruling out alternative diagnoses.

Electrodiagnostic studies can support a diagnosis of Parsonage-Turner syndrome when weak muscles are studied. Test sensitivity may be limited in early and mild cases. Typical findings include denervation and/or reinnervation in muscles supplied by affected nerves. Abnormalities in sensory nerve testing have been inconsistently reported, but when present, they support the diagnosis. Frequently, electrodiagnostic abnormalities are seen bilaterally, albeit asymmetrically, even when the clinical presentation is unilateral. While electrodiagnostic findings can support the diagnosis, limitations in sampling often lead to false-negative results in this disorder due to the patchy fascicular pattern of involvement. Specifically, electrodiagnostic examinations designed to evaluate for disorders like cervical radiculopathy or carpal tunnel syndrome may not include adequate sampling of commonly affected muscles in Parsonage-Turner syndrome, such as the serratus anterior and long thoracic nerve.

The primary role of imaging, including ultrasound and MR imaging, in the diagnosis of Parsonage-Turner syndrome is to exclude structural causes for the observed neurologic deficits, such as cervical disc disease, mass lesions, or postoperative hematoma. While this remains the primary purpose of imaging, several findings can also suggest the diagnosis of Parsonage-Turner syndrome. On MR imaging, the affected nerves typically demonstrate T2 hyperintensity, although the long thoracic nerve often does not demonstrate T2 hyperintensity even when affected. This may be an issue of resolution. With larger nerves, asymmetric fascicular enlargement can also occasionally be observed, consistent with the patchy, multifocal nature of the pathology. Hourglass constrictions of nerves can be observed in Parsonage-Turner syndrome as a bullseye sign, with peripheral T2 hyperintensity and central T2 hypointensity when imaging is orthogonal to the nerve.[6] After approximately 1 month, the muscles in the distribution of the affected nerves typically demonstrate T2 hyperintensity consistent with subacute denervation. With prolonged courses, atrophy and fatty infiltration can be observed in the muscles on T1-weighted sequences.[7] Similar findings can be observed using high-resolution ultrasound. Focal swelling and/or fascicular enlargement can often be identified. Later in the course of the disease, focal constriction and fascicular entwinement can also be observed. Muscle edema can be suggestive of early denervation change, although it is not a specific finding. However, later in the course of the disease, muscle atrophy in the distribution of the affected nerves can be identified on ultrasound.[7,8]

Questions

1. What are treatment options for acute Parsonage-Turner syndrome?
2. What care can be offered for patients with resultant scapular or shoulder region weakness and dysfunction?

Surgical Procedure

Parsonage-Turner syndrome is managed nonoperatively, although secondary nerve and/or orthopedic reconstruction can be considered in patients with incomplete recovery and resultant deficits.

Complications and Management

Pain Management

The acute pain of Parsonage-Turner syndrome can be managed with acetaminophen and nonsteroidal anti-inflammatory drugs, with consideration of short-term opioid therapy in cases of severe pain. Modalities like heat and electrical stimulation may also reduce pain.

Immunomodulation

Retrospective studies support a role for steroids in the acute phase, suggesting a higher likelihood of motor recovery within the first month and an overall greater likelihood of a good recovery.[3,4,9] Efficacy of steroids has yet to be established in large prospective studies or randomized trials; however, some experts recommend a short course of steroids at symptom onset for patients without contraindications. Some centers have trialed other immunotherapies, such as administration of intravenous immunoglobulin, especially when the disorder arises in the postoperative setting.[10–12] Further investigation of efficacy is needed.

Rehabilitation

Few data exist regarding physical and occupational therapy for patients with Parsonage-Turner syndrome, but the data available suggest that a multidisciplinary approach may be beneficial.[13] The goal of rehabilitation is to minimize the dysfunction and pain that can result from the weakness of shoulder girdle muscles and/or an unstable scapula. Physical therapy can address scapular positioning and coordination, endurance training of periscapular muscles, and activity modifications. It may take 2 to 3 years for a patient to reach a new functional baseline. It is important to counsel patients about the time involved and to utilize the time for making decisions about further reconstructive options.

Evidence and Outcomes

Due to limited prospective data, much about the natural history of Parsonage-Turner syndrome remains unclear. While some estimates suggest that 80% to 90% of patients recover fully within 3 years, other retrospective data suggest a less optimistic outlook.[14,15] At 2.5 years after diagnosis, a notable portion of patients (up to 50% to 66% in a retrospective study at a specialized center) report functional impairments in daily tasks, such as personal hygiene and grooming, household tasks, writing, and driving.[14] Correlations between shoulder pain, scapular dyskinesis, difficulties working above shoulder height, and increased fatigability support the hypothesis that underlying biomechanical factors, overuse, and pain may interact, creating a cycle of impairment leading to upper limb disability.[14] Good to excellent recovery can occur in a significant number of patients, but it is important to counsel patients that full recovery to premorbid levels is unlikely, and that, even with recovery back to normal strength, exercise intolerance is likely. Prognosis is also poorer with recurrent attacks and comorbid conditions.[1]

For refractory cases that have failed conservative management and demonstrate persistent deficits in key functional muscles, there are neural and orthopedic reconstruction options. These may include microneurolysis, decompression of involved nerves, nerve transfers, and tendon transfers. Further research in this area is needed, as outcomes have not been systematically studied.

Oral Boards Review—Management Pearls

1. Parsonage-Turner syndrome is a nonoperative condition.
2. Early evidence suggests a role for steroids administered in the acute phase.
3. Appropriate rehabilitation strategies aim at improving shoulder function in spite of decreased stability and/or weakness.

Pivot Points

1. If a postsurgical patient develops a peripheral neurologic deficit unrelated to the operative procedure, consider a diagnosis of Parsonage-Turner syndrome.
2. If a patient with Parsonage-Turner syndrome develops shortness of breath, especially nocturnally, consider a chest X-ray to evaluate for diaphragmatic involvement.
3. If the lesion localizes to the lower plexus, consider further workup for compressive or structural etiologies (e.g., lung cancer).

References

1. van Alfen N. Clinical and pathophysiological concepts of neuralgic amyotrophy. *Nat Rev Neurol*. 2011;7:315–322.
2. van Alfen N, van Eijk JJ, Ennik T, et al. Incidence of neuralgic amyotrophy (Parsonage Turner syndrome) in a primary care setting—a prospective cohort study. *PLOS ONE*. 2015;10:e0128361.
3. Van Eijk JJ, Groothuis JT, Van Alfen N. Neuralgic amyotrophy: an update on diagnosis, pathophysiology, and treatment. *Muscle Nerve*. 2016;53:337–350.
4. van Alfen N, van Engelen BG. The clinical spectrum of neuralgic amyotrophy in 246 cases. *Brain*. 2006;129:438–450.
5. Seror P, Stojkovic T, Lefevre-Colau MM, Lenglet T. Diagnosis of unilateral trapezius muscle palsy: 54 cases. *Muscle Nerve*. 2017;56:215–223.
6. Sneag DB, Saltzman EB, Meister DW, Feinberg JH, Lee SK, Wolfe SW. The MRI bullseye sign: an indicator of peripheral nerve constriction in Parsonage-Turner syndrome. *Muscle Nerve*. 2017;56(1):99–106.
7. Lieba-Samal D, Jengojan S, Kasprian G, Wober C, Bodner G. Neuroimaging of classic neuralgic amyotrophy. *Muscle Nerve*. 2016;54:1079–1085.
8. Aranyi Z, Csillik A, Devay K, et al. Ultrasonographic identification of nerve pathology in neuralgic amyotrophy: Enlargement, constriction, fascicular entwinement, and torsion. *Muscle Nerve*. 2015;52:503–511.
9. van Eijk JJ, van Alfen N, Berrevoets M, van der Wilt GJ, Pillen S, van Engelen BG. Evaluation of prednisolone treatment in the acute phase of neuralgic amyotrophy: an observational study. *J Neurol Neurosurg Psychiatry*. 2009;80:1120–1124.

10. Johnson NE, Petraglia AL, Huang JH, Logigian EL. Rapid resolution of severe neuralgic amyotrophy after treatment with corticosteroids and intravenous immunoglobulin. *Muscle Nerve*. 2011;44:304–305.
11. Moriguchi K, Miyamoto K, Takada K, Kusunoki S. Four cases of anti-ganglioside antibody-positive neuralgic amyotrophy with good response to intravenous immunoglobulin infusion therapy. *J Neuroimmunol*. 2011;238:107–109.
12. Naito KS, Fukushima K, Suzuki S, et al. Intravenous immunoglobulin (IVIg) with methylprednisolone pulse therapy for motor impairment of neuralgic amyotrophy: clinical observations in 10 cases. *Intern Med*. 2012;51:1493–1500.
13. Ijspeert J, Janssen RM, Murgia A, et al. Efficacy of a combined physical and occupational therapy intervention in patients with subacute neuralgic amyotrophy: a pilot study. *NeuroRehabilitation*. 2013;33:657–665.
14. Cup EH, Ijspeert J, Janssen RJ, et al. Residual complaints after neuralgic amyotrophy. *Arch Phys Med Rehabil*. 2013;94:67–73.
15. Tsairis P, Dyck PJ, Mulder DW. Natural history of brachial plexus neuropathy. Report on 99 patients. *Arch Neurol*. 1972;27:109–117.

Peripheral Nerve Biopsy

Miriana Popadich and Thomas J. Wilson

13

Case Presentation

A 66-year-old male presents with painful burning of the bilateral lower extremities accompanied by a rash, with waxing and waning symptoms over the last 2 to 3 years. He reports paresthesias in his lower extremities, particularly in his feet. During flares, his symptoms can ascend to the midthigh level and can also involve his hands. His periods of exacerbation are associated with lower limb edema that significantly limits his ability to walk. Early in the course of his disorder, he did not note any weakness, but he is now having gait difficulty. He is unclear if this is secondary to weakness. He has been treated with multiple prednisone tapers, with improvement in symptoms each time. His flares seem to be brought on by energy drink consumption or exercise. His past medical history is significant for hypertension, diabetes mellitus, and hypothyroidism. Comprehensive laboratory workup demonstrates a normal metabolic profile, normal thyroid function, hemoglobin A_{1c} in the normal range, and normal liver function tests. MR imaging of the lumbar spine demonstrates mild degenerative changes. His neurologist has requested a sural nerve biopsy.

Questions

1. What nerves are typically biopsied?
2. What evaluation should be performed prior to performing a nerve biopsy?

Assessment and Planning

The indications for nerve biopsy have decreased over the years, in part because of noninvasive genetic tests that are now available for a number of hereditary neuropathies. Nerve biopsy, however, still remains an important part of the diagnostic armamentarium in the evaluation of a number of diseases, including vasculitis, some hereditary neuropathies, toxic and metabolic neuropathies, inflammatory demyelinating conditions like chronic inflammatory demyelinating polyneuropathy (CIDP), and neoplastic and nonneoplastic infiltrative diseases, such as sarcoidosis, amyloidosis, neurolymphomatosis, and other metastatic tumor infiltration.

When considering a nerve biopsy, the surgeon should first assess whether the noninvasive or less invasive diagnostic options have been exhausted without yielding a diagnosis. The appropriate evaluation may include blood tests, cerebrospinal fluid studies, genetic tests, electrodiagnostic studies, imaging (including CT, MR imaging, and PET), autonomic testing, fat aspiration, and skin biopsy. The surgeon should also assess whether the diagnoses being considered can be made on the basis of a nerve biopsy. In the presented case, the neurologist is considering polyarthralgia, large- and small-fiber neuropathy, and vasculitis.

Obtaining a nerve biopsy, such as a sural nerve biopsy, allows examination of the axons and myelin and classification of the disorder into axonal neuropathy or demyelinating neuropathy. Furthermore, the nerve biopsy specimen allows examination of a number of other things that can aid in diagnosis. The blood vessels can be examined. The specimen can be examined for infiltrative cells or abnormal deposits. Plus, other important cells present in the specimen can be examined, including perineurial cells, mast cells, endothelial cells, pericytes, and lymphocytes.[1] Thus, the nerve biopsy can yield a plethora of information that can aid in making a diagnosis.

Questions

1. What are the considerations in determining what nerve to biopsy?
2. Who should be a part of the decision-making process when determining the biopsy target?

Oral Boards Review—Diagnostic Pearls

1. The surgeon should ensure that noninvasive and less invasive testing has been exhausted without yielding a diagnosis prior to considering a nerve biopsy.
2. Nerve biopsy allows examination of the axons and myelin to broadly classify neuropathies as axonal or demyelinating, but it also allows examination of a number of other cells present in the specimen, examination for infiltrative cells, and examination for abnormal deposits, all of which can aid in the diagnosis.

Pivot Points

1. The decision about which nerve to target for biopsy should be a team decision. It is important to coordinate and discuss with the patient's neurologist.
2. Clinical examination, electrodiagnostics, imaging findings, and potential diagnoses should all be considered when determining the nerve target and when determining whether to pursue a targeted fascicular biopsy or biopsy of a distal cutaneous nerve.

Decision-Making

Once a decision to pursue a nerve biopsy has been made, several other important decisions remain, including whether to perform the nerve biopsy alone or in conjunction with a muscle biopsy, whether to perform a whole nerve or a fascicular biopsy, which nerve to target, and which side or limb to target.

For most of these decisions, it is important to work in conjunction with the referring neurologist. In some cases, involving a rheumatologist (when one is involved in the patient's care) or radiologist (when nerves appear abnormal on imaging) in the decision-making process may be important. The first important decision is whether to perform nerve biopsy alone or in combination with a muscle biopsy. The list of potential diagnoses helps guide this decision, as some diagnoses will be aided by the addition of a muscle specimen. In one series of patients who underwent simultaneous muscle and nerve biopsy, definitive diagnosis was reached in 58% of the patients. In this group, the diagnosis was made on the basis of the muscle specimen alone in 27%, the nerve specimen alone in 60%, and both specimens in 13%.[2] In the right circumstances, when neuromuscular diseases are being considered, a muscle biopsy may be a useful addition to the nerve biopsy.

The next major decision is which nerve to target. This depends largely on the nerves involved in the pathologic process. The clinical examination, electrodiagnostic studies, and imaging studies guide this decision. The nerve most likely to be involved in the pathology should be targeted. In some highly selected cases, this may mean pursuing a targeted fascicular biopsy as the initial step, forgoing biopsy of a distal cutaneous nerve.[3] When utilized correctly, targeted fascicular biopsy has a high rate of diagnostic yield, surpassing that of the more traditional distal cutaneous nerve biopsy.[3] When whole-nerve biopsy of a distal cutaneous nerve is pursued, the most commonly targeted nerves are the sural and superficial peroneal nerves in the lower extremity and the superficial radial sensory nerve in the upper extremity. However, under the right circumstances, depending on which nerves are affected by the pathology, other nerves could be considered, including the saphenous nerve, lateral antebrachial cutaneous nerve, and medial antebrachial cutaneous nerve. The procedures for biopsy of the sural nerve and superficial radial sensory nerve are reviewed for the purposes of this chapter.

Finally, it is important to be aware of any special, nonroutine studies that are desired by the referring neurologist. Some tests may require special handling of the specimen. It is important to be aware of these requests to ensure appropriate handling of the specimen on the day of the operation and to ensure that any necessary special equipment, fixative solutions, etc., are available.

Surgical Procedure

Sural Nerve Biopsy

Sural nerve biopsy is performed under monitored anesthesia care with sedation and infiltration of local anesthetic. In pediatric or uncooperative patients, deep sedation or general anesthesia may be required. Preoperatively, prophylactic antibiotics are administered. The patient is positioned in a sloppy lateral position with a bump placed under the ipsilateral hip and the knee flexed. A 5-cm incision is planned between the lateral malleolus and the Achilles tendon, with the most caudal point of the incision just rostral to the lateral malleolus (Figure 13.1A). The operative site is then sterilely prepped and draped in the standard fashion.

The skin only is infiltrated with 1% lidocaine. After anesthesia is confirmed, the skin is incised. Dissection of the subcutaneous tissue is carried out; typically, the lesser saphenous vein is the first important structural landmark encountered. The

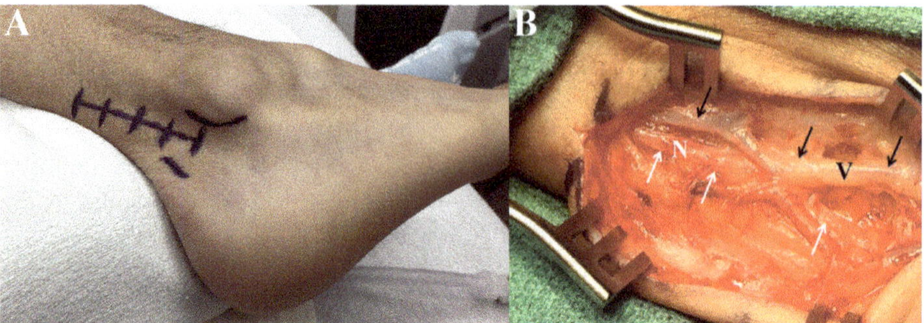

Figure 13.1. A, Planned incision for sural nerve biopsy. The incision is planned halfway between the Achilles tendon and lateral malleolus, beginning just rostral to the lateral malleolus and extending approximately 5 cm rostrally. B, Intraoperative photograph showing the sural nerve (N, white arrows), which can be located just posterior and deep to the lesser saphenous vein (V, black arrows).

sural nerve can usually be identified slightly posterior and deep to the lesser saphenous vein (Figure 13.1B). Once identified, the sural nerve is dissected free of the surrounding tissues for a length of at least 5 cm. Care is taken to avoid crushing, stretching, or coagulating the nerve in order to avoid artefacts that can reduce the diagnostic yield.

The specimen is taken by suture-ligating the nerve at the most proximal end of the incision, transecting the nerve 2 mm distal to the tie, and then transecting the nerve at the distal extent of the incision. Venous structures in this location can easily be confused with the sural nerve, so it is important to evaluate the specimen for the presence of fascicles. While it is not our routine practice, some centers send a small portion of the specimen for frozen section analysis to confirm the biopsy specimen is nerve tissue. The specimen is then processed according to the standard institutional protocol, taking care to follow any special handling instructions for the requested tests.

Some centers advocate repair of the nerve using a nerve conduit, autologous vein graft, or a fascicular turnover flap to allow potential recovery of the nerve.[4–6] We do not routinely perform any of these measures. The proximal cut end is buried as deep as possible to avoid the formation of a superficial neuroma. Hemostasis is then achieved. The wound is thoroughly irrigated with antibiotic-supplemented saline, and the wound is closed in layers.

The sural nerve is most accessible, as described, just posterior to the lateral malleolus at the level of the ankle. Alternatively, the sural nerve may be biopsied at the level of the gastrocnemius muscle belly inferior to the knee, particularly when a muscle biopsy is also desired, because this allows both muscle and nerve to be biopsied from the same incision.

Superficial Radial Sensory Nerve Biopsy

As in sural nerve biopsy, superficial radial sensory nerve biopsy is performed under monitored anesthesia care with sedation and infiltration of local anesthetic. In pediatric or uncooperative patients, deep sedation or general anesthesia may be required. Preoperatively, prophylactic antibiotics are administered. The patient is placed in the supine position, the shoulder is abducted to 90°, the elbow is placed halfway between pronation and supination, and the arm is placed on an arm table.

The key anatomic landmark in planning the incision is the brachioradialis muscle. The brachioradialis can be identified by asking the patient to flex the arm with the arm positioned midway between pronation and supination. A 5-cm incision is planned starting 2 cm proximal to the radial styloid between the tendons of the extensor carpi radialis longus and brachioradialis (Figure 13.2A). The operative site is then sterilely prepped and draped in the standard fashion.

The skin only is infiltrated with 1% lidocaine. After anesthesia is confirmed, the skin is incised. Dissection of the subcutaneous tissue reveals the tendons of the brachioradialis and extensor carpi radialis longus (Figure 13.2B). Gentle medial retraction of the brachioradialis tendon allows identification of the superficial radial sensory nerve. Care should be taken to avoid vascular injury, as the radial artery is in the vicinity of the nerve, on the deep side. The superficial sensory radial nerve should also not be confused with smaller, more superficial branches of the lateral antebrachial cutaneous nerve that may be encountered during the dissection. Once the superficial radial sensory nerve is identified, a 5-cm segment of the nerve is isolated.

The specimen is taken by suture-ligating the nerve at the most proximal end of the incision, transecting the nerve 2 mm distal to the tie, and then transecting the nerve at the distal extent of the incision. It is important to evaluate the specimen for the presence of fascicles. While it is not our routine practice, some centers send a small portion of the specimen for frozen section analysis to confirm the biopsy specimen is nerve tissue. The specimen is then processed according to the standard institutional protocol, taking care to follow any special handling instructions for the requested tests.

Some centers advocate repair of the nerve by various methods, but it is not our routine practice to do so. The proximal cut end is buried as deep as possible to avoid the formation of a superficial neuroma. Hemostasis is then achieved. The wound is thoroughly irrigated with antibiotic-supplemented saline, and the wound is closed in layers.

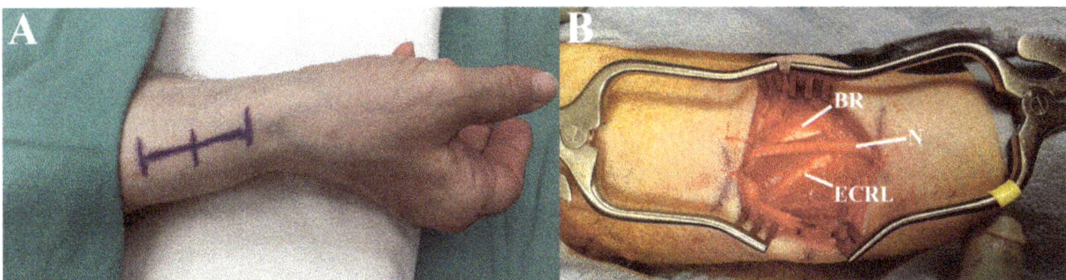

Figure 13.2. A, A 5-cm incision is planned starting 2 cm proximal to the radial styloid between the tendons of the extensor carpi radialis longus and brachioradialis. B, Intraoperative photograph showing the superficial radial sensory nerve (N) isolated between the brachioradialis (BR) and extensor carpi radialis longus (ECRL) tendons.

Oral Boards Review—Management Pearls

1. For sural nerve biopsy, an incision is made midway between the lateral malleolus and Achilles tendon, with the distal extent of the incision just rostral to the lateral malleolus. The sural nerve can typically be identified just posterior and deep to the lesser saphenous vein, a key structure to identify intraoperatively.
2. For superficial radial sensory nerve biopsy, an incision is made between the tendons of the brachioradialis and extensor carpi radialis longus, with the distal extent of the incision 2 cm proximal to the radial styloid. The nerve can be identified between the brachioradialis and extensor carpi radialis longus tendons by gently retracting the brachioradialis tendon medially. The radial artery is in the vicinity, and care should be taken to avoid vascular injury.
3. All nerve biopsy specimens should be examined for fascicles, as venous structures can easily be confused for nerves.

Aftercare

Postoperatively, the patient should expect to have permanent numbness in the distribution of the nerve that was biopsied. Occasionally, the patient may experience shocklike or "phantom" pains as the healing of the remaining nerve begins; however, this is rarely permanent. When it is severe, neuropathic pain medications, such as gabapentin or pregabalin, can be used.

Strenuous activity is limited until the wound is healed.

Questions

1. What is the typical diagnostic yield of biopsy of a distal cutaneous nerve (e.g., sural nerve or superficial radial sensory nerve)?
2. When should a targeted fascicular biopsy be considered?
3. What potential complications should be discussed with the patient preoperatively?

Complications and Management

Potential complications of distal cutaneous nerve biopsy include postoperative hematoma, wound infection, wound dehiscence, painful neuroma formation, chronic pain or paresthesias, and nondiagnostic biopsy. Wound infection may occur in up to 20% of patients.[7–10] Chronic pain and paresthesias are typically reported in up to a third of patients.[7,9,10] Some authors believe that repair of the biopsied nerve helps reduce these sensory disturbances.[4,5,11] We have found that the superficial radial sensory nerve seems to be more prone to painful neuroma formation than the sural nerve is, and this finding is echoed by others.[8] The most common complication is nondiagnostic biopsy. In most series, a nondiagnostic biopsy is obtained around 50% of the time, but it may occur as often as 70% of the time.[10,12] These potential complications, especially the possibility of a nondiagnostic biopsy, should be discussed with the patient preoperatively.

Oral Boards Review—Complication Pearls

1. Common complications of nerve biopsy include pain or bothersome paresthesias and nondiagnostic biopsy.
2. The typical reported rate of nondiagnostic distal cutaneous nerve biopsy is approximately 50%. This should be discussed preoperatively with the patient.
3. The superficial radial sensory nerve seems to be more prone to the development of painful neuromas than the sural nerve is.

Evidence and Outcomes

The reported diagnostic yield of nerve biopsy varies widely. Most series report the diagnostic yield to be about 50%, and this is what the authors typically quote to patients when discussing the procedure preoperatively.[10,13,14] Some series have reported up to 70% of biopsies as diagnostic, while others have reported up to 70% as nondiagnostic.[10,15]

In select patients, targeted fascicular biopsy may be a better approach, with a higher diagnostic yield than biopsy of a distal cutaneous nerve.[3,16,17] In one series, the diagnostic yield was nearly 85%.[3] In cases where there are electrodiagnostic changes and imaging abnormalities in the corresponding nerve, particularly when a dense deficit is already present, targeted fascicular biopsy may be the preferred choice.

While nerve biopsy in pediatric patients is certainly less common than in adult patients, there is evidence supporting its value. In one large series, a distinctive histopathologic diagnosis was arrived at in 33% of patients, while biopsy changed or refined the diagnosis in 58% of biopsied patients.[18]

References

1. Kanda T. Usefulness of sural nerve biopsy in the genomic era. *Neuropathology.* 2009;29:502–508.
2. Chen DJ, Prayson RA. Evaluation of simultaneous muscle and nerve biopsies for the diagnosis of neuromuscular diseases. *Ann Diagn Pathol.* 2014;18:282–285.
3. Capek S, Amrami KK, Dyck PJ, Spinner RJ. Targeted fascicular biopsy of the sciatic nerve and its major branches: rationale and operative technique. *Neurosurg Focus.* 2015;39:E12.
4. Flores LP. The use of autogenous veins for microsurgical repair of the sural nerve after nerve biopsy. *Neurosurgery.* 2010;66:238–243; discussion 243–234.
5. Ito T, Nakagawa R, Ishiura R, Yamamoto T, Narushima M. Nerve reconstruction after sural nerve biopsy with supermicrosurgical fascicular turnover flap. *J Plast Reconstr Aesthetic Surg* 2016;69:146.
6. Mikell CB, Chan AK, Stein GE, Tanji K, Winfree CJ. Muscle and nerve biopsies: techniques for the neurologist and neurosurgeon. *Clin Neurol Neurosurg.* 2013;115:1206–1214.

7. Gabriel CM, Howard R, Kinsella N, et al. Prospective study of the usefulness of sural nerve biopsy. *J Neurol Neurosurg Psychiatry*. 2000;69:442–446.
8. Hart MG, Santarius T, Trivedi RA. Muscle and nerve biopsy for the neurosurgical trainee. *Br J Neurosurg*. 2013;27:727–734.
9. Hilton DA, Jacob J, Househam L, Tengah C. Complications following sural and peroneal nerve biopsies. *J Neurol Neurosurg Psychiatry*. 2007;78:1271–1272.
10. Ruth A, Schulmeyer FJ, Roesch M, Woertgen C, Brawanski A. Diagnostic and therapeutic value due to suspected diagnosis, long-term complications, and indication for sural nerve biopsy. *Clin Neurol Neurosurg*. 2005;107:214–217.
11. Schoeller T, Huemer GM, Shafighi M, Gurunluoglu R, Wechselberger G, Piza-Katzer H. Microsurgical repair of the sural nerve after nerve biopsy to avoid associated sensory morbidity: a preliminary report. *Neurosurgery*. 2004;54:897–900; discussion 900–891.
12. Dyck PJ, Lofgren EP. Nerve biopsy. Choice of nerve, method, symptoms, and usefulness. *Med Clin North Am*. 1968;52:885–893.
13. Argov Z, Steiner I, Soffer D. The yield of sural nerve biopsy in the evaluation of peripheral neuropathies. *Acta Neurol Scand*. 1989;79:243–245.
14. Neundorfer B, Grahmann F, Engelhardt A, Harte U. Postoperative effects and value of sural nerve biopsies: a retrospective study. *Eur Neurol*. 1990;30:350–352.
15. Zhang YS, Sun AP, Chen L, Dong RF, Zhong YF, Zhang J. Nerve biopsy findings contribute to diagnosis of multiple mononeuropathy: 78% of findings support clinical diagnosis. *Neural Regen Res*. 2015;10:112–118.
16. Lyons MK. Nerve rootlet and fascicular biopsy in patients with hypertrophic inflammatory neuropathy. *Neurologist*. 2009;15:40–41.
17. Tracy JA, Rubin DI, Amrami KK, et al. Malignant peripheral nerve sheath tumor: the utility of fascicular biopsy and teased fiber studies. *J Clin Neuromuscul Dis*. 2012;14:28–33.
18. Ida CM, Dyck PJ, Dyck PJ, et al. Pediatric nerve biopsy diagnostic and treatment utility in tertiary care referral. *Pediatr Neurol*. 2016;58:3–11.

Section 2

Peripheral Nerve Pain Syndromes

Lateral Femoral Cutaneous Neuropathy—Meralgia Paresthetica

Srinivas Chiravuri

14

Case Presentation

A 40-year-old obese, diabetic man presents with severe thigh pain that is exacerbated by walking and standing. He demarcates the anterolateral thigh as the skin area with significant dysesthesias. The progressive pain and dysesthesias significantly decrease his quality of life. He denies any weakness. He denies any history of trauma, and prior evaluation failed to reveal any other medical condition (e.g., hypothyroidism), pelvic masses, or significant hip pathology. Behavior modification, resulting in improved diabetic control and weight loss, in addition to cessation of belt wearing, has not provided lasting relief. The patient has tried a variety of opioid and neuropathic pain medications that did not alleviate the pain and dysesthesias but resulted in significant adverse effects. He has undergone epidural steroid injections without relief and has otherwise failed conservative management.

On physical examination, he is well developed but obese (BMI 40). Allodynia is present over the skin of the anterolateral thigh. There are no palpable masses, but deep palpation slightly caudal and medial to the anterior superior iliac spine (ASIS) exacerbates the symptoms. Neither passive manipulation of the right hip joint nor resisted hip flexion results in pain. No tenderness to palpation is present in the gluteal cleft area around the posterior superior iliac spine or at the greater trochanter. Full active and passive range of motion of the patient's hips, knees, and ankles is present. Tinel test is positive slightly medial and caudal to the ASIS, with radiation of electric shocklike pain into the anterolateral thigh. No aberrations in motor strength or sensation (except for the anterolateral thigh) are present. Deep tendon reflexes are equal and symmetric at the bilateral patellar and Achilles tendons. Skin is clean, dry, and intact, without clubbing, cyanosis, or edema.

Questions

1. What is the most likely diagnosis?
2. What is the differential diagnosis?
3. Which diagnostic tests can be performed?

Assessment and Planning

This patient most likely is suffering from meralgia paresthetica (MP), otherwise known as lateral femoral cutaneous neuropathy. MP is a neurologic disorder characterized by a localized area of sensory symptoms, such as paresthesias, dysesthesias, numbness, and/or pain, in the anterolateral aspect of the thigh, which is the sensory distribution of the lateral femoral cutaneous nerve (LFCN). MP was first described by Hager in 1885 and was named by Roth in 1895, although it has been referred to as Bernhardt-Roth syndrome. MP most often occurs in 30- to 40-year-old individuals, with a reported incidence of 4.3 cases per 10,000 patient-years in the general population and 25 cases per 10,000 patient-years in diabetics.[1–3]

MP may be idiopathic or may result from trauma or iatrogenic injury (e.g., hip arthroplasty or bone graft harvest). The LFCN is a pure sensory nerve arising from the dorsal divisions of the L2 and L3 nerve roots. After emerging from the lateral border of the psoas major muscle, it follows a highly variable path, passing medial (most common) or lateral to the ASIS. The vast majority of the time, the nerve courses 2 cm or less medial to the ASIS, typically around 1 cm, although the course is highly variable.[4,5] It then travels between the fascia lata and iliacus to exit the pelvis. Typically it leaves the pelvis as a single branch medial to the sartorius and then divides into anterior and superior branches.[5] In most cases, the nerve exits beneath the inguinal ligament, but well- recognized variations include exiting above the inguinal ligament or piercing the ligament.[6]

The differential diagnosis for MP includes lumbar radiculopathy (typically L2 radiculopathy), intra-abdominal/intrapelvic lesions, and referred pain from the surrounding musculoskeletal structures. A systematic approach starting with the spine and proceeding to the peripheral nerves and surrounding potential pain generators can facilitate the careful consideration of each differential diagnosis.

Careful history and physical examination are necessary to establish the clinical diagnosis, but due diligence via imaging and electrodiagnostic studies (EDX) can eliminate causes other than idiopathic disease. MR imaging of the lumbar spine and EDX can evaluate lumbar radiculopathy as a potential cause. Intra-abdominal pathology, such as a primary tumor, metastasis, or other masses, can be sought with CT or MR imaging of the abdomen and pelvis. Other intra-abdominal pathology, such as diabetic amyotrophy (DA), can result in lumbosacral plexopathy. Typically, DA presents in older patients who have type 2 diabetes mellitus, with abrupt or subacute onset of hip and thigh pain, followed by weakness and muscle atrophy. DA often begins unilaterally but frequently progresses to bilateral involvement. Note that concomitant involvement of contiguous nerves, eventually leading to motor, reflex, and more widespread sensory loss, indicates a plexopathy rather than a single-nerve problem; the diagnostic workup should include a search for systemic vasculitis and undiagnosed diabetes. EDX help to localize the anatomic distribution of a lesion, differentiating a plexopathy from a mononeuropathy or a radiculopathy.

Hip pain and referred joint pain simulating the symptoms of MP can result from many conditions, including osteoarthritis (OA), rheumatoid arthritis, and trauma. The hip joint is a synovial ball-and-socket joint that permits movement in all directions, and it is innervated by branches from the femoral, obturator, and sciatic nerves. Patients with hip pathology present with groin pain that is provoked with internal rotation of the hip and range of motion. Referred pain from soft tissue structures around the hip, such as tendinopathies of the gluteus medius and minimus muscles, trochanteric bursitis, and iliotibial band syndrome, are also in the differential diagnosis. Joint imaging, orthopedic assessment, and image-guided diagnostic joint injections can differentiate primary joint pathology or referred musculoskeletal pain from idiopathic MP.

Once the differential diagnoses have been considered, definitive diagnosis of MP can be made with corroborating evidence from ancillary studies, such as EDX and ultrasound. EDX include nerve conduction studies (NCS) and electromyography (EMG) and can assist in determining the severity and extent, as well as timing and progression, of the neuropathy. NCS of the LFCN can be technically difficult and the symptomatic side must be compared with the asymptomatic side. EMG is normal with LFCN lesions, but the test is helpful in eliminating lumbar radiculopathy or plexopathy as the cause of the patient's symptoms. Finally, ultrasound-guided local anesthetic block of the LFCN can secure the diagnosis of MP. Ultrasound can also be helpful in identifying the anatomic location of the nerve and its branching pattern, and ultrasound can identify focal abnormalities in the nerve that suggest entrapment or injury.[7]

Oral Board Review—Diagnostic Pearls

1. MP is a clinical diagnosis, so a careful history and physical examination are necessary. Since the LFCN is a pure sensory nerve arising from the dorsal divisions of L2 and L3 with a highly variable path through the abdomen and pelvis, MP is characterized by isolated symptoms of pain, dysesthesias, and numbness in a circumscribed area over the anterolateral thigh, without motor weakness. A Tinel sign medial to the ASIS may be positive.
2. Idiopathic MP is more common in obese patients and those with diabetes. However, a variety of differential diagnoses from nerve root to peripheral nerve must be considered, including tumors, trauma, entrapment, and iatrogenic etiologies.
3. Ultrasound-guided diagnostic injections can result in amelioration of symptoms and can confirm the diagnosis. Anesthesia, temporary or permanent, over the skin of the anterolateral thigh without improvement in pain make the diagnosis of MP less likely.
4. Standard imaging of the LFCN is difficult. However, imaging of the surrounding joints and musculoskeletal structures can be useful. High-resolution ultrasound can be a valuable supplementary diagnostic modality.
5. The diagnostic value NCS of the LFCN is limited. However, EMG can differentiate between MP and spinal disorders or other nerve entrapment syndromes.

Decision-Making

The initial management of MP includes behavior modification, physical therapy, and pharmacotherapy. Behavior modification aims at weight loss and avoiding tight clothing and belts that cause external compression. Pharmacologic management includes oral medications, such as neuropathic pain medications (e.g., gabapentin, pregabalin, tricyclic antidepressants, duloxetine), anti-inflammatory medications, and topical agents, such as lidocaine cream or capsaicin. In addition, transcutaneous electrical nerve stimulation (TENS) may be helpful as part of the conservative treatment regimen. If the patient fails conservative management, and if the patient has had a positive response to a diagnostic injection, interventional and surgical options are reasonable. Interventional options include ultrasound-guided local anesthetic infiltration (with or without corticosteroids) around the LFCN, pulsed radiofrequency blockade of the LFCN, and neuromodulation by spinal cord stimulation or direct nerve stimulation. Surgical options include LFCN neurectomy or neurolysis.

Questions

1. What are the therapeutic options?
2. What interventional and surgical options exist?

Surgical Procedure

The most common surgical options for MP are neurolysis and neurectomy. No published data support the superiority of neurolysis or neurectomy as primary surgery, so preference for a surgical technique is unique to each surgeon and his/her experience.

With the patient supine, neurolysis can be achieved by decompression of the LFCN along its path from the ASIS through the inguinal ligament and along the medial sartorius as it emerges on its way to the skin of the anterolateral thigh. This option may be effective in patients with prior trauma or postsurgical neuropathy. The LFCN is a pure sensory nerve, which makes intraoperative stimulation useless. Regardless, we perform all of our peripheral nerve procedures under relaxant-free conditions. Neurectomy may yield better pain relief, but it results in anesthesia in the territory of the LFCN; to avoid postoperative formation of a painful neuroma, care must be taken to manage the proximal stump by resecting several centimeters of nerve, ligating the nerve stump, and allowing it to retract through the inguinal ligament into the retroperitoneal space.

To perform a neurectomy, an approximately 5-cm transverse incision is made 1 cm caudal to the ASIS and centered on the ASIS. The specific location of the incision can be altered depending on the location of the LFCN as determined by the preoperative ultrasound. The dissection is deepened until the inguinal ligament is identified. Next, the sartorial fascia is identified. The fascia is opened and dissection is carried out searching for the nerve. Once the nerve is identified, neurolysis is carried proximally to the point where the nerve exits the pelvis, typically below the inguinal ligament, although the nerve may pierce the inguinal ligament or exit above the inguinal ligament. In cases where the nerve exits below the inguinal ligament, the ligament is retracted to allow exposure of the intrapelvic LFCN. At this point, the LFCN is cut and a segment of the nerve is removed. The proximal stump is then tucked into the intrapelvic compartment. The wound is then copiously irrigated and is closed in layers.

Recently, a technique has been described for ultrasound-guided LFCN neurectomy, which may reduce the length of the incision, decrease operative time, better account for variable anatomy, and ensure that all branches of the nerve are accounted for.[8]

Interventional Techniques

Interventional options include ultrasound-guided local anesthetic infiltration (with or without corticosteroids) around the LFCN, pulsed radiofrequency blockade of the LFCN, and neuromodulation by spinal cord stimulation or direct nerve stimulation. Note that neuromodulation by nerve stimulation is not an option if the LFCN has undergone a prior transection. Injections with anesthetics and/or steroids may be temporarily or permanently effective as treatment, and/or they may be used for diagnosis.

To perform ultrasound-guided block of the LFCN, a high-frequency (7–12 MHz) linear-array ultrasound probe is placed immediately medial to the ASIS along the inguinal ligament, with the lateral end of the probe on the ASIS. The ultrasound probe is moved medially and inferiorly from this point. The fascia lata, fascia iliaca, sartorius, and tensor fascia lata are identified. The LFCN is identified as a small hypoechoic structure with a "honeycomb" appearance, and it is found below the fascia and above the sartorius muscle. Because the LFCN is a superficial structure, an in-plane approach is used with a shallow angle of approach. The skin is infiltrated with lidocaine, and the needle is inserted to reach the desired skin plane immediately medial and inferior to the ASIS. With ultrasound guidance, the LFCN can be blocked with a much lower dose of local anesthetic, as little as 0.3 mL of lidocaine. If no ultrasound guidance is available, LFCN block can be carried out with the patient in the supine position and a pillow under the knees to increase the patient's comfort. A point located 0.2 cm medial and 2 cm caudal to the ASIS is selected as the injection site. A "pop" is noted when a 22-gauge needle pierces the fascia lata. Injecting a volume of 2 to 5 mL of local anesthetic at this location can produce blockade of the LFCN. While local anesthetic infiltration is important for diagnostic purposes, corticosteroids can be added to the injected solution to reduce inflammation and potentially provide therapeutic benefit. Anesthesia in the distribution of the LFCN should be confirmed prior to assessing symptoms in order to ensure a successful diagnostic block.

To perform pulsed radiofrequency (RF) blockade of the LFCN, the nerve is identified using ultrasound as described above. Instead of a block needle, a radiofrequency needle (50 or 100 mm long with a 5-mm active tip) is inserted adjacent to the nerve. Stimulation at 50 Hz causes a tingling sensation down the thigh in the distribution of the LFCN. RF energy is applied as pulses of RF current (45 V) lasting for 120 seconds. The maximum temperature should not exceed 42°C, and the cycle can be repeated.

Neuromodulation

Direct nerve stimulation (rather than spinal cord stimulation) is the preferred neuromodulation modality unless the patient has bilateral pain or the nerve is not visible on ultrasound. The needle-insertion technique for a stimulation trial is the same as the technique described for the ultrasound-guided injection above, with the substitution of a 14-gauge Tuohy needle. A distinct pop is felt as the needle pierces the fascia lata. An electrical lead is placed, and after removal of the Tuohy needle, the lead is attached to the external generator in order to facilitate confirmation that stimulation produces paresthesia in the distribution of the LFCN. If the stimulation trial is successful, the patient then undergoes permanent implantation of the nerve stimulator.

Oral Board Review—Surgical Management Pearls

1. Surgical management by either neurolysis or neurectomy is plausible. No established published evidence supports the superiority of either technique, but consideration of the advantages and disadvantages of each technique is encouraged.
2. Interventional and neuromodulation techniques have added additional modalities to the treatment armamentarium for MP.
3. Intraoperative use of ultrasound helps to identify the LFCN in the context of its wide anatomic variability. If intraoperative ultrasound is not available, the LFCN is most easily located along the proximal medial border of the sartorius muscle.

Pivot Points

1. MP is optimally managed with multidisciplinary treatment.
2. Nonsurgical treatment should be attempted before interventional or surgical treatment modalities are applied.
3. When conservative management fails and LFCN nerve block is effective but temporary, a variety of surgical, interventional, and neuromodulation techniques are available.

Aftercare

Reiteration of the preoperative counseling regarding postoperative expectations for pain relief is useful, depending on which treatment the patient undergoes. For neurectomy or neurolysis, continuation of the existing medication regimen is recommended. When the positive effects of surgery subjectively improve the patient's symptoms, stepwise reduction of the medication dosage is reasonable. No immobilization is necessary postoperatively and routine activities can be continued. Neurolysis and neurectomy can typically be performed as outpatient procedures.

After neuromodulation by direct nerve stimulation, verification of appropriate pain coverage is followed by patient education regarding the use of the pulse generator and its components. After 2 to 3 weeks, the patient should return to the clinic for evaluation of the neuromodulation effects with the proceduralist and device specialist. Use of a pain diary is encouraged to track the patient's progress. The patient should carry a card that indicates that he has an implanted device.

Complications and Management

Potential general complications include wound infection, hematoma, and scar formation. Note that loss of sensation over the skin subserved by the LFCN is an expected result of neurectomy. Formation of a painful neuroma may require additional intervention. Damage to muscles or tendons and hernia formation are less common. Failure of surgery to relieve pain or recurrence of pain may occur. Complex regional pain syndrome can also develop postoperatively.

Available case reports do not mention significant complications or adverse effects with local infiltration and pulsed radiofrequency and hence no conclusions can be drawn. Neuromodulation by direct peripheral nerve stimulation is a relatively new procedure; complications that can occur include lead migration, unwanted stimulation of other body areas, lead erosion, generator failure, and skin breakdown over the leads or generator. Currently available peripheral nerve stimulation systems are not MRI-compatible and are therefore contraindicated if the patient requires serial MR imaging for other medical conditions.

Oral Board Review—Complications Pearls

1. Surgical management by neurolysis or neurectomy has different potential complications than neuromodulation.
2. A complication common to both surgical management and neuromodulation is failure to relieve the symptoms of MP. Furthermore, one intervention may preclude another; for example, neurectomy precludes the use of direct nerve stimulation.
3. Formation of a painful neuroma after neurectomy, resulting in recurrence of pain, may require additional surgery.

Evidence and Outcomes

No randomized controlled trials exist that compare surgical or interventional methods for treatment of MP. A recent study concluded there was insufficient evidence to recommend one surgical method over another.[9] Despite this, one prospective, nonrandomized study found that neurectomy reduced pain in a significantly higher number of patients than neurolysis did: neurectomy was successful in 93% of patients, whereas only 38% of neurolysis patients experienced pain relief.[10] Additional small case series have reported similar rates of pain reduction with LFCN neurectomy.[11] Some retrospective series have reported higher success rates (approximately 70% to

75%) for neurolysis.[12,13] The majority of patients are not bothered by the numbness in the LFCN distribution after neurectomy and even those bothered by the numbness prefer the numbness to the preoperative pain.[14,15] Also, although the evidence is drawn from small studies, the recurrence rate seems to be lower with neurectomy than with neurolysis.[15]

Pulsed radiofrequency neuromodulation has also been shown to be highly effective in small studies. One study reported 63% of patients were pain-free after the procedure, with an additional 27% of patients reporting significant pain relief. No significant complications were reported in the study.[16]

References

1. Harney D, Patijn J. Meralgia paresthetica: diagnosis and management strategies. *Pain Med.* 2007;8:669–677.
2. Parisi TJ, Mandrekar J, Dyck PJ, Klein CJ. Meralgia paresthetica: relation to obesity, advanced age, and diabetes mellitus. *Neurology.* 2011;77:1538–1542.
3. van Slobbe AM, Bohnen AM, Bernsen RM, Koes BW, Bierma-Zeinstra SM. Incidence rates and determinants in meralgia paresthetica in general practice. *J Neurol.* 2004;251:294–297.
4. Lee SH, Shin KJ, Gil YC, Ha TJ, Koh KS, Song WC. Anatomy of the lateral femoral cutaneous nerve relevant to clinical findings in meralgia paresthetica. *Muscle Nerve.* 2017;55:646–650.
5. Tomaszewski KA, Popieluszko P, Henry BM, et al. The surgical anatomy of the lateral femoral cutaneous nerve in the inguinal region: a meta-analysis. *Hernia.* 2016;20:649–657.
6. den Brave PS, Vas Nunes SE, Bronkhorst MW. Anatomical variations of the lateral femoral cutaneous nerve and iatrogenic injury after autologous bone grafting from the iliac crest. *J Orthop Trauma.* 2015;29:549–553.
7. Suh DH, Kim DH, Park JW, Park BK. Sonographic and electrophysiologic findings in patients with meralgia paresthetica. *Clin Neurophysiol.* 2013;124:1460–1464.
8. Henning PT, Wilson TJ, Willsey M, John JK, Popadich M, Yang LJ. Pilot study of intraoperative ultrasound-guided instrument placement in nerve transection surgery for peripheral nerve pain syndromes. *Neurosurg Focus.* 2017;42:E6.
9. Payne R, Seaman S, Sieg E, Langan S, Harbaugh K, Rizk E. Evaluating the evidence: is neurolysis or neurectomy a better treatment for meralgia paresthetica? *Acta Neurochir (Wien).* 2017;159:931–936.
10. de Ruiter GC, Kloet A. Comparison of effectiveness of different surgical treatments for meralgia paresthetica: results of a prospective observational study and protocol for a randomized controlled trial. *Clin Neurol Neurosurg.* 2015;134:7–11.
11. Berini SE, Spinner RJ, Jentoft ME, et al. Chronic meralgia paresthetica and neurectomy: a clinical pathologic study. *Neurology.* 2014;82:1551–1555.
12. Ducic I, Dellon AL, Taylor NS. Decompression of the lateral femoral cutaneous nerve in the treatment of meralgia paresthetica. *J Reconstr Microsurg.* 2006;22:113–118.
13. Siu TL, Chandran KN. Neurolysis for meralgia paresthetica: an operative series of 45 cases. *Surg Neurol.* 2005;63:19–23; discussion 23.

14. de Ruiter GC, Wurzer JA, Kloet A. Decision making in the surgical treatment of meralgia paresthetica: neurolysis versus neurectomy. *Acta Neurochir (Wien)*. 2012;154:1765–1772.
15. Emamhadi M. Surgery for meralgia paresthetica: neurolysis versus nerve resection. *Turk Neurosurg*. 2012;22:758–762.
16. Lee JJ, Sohn JH, Choi HJ, et al. Clinical efficacy of pulsed radiofrequency neuromodulation for intractable meralgia paresthetica. *Pain Physician*. 2016;19:173–179.

Saphenous Neuropathy

Anna Zdunczyk and Nora F. Dengler

15

Case Presentation

A 32-year-old woman presents with burning pain at the medial knee that is exacerbated by prolonged walking or running, quadriceps exercise, and flexion of the knee more than 100°. She notes dysesthesias in the medial knee and calf. The pain and dysesthesias significantly affect her daily life, particularly her ability to maintain her active lifestyle. She denies any history of trauma. She was previously evaluated by an orthopedic surgeon for these complaints and underwent a knee arthroscopy, which was negative. Aside from that, she has no surgical history. On physical examination, she has allodynia over the medial distal thigh. Palpation of the area around the adductor canal reveals some tenderness. The remainder of her neurologic examination is normal. MR imaging of the knee reveals no evidence of ligamentous, bony, or meniscal pathology.

Questions

1. What is the likely diagnosis?
2. What is the differential diagnosis?
3. Which diagnostic tests can be performed?
4. Is there an appropriate imaging modality?

Assessment and Planning

Based on the clinical presentation, the patient is diagnosed with saphenous neuropathy, an uncommon but painful entity. Saphenous neuropathy may arise spontaneously or secondary to trauma or a surgical procedure (e.g., knee arthroplasty or surgery for varices). The saphenous nerve is a sensory branch of the femoral nerve derived from the L1-L4 nerve roots. It branches medially distal to the inguinal ligament and enters the adductor (Hunter's) canal, bordered posteriorly by the adductor longus and magnus and anterolaterally by the vastus medialis. A fascial band derived from the medial intermuscular septum called the vastoadductor membrane forms the roof of the canal. The saphenous nerve pierces this fascial band to exit the canal and is vulnerable to mechanical shear at this point. A second site of entrapment is the penetration of fascial tissue between the sartorius and gracilis muscles more distally in the thigh. At the distal thigh, the nerve is in anatomic proximity to the femoral artery and its branches. Here, anatomic variations are reported.[1] The nerve passes the medial

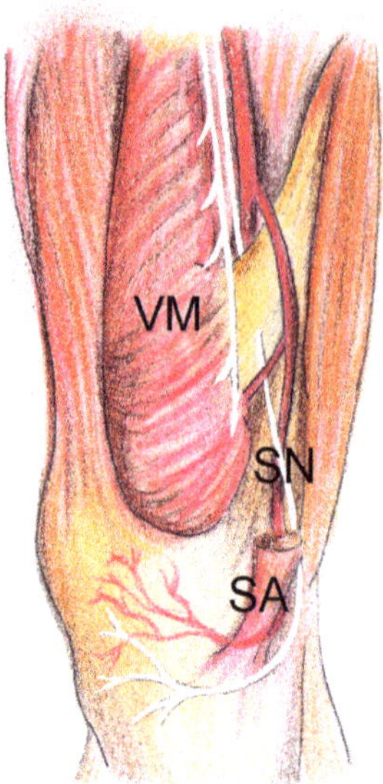

Figure 15.1. Saphenous nerve entrapment at the distal aspect of the thigh. The saphenous nerve pierces the vastoadductor fascia. Surgical anatomy includes the proximity of femoral nerve branches to the vastus medialis muscle (white, left of saphenous nerve) and branches of the femoral artery (red, on right). SA = sartorius muscle; SN = saphenous nerve; VM = vastus medialis muscle.

knee, giving off a large infrapatellar branch and then distributing superficial branches in the medial and frontal lower leg (Figure 15.1).

The differential diagnosis of anteromedial knee pain includes osteochondritis dissecans, nonspecific synovitis, patellofemoral disorder, complex regional pain syndrome, L3 or L4 radiculopathy, medial meniscal tear, local compression by tumor or ganglion, and pes anserine tendonitis. Venous insufficiency may also mimic symptoms of saphenous entrapment syndrome. A careful history and physical examination of the patient are crucial for diagnosis. A saphenous nerve block can be helpful for treatment and diagnosis.[2–5]

MR imaging of the knee helps to rule out many of the orthopedic disorders in the differential diagnosis. Knee arthroscopy can exclude internal derangement of the knee. High-resolution MR neurography allows detection of direct signs of nerve pathology (increased signal intensity and size of the nerve).[6,7] Neurosonography can also help localize nerve compression and indirect signs, such as nerve swelling.

Oral Boards Review—Diagnostic Pearls

1. A thorough history and physical examination are crucial for diagnosis. The burning character of the pain and presence of dysesthesia or hypesthesia in the medial aspect of the knee and the leg that can extend to the medial part of the foot and the hallux point to the diagnosis. A positive Tinel sign supports the suspected diagnosis. The motor examination will be normal.

2. Saphenous neuropathy has been reported after prolonged kneeling and in surfers who induce nerve compression by gripping a surfboard between their knees. Selective lesions of the infrapatellar branch may occur after a direct blow to the knee or after surgical procedures.
3. A therapeutic or diagnostic nerve block can be performed either approximately 10 cm proximal and 7 cm medial to the superior pole of the patella or guided by sonography. Pain diminution confirms a successful nerve block. Anesthesia in the distribution of the saphenous nerve without improvement in pain should make the diagnosis of saphenous neuropathy suspect.
4. Standard MR imaging of the saphenous nerve is challenging because of the nerve's small size. High-resolution MR images and specific protocols for nerve visualization are needed. Negative MR imaging does not rule out saphenous neuropathy. High-resolution ultrasound is an additional diagnostic tool, and it may be used for exact localization of the nerve lesion.
5. The diagnostic value of saphenous nerve conduction studies is limited due to potentially absent responses even in normal subjects and technical difficulties in patients with a larger body mass index. However, electromyographic studies help to differentiate between saphenous neuropathy and radiculopathy or other nerve compression syndromes.

Questions

1. What are the therapeutic options?
2. What kind of surgical strategies can be chosen? What are pros and cons for the different surgical options?

Decision-Making

The first therapeutic option usually consists of conservative management with physiotherapy and pharmacologic pain management using nonsteroidal anti-inflammatory drugs, neuropathic pain medications (e.g., gabapentin, pregabalin), and/or antidepressants (e.g., duloxetine, nortriptyline). Transcutaneous electrical nerve stimulation (TENS) may also be part of a conservative management strategy. A series of injections (bupivacaine and/or triamcinolone) may be helpful. However, the effects of both physiotherapy and injections are often short-lived.

After failed conservative management, surgery is a valid option. Surgical techniques include neurolysis, neurectomy, and neuromodulation (i.e., stimulation). Neurolysis is achieved by the decompression of the saphenous nerve in the adductor canal by splitting the fascia or by release of scar formation in the case of trauma or postsurgical neuropathy. Neurectomy is accompanied by hypesthesia in the saphenous nerve territory. Neurectomy can be an alternative primary procedure or a secondary approach after unsuccessful neurolysis. Special care needs to be taken to avoid painful neuroma formation in the stump. Symptomatic neuroma can be prevented by resection of 4 to 6 cm of nerve tissue and suturing the nerve ends into the vastus medialis muscle.[8] Neurectomy can be aided by the use of intraoperative ultrasound, which potentially reduces surgical time and improves postoperative results.[9]

Questions

1. What are the anatomic landmarks for surgery?
2. Which structures need to be protected to avoid perioperative morbidity?

Surgical Procedure

Surgery is performed under general anesthesia with the patient in the supine position and the involved lower extremity in a frog-leg position (i.e., slight external rotation of the hip and flexion of the knee). The femoral arterial pulse is palpated and a line is drawn from just lateral to the femoral pulse to the adductor tubercle on the medial knee. The line approximates the course of the femoral/saphenous nerve. An incision is made along the line, approximately over the adductor hiatus. After the skin incision, the vastus medialis and sartorius muscles are identified. The space between the muscles is then dissected, exposing the roof of the adductor canal. Careful dissection opening the vastoadductor membrane allows identification of the saphenous nerve. If neurolysis is to be performed, the nerve is decompressed from the entrance into the canal through its exit of the fascia. If neurectomy is to be performed, 4 to 6 cm of nerve is resected and the proximal end is buried in the vastus medialis. Special care needs to be taken to prevent damage to the motor branch innervating the vastus medialis muscle and the nearby vessels. At this point, the wound is copiously irrigated and the wound is closed in layers.

Oral Board Reviews—Management Pearls

1. Intraoperative use of electrophysiology (i.e., nerve stimulation) helps to identify the motor branch of the femoral nerve to the vastus medialis muscle, which should be protected.
2. Preoperative nerve sonography helps in surgical planning, helps to minimize the length of the incision, and helps to identify the femoral and genicular arteries. Use of intraoperative ultrasound may further decrease the size of the incision necessary to carry out the procedure and may improve postoperative outcomes by helping with identification of variable branching patterns of the saphenous nerve.

Pivot Points

1. Treatment of saphenous nerve entrapment is multidisciplinary.
2. Before surgical intervention is offered, a trial of conservative management with physiotherapy, pharmacologic pain management, and injections is recommended.
3. The different surgical options need to be discussed with the patient, including neurolysis, neurectomy, and neuromodulation.

Aftercare

A wound drain may be placed, depending on the surgeon's preference. Routine perioperative antibiotics are generally used but are not continued after surgery. Aftercare includes proper pain management. If the patient has a long history of chronic neuropathic pain, continuation of the existing medication regimen is recommended after surgery. If the patient reports a positive effect of surgery, a careful and stepwise reduction of the medical regimen is advised. Usually, straight immobilization of the knee is not necessary, but physical rest and local cooling may support the healing process and minimize postoperative wound pain. Typically, walking is allowed immediately postoperatively.

Complications and Management

General complications include wound infection or excessive scar formation. Loss of sensory function is a common complication after neurectomy. Damage to the motor branch of the femoral nerve innervating the vastus medialis muscle results in impaired knee extension and/or patellar luxation. Hypersensitivity of the scar area may be present. Postoperative hematoma, as well as damage to muscles, tendons, or vasculature of the medial thigh, can occur. Failure of surgery or relapse of pain may emerge. After neurectomy, formation of a painful neuroma is possible. Complex regional pain syndrome is rare postoperatively but is a risk.

Oral Board Reviews—Complications Pearls

1. A common complication is failure of surgery; improper patient selection due to misdiagnosis needs to be ruled out.
2. Scarring after neurolysis or neuroma formation after neurectomy that is accompanied by recurrence of pain is possible. Revision surgery and use of neuromodulating approaches are rescue options.

Evidence and Outcomes

A prospective randomized evaluation of treatment of saphenous nerve entrapment does not exist. Various case series describe success rates for surgical therapy of between 60% and 90%.[2,4] Patients with primary neurectomy have slightly better results than patients undergoing primary neurolysis.[5] However, recommendations based on high-quality evidence and long-term outcomes are missing.

References

1. Murayama K, Takeuchi T, Yuyama T. Entrapment of the saphenous nerve by branches of the femoral vessels. A report of two cases. *J Bone Joint Surg Am*. 1991;73:770–772.
2. Lippitt AB. Neuropathy of the saphenous nerve as a cause of knee pain. *Bull Hosp Jt Dis*. 1993;52:31–33.
3. Morganti CM, McFarland EG, Cosgarea AJ. Saphenous neuritis: a poorly understood cause of medial knee pain. *J Am Acad Orthop Surg*. 2002;10:130–137.

4. Romanoff ME, Cory PC Jr, Kalenak A, Keyser GC, Marshall WK. Saphenous nerve entrapment at the adductor canal. *Am J Sports Med.* 1989;17:478–481.
5. Worth RM, Kettelkamp DB, Defalque RJ, Duane KU. Saphenous nerve entrapment. A cause of medial knee pain. *Am J Sports Med.* 1984;12:80–81.
6. Damarey B, Demondion X, Wavreille G, Pansini V, Balbi V, Cotten A. Imaging of the nerves of the knee region. *Eur J Radiol.* 2013;82:27–37.
7. Donovan A, Rosenberg ZS, Cavalcanti CF. MR imaging of entrapment neuropathies of the lower extremity. Part 2. The knee, leg, ankle, and foot. *Radiographics.* 2010;30:1001–1019.
8. Lipinski LJ, Spinner RJ. Neurolysis, neurectomy, and nerve repair/reconstruction for chronic pain. *Neurosurg Clin N Am.* 2014;25:777–787.
9. Henning PT, Wilson TJ, Willsey M, John J, Popadich M, Yang LJ. Pilot study of intraoperative ultrasound-guided instrument placement in nerve transection surgery for peripheral nerve pain syndromes. *Neurosurg Focus.* 2017;42(3):E6.

Occipital Neuralgia

Orion Paul Keifer, Jr., Yarema B. Bezchlibnyk, Ashley Diaz, and Nicholas Boulis

16

Case Presentation

A 35-year-old female presents to a neurosurgical clinic for evaluation and treatment of chronic headaches. She reports that 5 years ago she was in a motor vehicle accident and since that time has had a headache every few days. The headache is characterized by sudden-onset, severe, unilateral, sharp, stabbing pain radiating from the upper cervical region and occiput to the vertex and lasting from a few seconds to minutes, occasionally associated with pain in the periorbital area. On several occasions within the last year, the pain has been severe enough to prompt a visit to the emergency department. The patient notes heightened sensitivity and pain whenever the back of her head or upper neck is touched or comes in contact with an object, which has led her to stop brushing her hair, wearing hats, and lying on pillows. Despite having been prescribed multiple medications by her primary care provider, including over-the-counter headache medications (e.g., naproxen and ibuprofen) and migraine prescription medications (e.g., ergot derivatives and triptans), no treatment has been effective in mitigating the pain. More recently, she was referred to a neurologist, who prescribed a trial of tricyclic antidepressants followed by gabapentin; both medications offered little relief in the severity or frequency of the headaches. Upon her referral to a neurosurgeon, careful examination reveals allodynia in the area of the lower occipital cranium and C1-C2 cervical region and a region of hyperesthesia over the back of her head. Otherwise, the neurologic and musculoskeletal exams are normal.

Questions

1. What is the likely diagnosis?
2. What criteria are used to establish the diagnosis?
3. What diagnostic tests can confirm or exclude this diagnosis?

Oral Boards Review—Diagnostic Pearls

Differentiating the various primary headache disorders is primarily based on a careful patient history and physical exam. Seldom are further tests definitively diagnostic. Key findings for each item in the differential diagnosis are:

1. Occipital neuralgia typically presents as paroxysmal lancinating pain in the distribution of the greater, lesser, and/or third occipital nerves. Tenderness to palpation and a Tinel sign over the nerves are important exam findings.
2. Migraine is characterized by unilateral, throbbing pain over the whole hemicranium that lasts for up to 72 hours. In addition, migraines typically have accompanying symptoms, such as nausea, vomiting, photophobia, and/or phonophobia. Common migraines do not have an aura, while classic migraines have an aura, which classically consists of a progressive, scintillating scotoma, although any transient neurologic disturbance is possible. Atypical forms of migraine also exist.
3. Cluster headaches, which have a stabbing quality, are exclusively unilateral and are almost exclusively localized to the periorbital region. Furthermore, the headaches last for 30 to 90 minutes and come in clusters a few times a day for weeks to months. Autonomic symptoms are prominent and include lacrimation, rhinorrhea, sweating, periorbital swelling, and complete or partial Horner's syndrome. Cluster headaches typically occur in middle-aged males.
4. Hemicrania continua is characterized by unilateral continuous (i.e., no pain-free interval) pain of the face and head of varying severity. As with cluster headaches, there are often accompanying autonomic symptoms. Most cases have a complete response to indomethacin treatment.
5. C2 neuralgia results from compression or inflammation of the C2 nerve root with various etiologies. Patients tend to report a throbbing occipital headache aggravated by motion and position. Associated symptoms, such as lacrimation and ciliary injection, may be observed, and the patient should be assessed for a prior history of chickenpox.
6. Tension headaches are daily or almost daily low-grade, nonpulsatile, dull, aching, pressure or constricting headaches that are usually bilateral but poorly localized. They typically have minimal associated symptoms, last 30 minutes to 7 days, and may be induced by stress, hunger, or eyestrain.
7. Temporal arteritis is an autoimmune disorder that results in constriction of the superficial temporal artery and its branches, leading to a unilateral, periorbital headache associated with monocular loss of vision. An elevated ESR suggests the diagnosis, which is confirmed by biopsy of the superficial temporal artery.

Assessment and Planning

The differential diagnosis for the presented case includes, in order of suspicion, occipital neuralgia, migraine, cluster headache, C2 neuralgia, tension headache, hemicrania continua, and temporal arteritis. Additionally, any form of neoplastic, congenital, or infectious process should be considered and ruled out as part of the workup.

Unlike migraine and tension headaches, occipital neuralgia is thought to be rare. However, because it is a relatively understudied entity, the epidemiologic characteristics of occipital neuralgia are unknown. Additionally, research suggests that a significant number of "migraineurs" may actually have misdiagnosed occipital neuralgia.[1] Such findings have spurred increased clinical and research interest in occipital neuralgia. From a pathophysiologic perspective, occipital neuralgia is thought to occur secondary to irritation of the greater, lesser, and/or third occipital nerves (C1-C3 origin). Approximately 90% of cases involve the greater occipital nerve (GON), with 10% attributed to the lesser occipital nerve (LON). Only a few cases involving the third occipital nerve (TON) have been reported to date. The GON arises from the dorsal primary ramus of C2, with an additional contribution from C3, and provides sensation to the medial portion of the posterior scalp as far anterior as the vertex and motor innervation to the semispinalis capitis. In contrast, the LON arises from the ventral primary ramus of C2, also with an additional contribution from C3. The LON courses superiorly along the posterior border of the sternocleidomastoid, providing sensation to the lateral portion of the scalp and the cranial surface of the auricle. Finally, the TON arises deep to the trapezius from the medial branch of the dorsal ramus of C3 and ascends medial to the GON to provide sensation to the skin over the rostral neck and the occiput near the external occipital protuberance. While occipital neuralgia may be described as idiopathic, a number of presumed causes have been identified in the literature, including trauma (especially motor vehicle accidents), aberrant vascular anatomy, and degenerative conditions. Rarer causes include neoplastic compression, Chiari malformation, temporal arteritis, and postherpetic neuralgia.

The International Headache Society has defined diagnostic criteria for occipital neuralgia (detailed in Table 16.1).[2] Diagnosis centers on the classic neuropathic pain symptom of severe lancinating pain in the distribution of the occipital nerves. Further corroboration is done with an anesthetic nerve block of the GON and/or LON to demonstrate temporary relief from pain. Nerve block can also concurrently assess the patient's tolerance to loss of sensation over the scalp (a common and sometimes poorly tolerated sequela of interventions). While imaging is not required to fulfill the diagnostic criteria, it is useful to exclude other diagnoses and can help to determine the etiology of occipital neuralgia. For example, in older patients, open-mouth X-ray can evaluate the C2 region for arthritic or degenerative changes. In addition, other processes (e.g., neoplastic or degenerative disease) can be evaluated by CT or MR imaging of the craniocervical junction. CT angiography, MR angiography, and ultrasound can be used to identify the relationship of the nerves and vessels, including the adjacent occipital artery, to rule out vascular compression.

The patient presented here responded to an anesthetic block of the GON, which helped confirm the diagnosis of occipital neuralgia. Imaging did not show any particular anatomic abnormalities that explained the etiology of her occipital neuralgia. After a careful discussion of the different treatment options available, the patient opted for treatment with occipital nerve stimulation. She underwent a trial of neurostimulation of the GON, which resulted in a drastic reduction in the severity and frequency of her episodes of occipital neuralgia. Following the trial stimulation,

Table 16.1.
Description of, and Diagnostic Criteria for, Occipital Neuralgia, from the International Headache Society

Description	Unilateral or bilateral paroxysmal, shooting or stabbing pain in the posterior part of the scalp, in the distribution of the greater, lesser, or third occipital nerve, sometimes accompanied by diminished sensation or dysesthesia in the affected area and commonly associated with tenderness over the involved nerve(s).
Diagnostic Criteria	A. Unilateral or bilateral pain fulfilling criteria B–E B. Pain is located in the distribution of the greater, lesser, and/or third occipital nerves C. Pain has two of the following three characteristics: 1. Recurring in paroxysmal attacks lasting from a few Rseconds to minutes 2. Severe intensity 3. Shooting, stabbing or sharp in quality D. Pain is associated with both of the following: 1. Dysesthesia and/or allodynia apparent during innocuous stimulation of the scalp and/or hair 2. Either or both of the following: a) Tenderness over the affected nerve branches b) Trigger points at the emergence of the greater occipital nerve or in the area of distribution of C2 E. Pain is eased temporarily by local anesthetic block of the affected nerve F. Not better accounted for by another ICHD-3 diagnosis

Source: Headache Classification Committee of the International Headache Society. The international classification of headache disorders, 3rd edition (beta version). *Cephalalgia.* 2013;33:629–808.

she opted for the permanent, bilateral electrode implantation, and she has continued to be nearly pain free.

Questions

1. What is the relevant anatomy of the structure(s) likely to be involved in this condition, and how does one distinguish neuralgia involving these structures?
2. What are the first- and second-line therapies in the management of occipital neuralgia?
3. What are the indications and contraindications for surgical intervention?

Decision-Making

Unlike more common primary headache and craniofacial pain entities, occipital neuralgia does not have a standard of care. However, the natural course of decision-making for patients tends to proceed from the least aggressive treatment to the most aggressive intervention. Initial conservative treatment includes rest, warm or cold compresses, massage, and physical therapy. Anti-inflammatory medications and muscle relaxants may be used to reduce acute pain. More chronic pharmacologic therapies include tricyclic antidepressants and antiepileptics, although their use has not been rigorously researched in a controlled fashion. Patients who fail these treatments may be candidates for local anesthetic occipital nerve block, corticosteroid injection, and/or botulinum toxin type A injection. While these interventions tend to be effective, their effects are short-lived and require re-injection. Furthermore, occipital neuralgia may become refractory to these interventions over time. Patients who experience suboptimal pain control or whose disease becomes refractory to these interventions may be referred to a neurosurgeon for more aggressive interventions.

Because no single procedure has emerged as superior, the neurosurgical repertoire of treatments for occipital neuralgia remains relatively broad. In general, surgical methods can be divided into nerve-destructive and nerve-sparing procedures. The destructive methods may be used to create lesions anywhere along the nerve pathway, including the spinal root (i.e., cervical dorsal rhizotomy), dorsal ganglion (i.e., C2 ganglionectomy), or the peripheral nerve itself (i.e., GON neurectomy). The methods used to ablate the neural structures include surgical transection and radiofrequency lesioning (most often in the purview of a pain specialist). The strength of the ablative methods lies in the strong history of the techniques, including refinements in the methods to mitigate associated complications. The main drawbacks of ablative procedures are the permanent nature of their effects and the inability to titrate their use over time. Rescue therapies for failed interventions are relatively limited. Destructive approaches are highly invasive and require a high degree of technical skill.

Neuromodulation (e.g., occipital nerve stimulation and high cervical spinal cord stimulation) and various decompressive/joint stabilization procedures (vascular and musculoskeletal) are nerve-sparing surgical treatments. Occipital nerve stimulation has the benefits of being reversible, nondestructive, and titratable over time. Furthermore, it is customary to conduct a trial with temporary placement of stimulating electrodes prior to the implantation of a permanent system, allowing for testing of the treatment before its full implementation. However, the treatment is not universally successful, and the neurostimulation systems are expensive and require ongoing battery replacement. Appropriate decompressive techniques depend on the source of compression. Occipital neuralgia that is secondary to degenerative atlantoaxial instability in the elderly is one example.[3,4] In this case, the resulting C2 nerve compression is ameliorated with joint fixation and stabilization (albeit fixation can also lead to occipital nerve irritation and de novo postoperative neuralgia). Similarly, there are a few case reports of muscular, vascular, and scar compression of the nerve leading to symptoms that have improved with decompression.[5–9] These remain a minority of cases.

Questions

1. What factors influence a recommendation for ablative versus nerve-sparing procedures in a given patient with occipital neuralgia?
2. What surgical procedures can be paired in primary rescue for failed treatment or recurrent pain?

Surgical Procedures

Surgical procedures for occipital neuralgia may be undertaken either unilaterally or bilaterally, based on the clinical presentation. Typically, the bilateral version of the surgery is a mirror of the unilateral surgery, with obvious associated changes (e.g., full versus hemilaminectomy). Significant differences between unilateral and bilateral surgery are discussed under the relevant procedures. Although practices may vary, general anesthesia is preferentially used in nearly all procedures, since patients are generally positioned prone. The patient's head is typically placed in three-point fixation with a Mayfield head holder. All bony prominences are appropriately padded, sequential compression devices are placed on the legs for thromboembolism prophylaxis, and the appropriate preoperative antibiotics are administered. Before incisions are made, the area is infiltrated with local anesthetic.

In all cases, localization is critical. Using anatomic landmarks, the GON is most reliably identified 3 to 6 cm lateral to the external occipital protuberance; the occipital artery runs lateral to the nerve. Palpation of arterial pulsations may be useful in confirming the anatomy of the nerve or a Doppler probe may be used to identify the artery as a guide to the location of the nerve. The LON is typically identified lateral to the GON along the superior nuchal line, at a point approximately one third of the distance between the mastoid and the external occipital protuberance or 3 cm medial and posterior to the mastoid tip. The TON is medial to the GON, 0 to 0.5 cm off the midline.

Ablative Procedures

Radiofrequency Ablation

Radiofrequency ablation is a minimally invasive, percutaneous technique for lesioning a given peripheral nerve. The patient is typically placed in the seated position, with the posterior neck and suboccipital region prepped and draped. The procedure is performed with the patient awake, to allow for monitoring of paresthesias. Depending on the surgeon, local anesthetic may or may not be used. If the intent is to use the ablative needle to confirm the nerve with stimulation, then local anesthetic is not used, in order to facilitate stimulation-induced paresthesias. Accurate localization of the GON, LON, or TON is imperative for effective application of radiofrequency pulses. Nerve localization often involves the manual palpation of specific anatomic landmarks, as described above, followed by adjuvant techniques to further refine localization, including nerve stimulation and/or ultrasound detection of the occipital artery and nerve. Once the nerve has been localized, a specially designed high-gauge needle connected to a lesion generator is inserted in the proximity of the nerve to be ablated, with or without ultrasound guidance. The nerve is then stimulated at sublesional intensities to confirm correct placement (50 Hz, < 0.5 V) and to rule out stimulation of motor branches (2 Hz). After confirmation of correct positioning, the frequency, voltage, and pulse-burst settings are increased to ablative levels (e.g., 2 Hz, 45 V, 20 milliseconds, 240 seconds). Temperature levels are monitored throughout the procedure, with the nerve being lesioned for 90- to 120-second intervals at 42°C. Pressure is applied at the needle insertion site and the area is cleaned and bandaged.

Cervical Dorsal Rhizotomy

Several variants of the cervical rhizotomy have been described in the literature (e.g., intradural versus extradural, complete versus partial). The procedure described here is partial intradural cervical dorsal rhizotomy; for the complete version, the entire dorsal rootlet is lesioned.

The patient is given general anesthesia with orotracheal intubation and is placed in a prone position with the head secured by three-point pin fixation to allow access to the C1-C3 region of the spinal column. The patient is prepped and draped in a standard fashion, with the occiput to the C4 spinous process left in the field. The extent of the exposure varies, although typically a midline cervical incision is made extending from C1 to the spinous process of C3. To facilitate the exposure of the lamina, the paraspinal muscles are separated from the bone in a subperiosteal fashion with Bovie electrocautery and a periosteal elevator. The muscles are then retracted for visualization of, and access to, the laminae. A full C1-C2 laminectomy or hemilaminectomy is performed to expose the underlying dura. Depending on the exposure desired, a C3 laminotomy may or may not be performed. After meticulous hemostasis has been obtained, the dura is incised and is tacked to the overlying muscle in a tented fashion to maximize exposure and minimize CSF contamination. A surgical microscope is then used to visualize the nerves arising from the C2 and C3 rootlets as they proceed to their exit foramina, as well as any intercalating rootlets from C1 and/or C4 contributing to the nerves. The dorsal rootlets are then identified. This is facilitated by visualization of the dentate ligament, which splits the dorsal and ventral rootlets. The rootlets are then separated from any adjacent blood vessels with microsurgical instruments; care is also taken to avoid any branches contributing to the ascending spinal accessory nerve. The rootlets are then separated into two portions (for partial rhizotomies). One portion (one half of the rootlets) is then coagulated with bipolar electrocautery and is sectioned with a microsurgical blade. After lesioning, the dura is closed in a watertight fashion. The muscle, fascial planes, and skin are closed in layers.

C2 Ganglionectomy

The patient is administered general anesthesia with orotracheal intubation and is placed in a prone position. The head is secured with three-point pin fixation, with the neck slightly flexed. The patient is prepped and draped in a standard fashion, with the area from the occiput to the C4 spinous process left in the field. A midline cervical incision is made extending from C1 to the spinous process of C3. To facilitate the exposure of the laminae and lateral masses, the paraspinal muscles are separated from the bone in a subperiosteal fashion with Bovie electrocautery and a periosteal elevator. Once the laminae and lateral masses are exposed, an operative microscope is brought in for the remainder of the procedure. Exposure of the C2 ganglion proceeds by careful dissection within the atlantoaxial interlaminar space, working laterally from the thecal sac just inferior to the arch of C1 until the epidural venous plexus that surrounds the dorsal aspect of the ganglion is identified and removed. During exposure of the ganglion, care should be exercised in identifying and avoiding the vertebral artery. Once the plexus has been removed, full visualization of the ganglion may require a C1 laminotomy; the ganglion may be identified as an area of increased circumference proximal to the primary rami of C2, approximately 2 to 4 mm lateral to the dural exit of the C2 nerve root. Once the ganglion has been identified, each end of the ganglion (e.g., dural epidural sleeve around the dorsal rootlets and the dorsal and ventral primary rami) must be dissected to facilitate ganglion removal. The tissue just proximal and distal to the ganglion is coagulated with bipolar cautery and a scalpel is used to excise the ganglion. Once the ganglion is removed, inspection for bleeding or CSF leakage is necessary. The muscle, fascial planes, and skin are closed in layers in a standard fashion.

GON and LON Neurectomy

GON and LON neurectomy was one of the first surgeries performed for the treatment of occipital neuralgia. While it is currently out of favor in lieu of some of the other surgical procedures, it may be performed in conjunction with decompressive operations.

Patients are usually placed under general anesthesia with endotracheal intubation. The patient is positioned prone, with the head in a horseshoe head holder. The scalp is shaved above the superior aspect of the nuchal line. Ultrasound is then used to detect the occipital artery and the adjacent GON, which is delineated with a marking pen. The area is prepped and draped in a standard fashion. A skin incision is made at sufficient depth to expose the fascia overlying the GON and the occipital artery. The nerve and artery are then carefully separated, and external neurolysis is performed over approximately 4 cm of the GON to free it from the surrounding tissue. A 3-cm length of nerve is then excised. Depending on the clinical picture, the LON may also be explored, dissected, and excised in a similar fashion. The proximal ends of the nerves should be placed deep in the surrounding musculature with imbrication of muscle around the stump to mitigate reinnervation of the skin. The skin is then closed in a standard fashion.

Nerve-Sparing Procedures

Decompression

There are several proposed "compressive" etiologies that can account for the occurrence of occipital neuralgia. An exhaustive detailing of the decompressive surgical procedures is beyond the immediate scope of this chapter. Perhaps the most common compressive etiology for occipital neuralgia, especially in elderly patients, is atlantoaxial joint instability. Surgical solutions are typically aimed at C1-C2 fixation, with the goal of re-establishing stability. Concurrent neurectomy and ganglionectomy may be considered at the time of the fixation procedure, both as a treatment for preoperative occipital neuralgia and as a preventive maneuver for the development of postoperative neuralgia (e.g., secondary to screw placement or scar-related compression). Similarly, some occipital neuralgia has been attributed to compression by musculature, vasculature, or scarring from a previous surgery. In these cases, relief has been attained by removing the compressive entity.

Neurostimulation

Occipital Stimulation

Multiple procedures have been described for occipital nerve stimulation in the treatment of occipital neuralgia. Common to all of them is the placement of electrode leads in the vicinity of the occipital nerve, with either direct or indirect confirmation based on intraoperative anatomy or imaging, respectively. The electrode may be placed alongside the nerve, wrapped around the nerve, or perpendicular to the nerve. It is important to note that most authors strongly recommend a trial of occipital nerve stimulation, typically 1 to 2 weeks in duration, prior to implantation of a permanent system. Over the course of the trial, the patient may adjust various parameters of stimulation to help establish whether the occipital neuralgia is treated satisfactorily by this intervention.

Anesthesia with local anesthetic and conscious sedation, monitored anesthesia care, and general anesthesia have all been described for placement of trial stimulation leads, although procedures conducted in the prone position are almost always done under general anesthesia to ensure control to the patient's airway. The placement of permanent leads is often performed under general anesthesia due to the need for multiple incisions and the pain associated with tunneling the electrodes subcutaneously to the site where the implantable pulse generator (IPG) will be located. Positioning depends on the technique selected and on the laterality of the occipital neuralgia. Although a variety of techniques exist, the authors' technique for permanent lead placement is described here. For unilateral procedures, the patient is placed on the operating table in the supine position with a bump under the ipsilateral shoulder. The head is turned to the contralateral side, so that the ipsilateral pinna is parallel to the ground, and is positioned on a donut headrest. An electric razor is then used to clip the hair in a large patch extending from the postauricular region across the occiput to the midline of the head. For bilateral procedures, each side may be implanted in turn as above. Alternatively, the patient may be placed in a prone position, with the head placed in a radiolucent headrest or pin fixation. For placement of trial leads, a stab incision is fashioned at the tip of the ipsilateral mastoid. If bilateral temporary leads are to be implanted in the prone position, stab incisions are fashioned at the level of C1, 1 cm lateral to and on either side of midline. The procedure is otherwise identical to the unilateral procedure, except that the Tuohy needle is aimed toward the ipsilateral mastoid. For placement of permanent leads, a curvilinear incision is planned approximately 2 cm behind the pinna and just posterior to the mastoid, extending from the mastoid tip superiorly for approximately 3 cm, to just above the root of the mastoid process. A second 5-cm incision is planned 3 cm below the ipsilateral clavicle. These incisions are infiltrated with local anesthetic and are opened with a scalpel. The postauricular incision is carried down to periosteum, while the infraclavicular incision is carried down to the pectoralis fascia, where a suprafascial pocket large enough to accommodate the pulse generator is created.

To place the neurostimulator lead, a Tuohy needle is gradually bent by hand until it is gently curved in the direction of the bevel. This needle is then placed at the tip of the mastoid within either the stab incision or the curvilinear incision

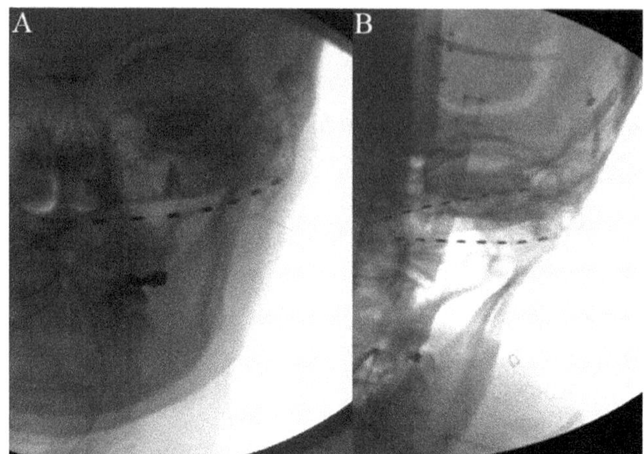

Figure 16.1. Intraoperative fluoroscopic images showing the final placement of one 8-contact electrode (A) and two 8-contact electrodes for extended coverage (B).

and is passed in the epifascial plane subcutaneously toward the midline, with the tip directed toward C1. Intraoperative anteroposterior (AP) fluoroscopy is used to guide the insertion and to confirm the final position of the needle. Visualization of all skin overlying the electrode is imperative to ensure that penetration of the skin by the introducer needle has not occurred. The stylet is then removed and is replaced with a quadripolar or octopolar neurostimulating electrode. The internal stylet of the electrode is then removed, along with the Tuohy needle, leaving the electrode in place (Figure 16.1).

At this time, some neurosurgeons will lighten sedation (if the patient is not under general anesthesia) to test for stimulation-induced paresthesias and to adjust the position of the electrodes accordingly. For trial leads, the electrode is secured in place at the skin using a purse-string stitch. Permanently placed leads are secured within the postauricular incision using a rubber sleeve that is placed around the lead and is sutured to the periosteum. A strain-relieving loop is then fashioned and affixed to the periosteum at multiple sites. For treatment of unilateral occipital neuralgia, the authors have also used paddle leads placed in the perifascial plane. These leads provide an excellent array of contacts and are far less prone to lead migration. Alternatively, paddle leads have been placed in a similar fashion through open surgery (Figure 16.2).[10]

To connect permanently placed leads to an infraclavicular IPG, the tunneling instrument provided by the manufacturer, fitted with a plastic straw, is passed subcutaneously from the postauricular incision down to the infraclavicular incision. The trocar is then removed, and the end of the electrode is passed through the plastic straw down to the infraclavicular pocket. The straw is then removed and the electrode is connected to the IPG. The IPG is placed within the infraclavicular pocket, with the redundant length of wire looped behind it, and is secured to the pectoralis fascia with sutures. When a midline approach is used for lead placement, a gluteal or flank IPG pocket is generally utilized. Prior to closure of the incisions in layers, the programmer is used to perform an impedance check, and all wounds are copiously irrigated with antibiotic-impregnated normal saline. Optional postoperative multiview head X-rays can be performed to confirm positioning (Figure 16.2).

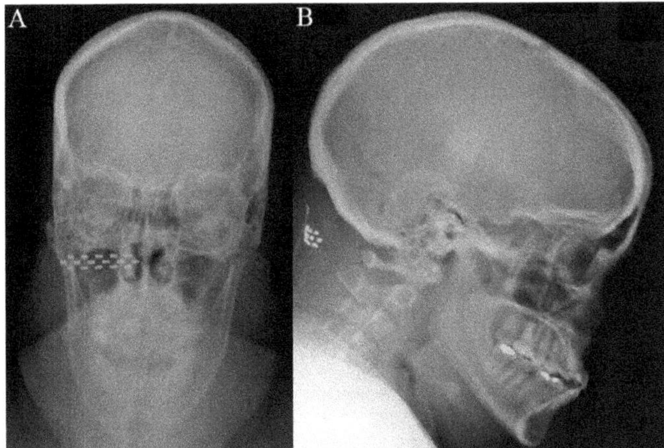

Figure 16.2. Anteroposterior (A) and lateral (B) head X-rays showing the placement of a 5-6-5 paddle-style electrode.

High Cervical Spinal Cord Stimulation

High cervical spinal stimulation is an alternative to occipital nerve stimulation, with the target consisting of the dorsal roots of C2 and C3. As with occipital nerve stimulation, a trial consisting of 1 to 2 weeks of stimulation is highly recommended prior to implantation of a permanent system. Again, various parameters of stimulation may be adjusted to help establish the efficacy of this intervention in treating the symptoms of occipital neuralgia.

The trial leads are typically implanted percutaneously. The patient is positioned prone, with the head fixed in pins using a Mayfield clamp; therefore, these procedures are typically performed under general anesthesia. Fluoroscopy is then used to identify the C5-C6 interlaminar space, and the lateral aspect of the contralateral pedicle of C7 is marked on the patient's skin. Local anesthetic is instilled in this area, and a stab incision is made. A Tuohy needle is then advanced to the C5-C6 interlaminar space, directed just shy of midline. It is then carefully advanced into the epidural space, after which the stylet is removed, and a neurostimulator lead is passed superiorly in the contralateral lateral recess. The lead must be placed as high as possible, with the tip resting at the most superior terminus of the epidural space under the C1 posterior arch. A stitch is then placed around the neurostimulating lead at the exit site. Proper placement is confirmed postoperatively with paresthesias in the distribution of the occipital nerve.

Permanent leads may be placed in a similar fashion in the case of tubular octopolar leads, with the only difference being that the stab incision is somewhat more extensive in order to accommodate a subcutaneous anchoring stitch and a strain-relieving loop at this site. The terminal end of the lead is then passed subcutaneously to an IPG implanted most commonly in the gluteal region.

Alternatively, paddle leads may be placed via an open procedure. This procedure may be indicated in patients who have experienced repeated migration of tubular leads or in patients experiencing unpleasant recruitment of surrounding muscle and/or motor nerve stimulation. A midline cervical incision is made extending from C4 to C7, with the paraspinal muscles being separated from the bone in a subperiosteal fashion with Bovie electrocautery and a periosteal elevator. The muscles are then retracted to visualize and access the C5 and C6 laminae. The interspinous ligament between C5 and C6 is removed, along with a portion of the C5 spinous process. To gain access to the epidural space, a hemilaminectomy of C6 is completed, with the intervening ligamentum flavum being removed with Kerrison rongeurs and curettes. The paddle lead is then passed superiorly under fluoroscopic guidance as far as possible, with the tip resting just under the C1 posterior arch at the midline. Often the distal end of the lead is sutured to the ligamentum flavum at C5-C6 to prevent lead migration inferiorly.

Oral Boards Review—Management Pearls

1. Identification of the involved neural structures is critical in making the diagnosis of occipital neuralgia and in establishing the nerve(s) to be treated. A focused history should include the distribution of the patient's pain, the location from which any radiating pain originates, and the presence of any associated numbness or dysesthesias. A careful physical examination should assess the dermatomal distribution of any numbness or dysesthesias, as well as assess for focal tenderness. In addition, the physician should assess for any aggravating or alleviating postures of the head and neck.
2. Intraoperative confirmation of the involved nerve is essential to treatment efficacy, whether by direct or indirect measures. Using anatomic landmarks, the GON is located 3 to 6 cm lateral to the external occipital protuberance, while the LON is located 3 cm medial and posterior to the mastoid tip. The TON is located 0 to 0.5 cm off the midline. Additionally, the occipital artery courses adjacent to the GON and may be identified with intraoperative Doppler ultrasonography or may be observed directly through a cutdown procedure. Finally, intraoperative fluoroscopy may be used to confirm appropriate placement of the neurostimulating leads, which should pass just over top of the fascia. Leads targeting the GON should pass from the level of the posterior arch of C1 to the root of the mastoid, while leads targeting the LON should pass from the level of the posterior arch of C1 to the tip of the mastoid.

Pivot Points

1. The absence of a response to local anesthetic block should raise concern for a diagnosis other than occipital neuralgia.
2. All patients being considered for surgical management of pain should be screened for neuropsychological issues. A patient who has a strong psychological component to his or her pain should be treated surgically only under exceptional circumstances.

3. Patients with comorbidities that significantly impair wound healing, including immunologic disorders or a history of recurrent infections, or conditions that compromise skin integrity in and around the surgical area, such as a history of dermatologic malignancy or radiation, are best managed with ablative procedures.
4. Occipital nerve stimulating leads should be trialed for 1 to 2 weeks before the implantation of a permanent system.

Aftercare

In all cases, it is essential to restart the patient's preoperative analgesic regimen immediately postoperatively; additional narcotic pain medicine should be prescribed for postoperative breakthrough pain. Immediate postoperative care is geared toward ruling out complications, while follow-up typically includes clinic visits in 2 and 6 weeks to evaluate the surgical site and to assess the patient's pain level. The patient is also encouraged to visit a pain specialist for management of the pain medication regimen over time, as well as for long-term vigilance for recurrence of the patient's pain or occurrence of delayed complications, including deafferentation pain.

Complications and Management

Ablative Procedures

A known side effect of all ablative procedures is numbness on the occipital portion of the scalp. Typically, patients are able to adapt to the persistent numbness; however, some patients find it disabling. Unfortunately, there are limited options for management of numbness. A relatively rare complication associated with numbness is the occurrence of deafferentation pain, characterized by hyperpathia and allodynia in the C1-C3 dermatomes. Typically, patients are offered either neuromodulation or ganglionectomy for deafferentation syndrome, although there is limited evidence on effectiveness.

Radiofrequency Ablation

Given the minimally invasive nature of the radiofrequency ablation procedure, there are few associated complications apart from those described above. However, injury to the occipital artery may occur, leading to an expansile hematoma, rarely requiring surgical evacuation. Recurrence of occipital neuralgia after radiofrequency ablation is relatively common, prompting an additional round of radiofrequency treatment.[11]

Cervical Rhizotomy

Potential serious neurologic complications of cervical rhizotomy include injury to cranial nerves (the spinal accessory nerve is particularly at risk) and to the spinal cord. In the worst case, this may lead to high-level quadriplegia and associated difficulty with spontaneous ventilation.

Hemorrhagic complications include the rare spinal epidural hematoma, which typically presents as rapidly progressive myelopathy. This should prompt emergent neuroimaging or operative exploration, depending on the rapidity and severity of the decline.

Arachnoiditis or inflammation leading to scarring in the region of the surgery may occasionally occur and can present as an expansile lesion leading to neuropathic pain, radiculopathy, and, in severe cases, progressive myelopathy.

A CSF leak may result from failure to achieve watertight closure of the dura. This may present as the leakage of clear to blood-tinged fluid from the incision site in association with positional headaches and/or nausea. Initial treatment consists of oversewing the incision, with or without CSF diversion with serial lumbar punctures or the placement of a lumbar drain. Persistent leakage despite these measures should prompt surgical exploration to identify and correct the dural defect, since potential complications of a persistent CSF leak include bacterial meningitis. Pseudomeningoceles may arise in the region of the surgical site and are mostly benign, apart from cosmetic concerns. Therefore, elective operative correction is typically considered on a case-by-case basis. Rarely, pseudomeningoceles may compress neural structures, causing myelopathy and may require decompression and repair of the underlying dural defect.

C2 Ganglionectomy

The complications of ganglionectomy parallel those of cervical rhizotomy. Additionally, injury to the vertebral artery may rarely occur, potentially leading to arterial dissection or intraoperative hemorrhage. Postoperative changes in neurologic status, whether transient or persistent, should prompt vascular imaging, including a CT angiogram and/or formal angiogram. Treatment depends on the clinical and radiologic findings. Options include antiplatelet or anticoagulant medications or endovascular procedures. Direct injury causing intraoperative arterial bleeding should be managed by rapid compression over the site of the bleed, followed by exposure of the vertebral artery above and below the injury to obtain proximal and distal control in order to effect an intraoperative repair, or, if this is not feasible, sacrifice of the vessel with or without bypass.

Neurectomy

As with radiofrequency ablation, complications include injury to the occipital artery potentially requiring surgical evacuation. A complication unique to the neurectomy procedure is the development of a postoperative neuroma, which is often painful to the touch. A neuroma can be treated surgically, and the risk of developing a neuroma is thought to be mitigated by neuralization (embedding of nerve into muscle) of the proximal end of the transected nerve.

Nerve-Sparing Procedures

Decompression

Complications are entirely dependent on the procedure performed.

Neurostimulation

The most common complaint with neurostimulation is lack of efficacy, the frequency of which varies, with between 20% and 40% of patients reporting no or minimal effect.[12–14] Placement of the trial leads themselves is typically well tolerated, although temporary lead migration or infection requires expeditious removal in a procedure that may be done on an outpatient basis.

In the placement of occipital nerve stimulating leads, injury to the occipital artery may occur, potentially requiring surgical evacuation. Furthermore, injury to the nerve itself may occur, resulting in a neuroma, which could further incite pain.

For high cervical spinal cord stimulation, the terminus of the spinal epidural space just under the posterior arch of C1 often impedes optimal placement of the electrode, resulting in no, or weak, paresthesias in the distribution of the occipital nerve. Inadvertent puncture of the dura is a relatively common complication of percutaneous lead implantation, with persistent CSF fistulae occurring in approximately 3% of patients.[15] Other complications include those that may occur with any open procedure on the cervical spinal cord, including injury to the spinal cord or postoperative spinal epidural hematoma.

The placement of permanently implanted stimulator leads is typically well tolerated. In the case of occipital nerve stimulation, passing the extension wire subcutaneously via the neck may result in injury to the external jugular vein. Typically, this is managed with manual compression at the site of injury. Very rarely, injury to deeper vascular structures may occur, and this should be managed with direct compression and dedicated vascular imaging.

The most common perioperative complications are hardware failure, lead migration, skin erosion, wound dehiscence, and infection. These may occur anywhere over the course of the implanted system, including the stimulating leads, extension leads, and IPG. Management typically entails repair or replacement of defective components or explantation of the system, with intraoperative cultures and postoperative antibiotic therapy in the case of infection. Once the infection is cleared (typically after 6 weeks of antibiotic therapy), the system may be re-implanted at the discretion of the patient and surgeon.

Oral Boards Review—Complications Pearls

1. For cervical dorsal rhizotomy, ganglionectomy, or procedures with epidural lead placement, any progressive postoperative neurologic impairment should raise concern for a spinal epidural hematoma. Emergent neuroimaging or, if the progression is sufficiently rapid, emergent operative exploration, is indicated in these cases.
2. For ganglionectomy procedures, the presence of postoperative cranial nerve deficits, vertigo, ataxia, and/or long-tract signs should raise concern for a vertebral artery dissection. Emergent neuroimaging with CT angiography or formal angiogram is indicated, with concomitant aspirin, heparin, or endovascular repair dictated by the particular findings of the studies.
3. For neurectomy procedures, the presence of a painful or prominent postoperative neuroma is a relative indication for surgical exploration and excision.
4. For neurostimulation procedures, any erythema, tenderness, and swelling overlying the neurostimulating lead or IPG should immediately raise

concern for a hardware infection, which requires urgent explantation, cultures of the infected site and hardware, and broad-spectrum antibiotics pending speciation and sensitivities.

5. A relatively rare complication associated with ablative procedures is the occurrence of deafferentation pain, characterized by hyperpathia and allodynia in the C1-C3 dermatomes. Typically, patients are offered either neuromodulation or ganglionectomy for deafferentation syndrome.

Evidence and Outcomes

Evidence for surgical procedures in the treatment of medically refractory occipital neuralgia is generally based on anecdotal reports, retrospective studies, and small case series. Very few randomized, controlled trials (RCTs) have been conducted, and these have typically been directed toward treatment of migraine rather than occipital neuralgia. Thus, the results of these studies should be interpreted with caution. The lack of research is likely secondary to occipital neuralgia being relatively uncommon.

Radiofrequency Ablation

A number of case series on radiofrequency ablation have demonstrated a success rate of approximately 55%, with success defined as ≥ 50% improvement in pain at 3 to 6 months postoperatively.[16] In addition, a recent RCT assessed the efficacy of radiofrequency ablation compared to steroid injections in patients with migraines and occipital neuralgia. At 6 weeks after the procedure, 61% of patients treated with radiofrequency ablation had a positive outcome, compared to 36% of those treated with steroids. At 6 months, the rates declined to 26% and 8%, respectively. In a subgroup analysis, patients with occipital neuralgia fared worse than migraineurs.[17]

Cervical Dorsal Rhizotomy

Cervical dorsal rhizotomy is uncommonly performed for occipital neuralgia. However, a large, single-institution retrospective study recently reported that 64% of patients experience excellent pain relief 5 years postoperatively, with an additional 20% of patients reporting partial relief.[18]

C2 Ganglionectomy

The evidence for C2 ganglionectomy is generally limited to small, single-institution case series. These demonstrate substantial reduction of pain in the majority of patients immediately postoperatively, although long-term results are more circumspect, with excellent or moderate results in 50% to 60% of patients.[19,20] Typically, pain of traumatic origin responds better than pain from other etiologies.

Occipital Nerve Neurectomy

Peripheral neurectomy is associated with a 70% success rate in appropriately selected patients, typically those with pain caused by trauma and pain limited to a single nerve distribution that is completely relieved by a local anesthetic block.[21]

Decompression

Outcomes of decompression depend on the procedure performed. However, a recent systematic review indicates a success rate of 68% to 100%, with a pooled analysis yielding an overall success rate of 86%, in achieving at least a 50% reduction in pain.[16]

Neurostimulation

A number of retrospective chart reviews and small, uncontrolled prospective case series support the use of neurostimulation, either occipital nerve stimulation or high cervical stimulation, for the treatment of occipital neuralgia. The reported efficacy varies from 50% to 100% improvement of pain in patients who proceed to permanent neurostimulator implantation after a successful trial, with a recent systematic review yielding an overall success rate of 68% for occipital nerve stimulation.[16,22–24] Similar success rates have been noted in patients undergoing permanent implantation for high cervical spinal cord stimulation.[15]

References

1. Anthony M. Headache and the greater occipital nerve. *Clin Neurol Neurosurg.* 1992;94:297–301.
2. Headache Classification Committee of the International Headache Society. The international classification of headache disorders, 3rd edition (beta version). *Cephalalgia.* 2013;33:629–808.
3. Ehni G, Benner B. Occipital neuralgia and C1-C2 arthrosis. *N Engl J Med.* 1984;310:127.
4. Post AF, Narayan P, Haid RW Jr. Occipital neuralgia secondary to hypermobile posterior arch of atlas. Case report. *J Neurosurg.* 2001;94:276–278.
5. Cornely C, Fischer M, Ingianni G, Isenmann S. Greater occipital nerve neuralgia caused by pathological arterial contact: treatment by surgical decompression. *Headache.* 2011;51:609–612.
6. Gille O, Lavignolle B, Vital JM. Surgical treatment of greater occipital neuralgia by neurolysis of the greater occipital nerve and sectioning of the inferior oblique muscle. *Spine (Phila PA 1976).* 2004;29:828–832.
7. Kutlay M, Cemil B, Kaya S, Topuz K, Demircan MN. A rare case of occipital neuralgia secondary to ball bullet gunshot wound. *Cent Eur Neurosurg.* 2010;71:224–226.
8. Lucchesi C, Puglioli M, Gori S. Occipital neuralgia: a symptomatic case caused by an abnormal left vertebral artery. *Neurol Sci.* 2013;34:243–245.
9. White JB, Atkinson PP, Cloft HJ, Atkinson JL. Vascular compression as a potential cause of occipital neuralgia: a case report. *Cephalalgia.* 2008;28:78–82.
10. Oh MY, Ortega J, Bellotte JB, Whiting DM, Alo K. Peripheral nerve stimulation for the treatment of occipital neuralgia and transformed migraine using a C1-2-3 subcutaneous paddle style electrode: a technical report. *Neuromodulation.* 2004;7:103–112.
11. Huang JH, Galvagno SM Jr, Hameed M, et al. Occipital nerve pulsed radiofrequency treatment: a multi-center study evaluating predictors of outcome. *Pain Med.* 2012;13:489–497.
12. Finiels PJ, Batifol D. The treatment of occipital neuralgia: review of 111 cases. *Neurochirurgie.* 2016;62:233–240.

13. Johnson MD, Burchiel KJ. Peripheral stimulation for treatment of trigeminal postherpetic neuralgia and trigeminal posttraumatic neuropathic pain: a pilot study. *Neurosurgery.* 2004;55:135–141; discussion 141–142.
14. Slavin KV, Nersesyan H, Wess C. Peripheral neurostimulation for treatment of intractable occipital neuralgia. *Neurosurgery.* 2006;58:112–119; discussion 112–119.
15. Chivukula S, Tempel ZJ, Weiner GM, et al. Cervical and cervicomedullary spinal cord stimulation for chronic pain: efficacy and outcomes. *Clin Neurol Neurosurg.* 2014;127:33–41.
16. Ducic I, Felder JM III, Fantus SA. A systematic review of peripheral nerve interventional treatments for chronic headaches. *Ann Plast Surg.* 2014;72:439–445.
17. Cohen SP, Peterlin BL, Fulton L, et al. Randomized, double-blind, comparative-effectiveness study comparing pulsed radiofrequency to steroid injections for occipital neuralgia or migraine with occipital nerve tenderness. *Pain.* 2015;156:2585–2594.
18. Gande AV, Chivukula S, Moossy JJ, et al. Long-term outcomes of intradural cervical dorsal root rhizotomy for refractory occipital neuralgia. *J Neurosurg.* 2016;125:102–110.
19. Lozano AM, Vanderlinden G, Bachoo R, Rothbart P. Microsurgical C-2 ganglionectomy for chronic intractable occipital pain. *J Neurosurg.* 1998;89:359–365.
20. Wang MY, Levi AD. Ganglionectomy of C-2 for the treatment of medically refractory occipital neuralgia. *Neurosurg Focus.* 2002;12:E14.
21. Sharma RV, Pawar SJ, Lad SD, Mahapatra AK. Current status of peripheral neurectomy for occipital neuralgia. *Neurosurg Q.* 2005;15:232–238.
22. Rasskazoff SY, Slavin KV. Neuromodulation for cephalalgias. *Surg Neurol Int.* 2013;4:S136–150.
23. Sweet JA, Mitchell LS, Narouze S, et al. Occipital nerve stimulation for the treatment of patients with medically refractory occipital neuralgia: Congress of Neurological Surgeons systematic review and evidence-based guideline. *Neurosurgery.* 2015;77:332–341.
24. Vanelderen P, Rouwette T, De Vooght P, et al. Pulsed radiofrequency for the treatment of occipital neuralgia: a prospective study with 6 months of follow-up. *Reg Anesth Pain Med.* 2010;35:148–151.

Neuropathic Groin Pain

Stacy N. Wong and Line G. Jacques

17

Case Presentation

A 57-year-old man presents with chronic, refractory left groin and left-sided testicular pain. He underwent laparoscopic bilateral inguinal hernia repair with mesh 10 months earlier and 6 months earlier he had exploratory reoperation for scar tissue debridement. At the time of reoperation, the mesh was not found to be in contact with the nerve. The patient complains of persistent "squeezing" pain from the left of his umbilicus to his left testicle. He reports severe stabbing and electrical pain in his left testicle when the cremaster muscle is engaged for scrotal temperature regulation. There is left inguinal numbness at the site of his hernia repair incision. He denies urinary and bowel incontinence. He reports normal sensation in his penis and scrotum. His pain management specialist ordered an ultrasound, which was negative for recurrent hernia and infection. The patient is currently taking duloxetine, oxycodone, and pregabalin, with minimal relief of pain. He previously tried gabapentin but ultimately discontinued its use because of its adverse effects.

On exam, the patient is well developed and moderately overweight (BMI 34). His abdomen is soft, without distension or palpable masses. There is no tenderness to palpation. He does not display rebound tenderness or guarding. All deep tendon reflexes are 2+ bilaterally. There is no Tinel sign at the site of the incision. The remainder of the neurologic examination is normal.

Questions

1. What is the likely diagnosis?
2. What is the most appropriate imaging modality?
3. What are the most appropriate anatomic areas to image, and why?
4. What is the appropriate timing for the diagnostic workup?

Assessment and Planning

The patient is referred to a neurosurgeon for postherniorrhaphy chronic groin pain. Chronic groin pain occurs in up to 50% of patients undergoing inguinal hernia repair.[1] Postherniorrhaphy groin pain lasting more than 8 weeks is typically found to be neuropathic. Other diagnoses that should be considered and ruled out include mesh infection/displacement, recurrent hernia, and osteitis pubis.[2] In this case, the pain pattern is most consistent with ilioinguinal neuropathy. The three most common nerves involved in postherniorrhaphy neuropathic groin pain are the ilioinguinal nerve, iliohypogastric nerve, and genital branches of the genitofemoral nerve.[3,4] Injury to these nerves typically occurs secondary to crush, cautery, stretch, or irritation by sutures or staples.[2] The classic diagnostic triad includes pain originating near the scar and radiating to the groin, sensory symptoms in the distribution of the involved nerve, and pain relieved by the injection of local anesthetic around the involved nerve.[5,6] However, while a positive response to injection of local anesthetic is considered a positive diagnostic sign, the lack of a response does not rule out the condition.[2]

Non-neuropathic causes of the patient's pain should be excluded first. This is typically accomplished with imaging, either ultrasound or MR imaging, but this evaluation should be deferred to the general surgeon. Once non-neuropathic causes have been excluded, neuropathic groin pain is best evaluated with a thorough physical examination supplemented with imaging. Specifically, MR neurography of the pelvis can be helpful in identifying neuromas and focal injuries within the lumbosacral plexus and groin nerves. In the present case, the patient underwent abdominal ultrasound and CT, which were both negative for recurrent hernia and infection. Absence of a Tinel sign at the site of the incision suggests that the nerve is neither injured by the mesh nor is there a neuroma at the surgical site.

Oral Boards Review—Diagnostic Pearls

1. Risk factors for persistent pain after herniorrhaphy include:[7]
   - Younger age (patients less than 40 years old are more likely to report chronic pain than patients over 60)
   - Higher BMI
   - Pre-existing pain disorders
   - Work status
   - Postoperative complications
   - Female sex
   - Recurrent hernia repair
   - Psychological factors (low preoperative optimism, less sense of control)
2. The classic diagnostic triad for postherniorrhaphy neuropathic groin pain is:
   - Pain originating near the scar and radiating to the groin
   - Sensory symptoms in the distribution of the involved nerve (e.g., dysesthesia, hyperesthesia, or hypesthesia)
   - Pain relieved by the injection of local anesthetic around the involved nerve(s)

Questions

1. How do the clinical and radiologic findings influence surgical planning?
2. What is the most appropriate timing for intervention in this patient?
3. How should surgery be approached in a patient with refractory neuropathic groin pain?

Decision-Making

There are multiple algorithms for the management of patients with chronic groin pain; however, the philosophy of treatment aligns with the World Health Organization's pain ladder, and the clinicians' treatment progression should begin with the least invasive interventions. Initial management is typically medical, with tricyclic antidepressants, neuropathic pain medications, such as gabapentin or pregabalin, or narcotic pain medications. Behavioral therapy can also be helpful. Local injection of steroids should be tried before considering surgical therapy. With refractory pain, radiofrequency ablation, surgical neurectomy, or neuromodulation/neurostimulation should be considered.[4,6,8–10]

Given the failure of conservative pain management in the present patient, it is reasonable to explore surgical options, either neuromodulation or neurectomy. Neuromodulation or neurostimulation is available in different modalities, including conventional neurostimulation and, more recently, dorsal root ganglion (DRG) stimulation. Conventional spinal cord stimulation (SCS) for groin pain involves placing implantable lead(s) at or around the T11-T12 spinal level (lateral to the midline, coinciding with the side of the patient's pain) in order to cover the nerves of the groin. Conventional stimulation at this level may cause unwanted paresthesias or discomfort in the leg and buttocks due to the size and shape of the electrical field. Stimulation sensation may also be influenced by CSF thickness and lead migration. In contrast, DRG stimulation in the setting of groin pain offers several advantages by providing focused pain management, due to the unique lead design, unconventional stimulation parameters, and locations for the lead placement. Since the lead is placed along the DRG in the neural foramen, there is limited space for the lead to migrate and CSF thickness does not influence undesirable paresthesias.[11] In the setting of groin pain, the DRG lead is positioned at L1 or L2 in order to target only the nerves of the groin, thereby providing pain relief without additional unwanted paresthesias in the leg or buttock. For the patient presented, DRG stimulation is an appropriate choice given that the goal is to target and specify the nerve root that innervates the ilioinguinal nerve.

An alternative surgical approach is triple neurectomy (of the ilioinguinal, iliohypogastric, and genitofemoral nerves). Traditionally, this procedure has been performed as a two-stage operation; the first stage through the inguinal region for ilioinguinal and iliohypogastric neurectomy and the second stage through a flank incision for genitofemoral neurectomy.[8] More recently, a laparoscopic approach for triple neurectomy has been described.[4]

Surgical Procedure

Laparoscopic Triple Neurectomy

Understanding the anatomy of the ilioinguinal, iliohypogastric, and genitofemoral nerves in the retroperitoneal space is important for surgical success. The two key surgical landmarks in laparoscopic triple neurectomy are the psoas muscle and the point of penetration of the genitofemoral nerve into the psoas muscle. The iliohypogastric and ilioinguinal nerves emerge from between the psoas muscle and the quadratus lumborum, running lateral to the course of the genitofemoral nerve. The nerves can be distinguished by identifying the point at which the iliohypogastric nerve penetrates the transversalis muscle.

The procedure is performed under general endotracheal anesthesia with the patient positioned in the lateral decubitus position and the affected side up. The table is flexed maximally. The neurectomy is performed in conjunction with an experienced laparoscopist. An incision is made caudal to the tip of the 12th rib in order to gain access to the retroperitoneal space. Once entrance into the retroperitoneal space is digitally confirmed, a port and retroperitoneoscope are introduced. Three additional ports are then placed under direct visualization; the first in the anterior axillary line above the iliac crest, the second in the anterior axillary line just anterior to the 11th rib, and the third anterior to the second port in the midclavicular line. A 30° retroperitoneoscope is typically utilized.

The genitofemoral nerve is first identified by sweeping the fascia off the surface of the psoas muscle to expose the nerve as it runs along the surface of the muscle. After the branch point, the genital branch will run medial to the femoral branch. Both branches should be identified. Once they are all identified, either the common trunk or both branches individually are divided, with resection of a portion of the nerve that can be examined ex vivo to confirm the presence of nerve fascicles. Next, the ilioinguinal and iliohypogastric nerves are identified at the point of exit between the psoas and the quadratus lumborum. These nerves may emerge as a common trunk or as separate branches. When they are separate branches, the iliohypogastric nerve runs lateral and cephalad to the ilioinguinal nerve. Both branches must be identified to ensure surgical success. Once both are identified, transection is undertaken at the level of the common trunk or both branches can be transected individually. Again, a section of each nerve is removed for examination. The insufflation pressure is then reduced and each incision is closed.[4]

DRG Stimulation

The surgical treatment of groin pain via traditional epidural spinal cord stimulation is very difficult to achieve.[12] DRG stimulation is a reversible, nonablative option.[11,13] The patient is screened for suitability for neuromodulation with a thorough clinical evaluation, quality of life questionnaires, VAS pain scores, and pain mapping. A psychological evaluation is performed prior to surgery to exclude any contraindications to the therapy.

In the operating room, under monitored anesthetic care with heavy sedation, the patient is placed in the prone position with abdominal support to limit the amount of lordosis. A DRG lead is placed in the epidural space at the foraminal level and intraoperative stimulation is performed in order to verify the accurate placement of the lead (Figure 17.1). Fluoroscopy is used to ensure the correct position of the lead. After a positive trial, the pulse generator will be implanted according to the body habitus. DRG stimulation is performed as an outpatient procedure.

Aftercare

After recovery in the postanesthesia care unit, the clinical specialist for the DRG device will activate the stimulator, verify appropriate pain coverage, and discuss the use of the pulse generator and its components with the patient. The patient will typically

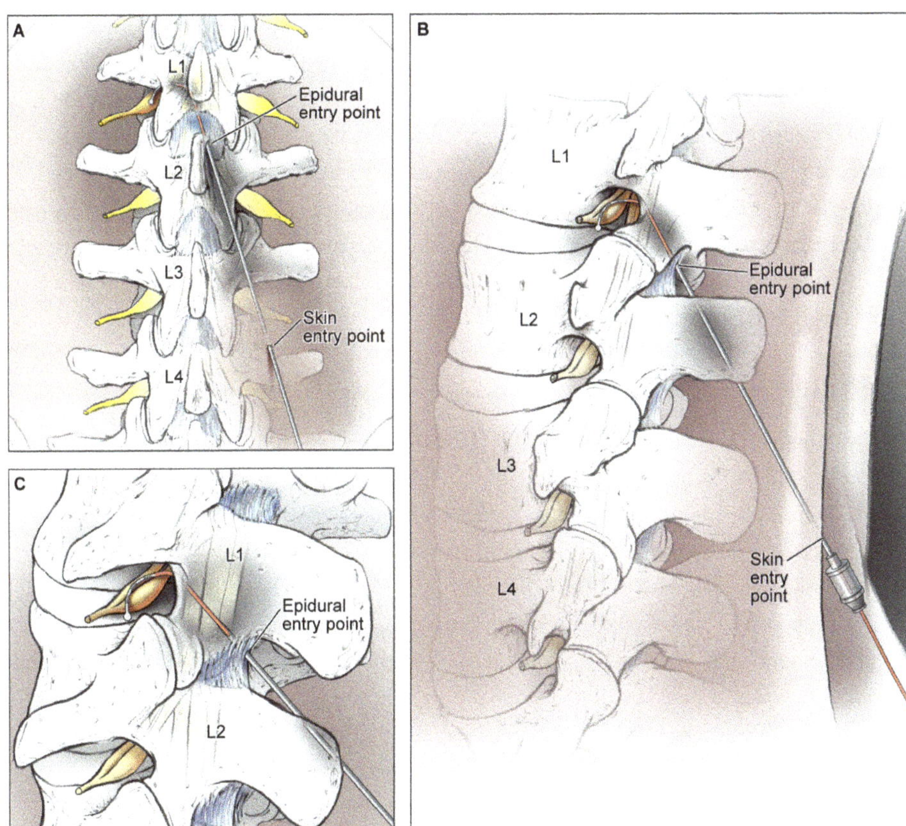

Figure 17.1. A, Access for percutaneous insertion of the dorsal root ganglion (DRG) lead is achieved through a contralateral, paramedian approach. The skin puncture is typically two spinal levels below the intended epidural entry point, in this case at the midline of L1-L2. B, The lead's contact points are placed on the superior dorsal aspect of the DRG. C, Magnified view of the neural foramen showing the optimal lead position in the superior dorsal aspect of the foramen. Lead position is confirmed with fluoroscopy.

return in 2 to 3 weeks for follow-up evaluation of progress with the neurosurgeon and the device specialist. The patient is urged to maintain a pain diary to record progress and effectiveness of the device. Patients should also be encouraged to obtain a medical alert bracelet in order to notify other health care providers of the presence of the implantable device and of precautions that may need to be taken prior to additional future treatment(s). Management of device programming is provided by the clinical device specialist of the DRG manufacturer, although ideally hospitals and clinics providing DRG stimulation will have their clinicians trained to deal with patient programming issues in order to provide optimal care for patients.

Complications and Management

As with any surgical procedure involving an implantable device, a number of complications can occur, including bleeding, infection, allergy to the device, rejection of the device, nerve root injury, cerebrospinal fluid leak, and pain at the surgical site.

DRG stimulation is a relatively new procedure; therefore, data on complications and management need to be gathered through future prospective studies. In general, the complications associated with any implanted neurostimulation device include migration of the stimulator lead(s), cerebrospinal fluid leak, undesirable stimulation of an unaffected body region due to the development of scar tissue or postural changes, loss of effectiveness over time, pulse generator failure, and skin breakdown over the pulse generator or lead wires. Currently, the DRG stimulation hardware is not compatible with MR imaging; therefore, DRG therapy is contraindicated for patients who require serial MR imaging.

References

1. Cunningham J, Temple WJ, Mitchell P, Nixon JA, Preshaw RM, Hagen NA. Cooperative hernia study. Pain in the postrepair patient. *Ann Surg*. 1996;224:598–602.
2. Hakeem A, Shanmugam V. Current trends in the diagnosis and management of post-herniorraphy chronic groin pain. *World J Gastrointest Surg*. 2011;3:73–81.
3. Reinpold W, Schroeder AD, Schroeder M, Berger C, Rohr M, Wehrenberg U. Retroperitoneal anatomy of the iliohypogastric, ilioinguinal, genitofemoral, and lateral femoral cutaneous nerve: consequences for prevention and treatment of chronic inguinodynia. *Hernia*. 2015;19:539–548.
4. Song JW, Wolf JS Jr, McGillicuddy JE, Bhangoo S, Yang LJ. Laparoscopic triple neurectomy for intractable groin pain: technical report of 3 cases. *Neurosurgery*. 2011;68:339–346; discussion 346.
5. Starling JR, Harms BA. Diagnosis and treatment of genitofemoral and ilioinguinal neuralgia. *World J Surg*. 1989;13:586–591.
6. Starling JR, Harms BA, Schroeder ME, Eichman PL. Diagnosis and treatment of genitofemoral and ilioinguinal entrapment neuralgia. *Surgery*. 1987;102:581–586.
7. Liem L, Mekhail N. Management of postherniorrhaphy chronic neuropathic groin pain: a role for dorsal root ganglion stimulation. *Pain Pract*. 2016;16:915–923.
8. Amid PK. Causes, prevention, and surgical treatment of postherniorrhaphy neuropathic inguinodynia: triple neurectomy with proximal end implantation. *Hernia*. 2004;8:343–349.
9. Mitra R, Zeighami A, Mackey S. Pulsed radiofrequency for the treatment of chronic ilioinguinal neuropathy. *Hernia*. 2007;11:369–371.
10. Stulz P, Pfeiffer KM. Peripheral nerve injuries resulting from common surgical procedures in the lower portion of the abdomen. *Arch Surg*. 1982;117:324–327.
11. Schu S, Gulve A, El Dabe S, et al. Spinal cord stimulation of the dorsal root ganglion for groin pain—a retrospective review. *Pain Pract*. 2015;15:293–299.
12. Barolat G, Massaro F, He J, Zeme S, Ketcik B. Mapping of sensory responses to epidural stimulation of the intraspinal neural structures in man. *J Neurosurg*. 1993;78:233–239.
13. Zuidema X, Breel J, Wille F. Paresthesia mapping: a practical workup for successful implantation of the dorsal root ganglion stimulator in refractory groin pain. *Neuromodulation*. 2014;17:665–669; discussion 669.

Section 3

Peripheral Nerve Tumors

Nerve Sheath Tumors—Schwannomas and Neurofibromas

Christian Heinen and Thomas Kretschmer

18

Case Presentation

A 45-year-old man presented with a growing mass in the left medial thigh. He noticed painful tingling sensations on contact only but no permanent sensory deficit or weakness. The paresthesias originated from the mass and radiated down the medial lower leg to the medial malleolus. There was no history of other masses in the patient or his family. He noted slow growth of the mass over 2 to 3 years. At first, a lipoma was suspected. He was then referred to our peripheral nerve clinic. On physical examination, the patient exhibited no neurologic deficits and no skin abnormalities. Percussion or manipulation of the mobile, walnut-sized mass yielded a positive Tinel sign, with paresthesias in the medial thigh and lower leg. MR imaging revealed a clearly delimited, fusiform mass arising from the saphenous nerve, with homogeneous contrast enhancement and peripheral T2 hyperintensity combined with central T2 hypointensity.

Questions

1. What are the likely diagnoses?
2. Which imaging modality is best suited for further investigation?
3. Is time of the essence, and why?

Assessment and Planning

A peripheral nerve sheath tumor (PNST) is suspected due to the clinical presentation in conjunction with imaging of a fusiform mass in the course of a peripheral nerve. The differential diagnosis includes schwannoma and neurofibroma, which are the most frequently encountered types of PNST. PNSTs account for approximately 10% of all soft tissue tumors.[1] Sporadic PNST has to be differentiated from PNST associated with a genetic disorder, as in neurofibromatosis (NF) 1 or 2 or schwannomatosis. While the incidence is 2 in 100,000 for sporadic PNST, in NF1 and NF2 or schwannomatosis, the incidence of PNST reaches 100%.[2] In addition, malignancy occurs in sporadic PNST with an incidence of 0.001%. With a 10% lifetime risk of malignant transformation of PNST, patients with NF1 bear a much higher risk.[3] Therefore, the clinical history, family history, and a thorough physical examination, including whole-body skin inspection, are crucial.

Both schwannomas and neurofibromas grow within the epineurium. However, these entities are distinct with respect to their relation to the fascicular topography of the nerve. Schwannomas usually arise from one fascicle, which loses function over time. In contrast, neurofibromas typically involve more than one fascicle. While difficult to distinguish on imaging, these tumors display different features on histopathology.

The typical presentation of a benign PNST is a slowly growing mass causing pain or paresthesias on contact. Spontaneous pain is the exception and should raise concern about malignancy. A neurologic deficit as a first symptom is rare (2%–5%); if it is present in conjunction with tumor size > 5 cm or rapid growth, malignant transformation should be suspected.[4] On examination, benign PNSTs are typically mobile. A fixed mass indicates a more aggressive growth pattern. A positive Tinel sign over the mass is common.

The gold standard for imaging evaluation is contrast-enhanced MR imaging. On T1-weighted MR imaging, benign PNSTs typically have distinct borders and are isointense to slightly hypointense to skeletal muscle, but they demonstrate avid, homogeneous contrast uptake (Figure 18.1). On T2-weighted images, the lesion is typically hyperintense. Several radiologic signs can be present (but are not universally present), including the target sign and split fat sign. The target sign is the appearance of the lesion with a rim of T2 hyperintensity surrounding central T2 hypointensity. The split fat sign is best appreciated on T1-weighted images, where a thin rim of fat is present around the lesion. Basically, any lump being considered for surgery warrants evaluation with MR imaging.

Recently, high-resolution ultrasound has gained importance in peripheral nerve visualization (Figure 18.2).[5] A high-frequency probe can differentiate the intact nerve portion and even uninvolved fascicles from tumor and tumor-bearing fascicles, which can be useful for surgical planning, especially for large PNSTs. However, no modality is able to reliably differentiate schwannoma from neurofibroma or benign PNST from malignant PNST.

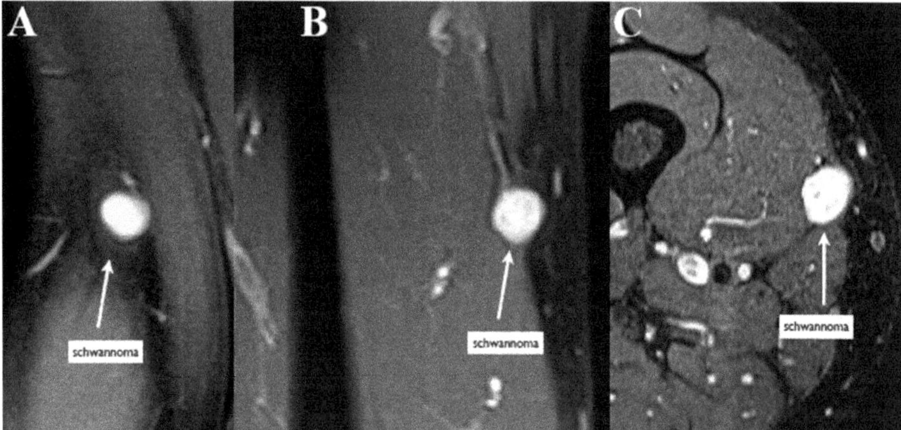

Figure 18.1. Sagittal (A), coronal (B), and axial (C) T1-weighted, post-gadolinium MR images showing a well-circumscribed mass with avid contrast enhancement consistent with a benign nerve sheath tumor.

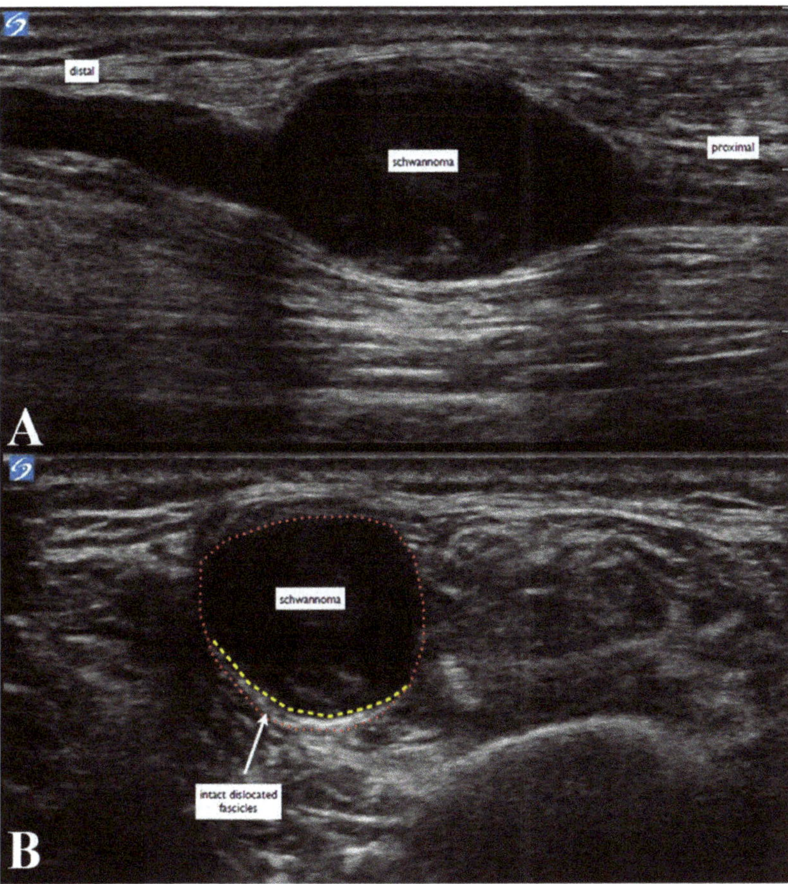

Figure 18.2. Longitudinal (A) and transverse (B) high-resolution ultrasound images showing a well-circumscribed tumor displacing intact normal fascicles, consistent with a benign nerve sheath tumor.

Oral Boards Review—Diagnostic Pearls

1. Clinical history, family history, and a thorough physical examination, including whole-body skin inspection, are crucial.
2. NF1, NF2, and schwannomatosis have to be ruled out.
3. The main clinical feature of a PNST is a palpable mass (or mass visualized on imaging) within the course of a nerve.
4. If a PNST is suspected, MR imaging is mandatory, and high-resolution ultrasound can help in surgical planning.
5. Spontaneous pain, rapid growth, size > 5 cm, and a fixed mass should raise concern about malignancy.

Questions

1. What are the typical imaging findings with a benign PNST?
2. What are the indications for surgical resection of a benign PNST?
3. What is the goal of surgery?

Decision-Making

Indications for surgical resection include symptomatic lesions (typically pain), tissue diagnosis, definitive treatment of the tumor to decrease or eliminate the need for follow-up, and resection while the tumor is small in an area where resection of a larger tumor could present difficulties and additional risk. Function-sparing, microsurgical enucleation of both schwannomas and neurofibromas represents the appropriate treatment when surgery is undertaken. Decision-making about patients with NF and schwannomatosis is multifactorial, given the lack of possible surgical cure. For small, solitary PNSTs that are asymptomatic and that do not have features concerning for malignancy, observation with serial imaging and clinical examinations is reasonable.

When surgery is undertaken, regardless of whether the pathology is schwannoma or neurofibroma, treatment should be function-sparing, microsurgical enucleation of the tumor. When an intraoperative microscope, electrical stimulation, and careful dissection are used, complication rates can be kept below 5% and recurrence is rare.[1,6] Given the low complication rate, surgery should strongly be considered if patients report pain or sensorimotor impairment secondary to the PNST, and even when the lesion is cosmetically unappealing. When there is concern about malignancy, the authors prefer open microsurgical biopsy, but this is controversial, and other surgeons use percutaneous needle biopsy. Fascicle-sparing dissection and tumor removal require expertise. Potential complications, such as motor weakness, sensory impairment, and new-onset pain, need to be thoroughly discussed with the patient prior to surgery. In general, removal can be accomplished with no or minimal morbidity in experienced hands. Neurofibromas are said to be slightly more difficult to remove, as more fascicles are involved.

Pain at rest and quickly growing masses with rapid neurologic deterioration or deficits may suggest malignant transformation and should alert the physician. In such cases, assessment, overall strategy, and the surgical approach are different. Time is of the essence. A percutaneous biopsy or an open incisional biopsy under monitoring, as the authors prefer, can be undertaken, followed by staged radical removal of the affected nerve and the surrounding tissue if malignancy is confirmed histopathologically. In these cases, function cannot be spared. Again, extensive preoperative counseling of the patient, including all possible scenarios, is mandatory.

Surgical Procedure

For benign PNSTs, the operation is carried out under relaxant-free, total intravenous anesthesia, enabling intraoperative electrophysiologic monitoring. Positioning of the patient should allow for easy access to, and exposure of, the whole tumor, including the normal nerve both proximal and distal to the tumor-bearing segment. Initial dissection should uncover the entire tumor. Proximal and distal control of the nerve should be achieved by identifying and looping the normal nerve proximal and distal to the tumor. After the surgeon has obtained proximal and distal control, the epineurium is stimulated under microscope or loupe magnification to identify a nonresponding, fascicle-free area that can be used as a safe corridor into the tumor. In selected cases, intraoperative ultrasound can help to visualize internal topography prior to epineuriotomy. The incision is lengthened into a longitudinal epineuriotomy to reveal the space between the interfascicular epineurium and the outer aspect of the tumor capsule. Transverse nerve incisions are contraindicated, as they jeopardize healthy fascicles. In cases where fascicle identification at the tumor equator is difficult (e.g., with large schwannomas), starting dissection at the poles in the transitional area from nerve to tumor helps to identify the tumor-bearing fascicle as well as the course of normal fascicles. The altered tumor-bearing fascicle is followed, and thus a more easily identifiable layer for further dissection is created. Differentiating the interfascicular epineurium from the true capsule can be difficult. This is an important distinction, however. Dissecting between the interfascicular epineurium and true capsule will allow the normal fascicles to be dissected away from the tumor. If dissection is done within or outside of the interfascicular epineurium, the normal fascicles will not fall away from the tumor and may be harmed.

Continuing to dissect the normal fascicles away from the tumor circumferentially allows isolation of the tumor and its input and output fascicles that are intrinsic to the tumor. For schwannomas, a single fascicle is typically identified as the input and output fascicle. For neurofibromas, there are often multiple input and output fascicles. In cases of neurofibromas, it is important to spend time performing an interfascicular dissection at the poles to be sure fascicles that are extrinsic to the tumor are properly identified and are not improperly thought to be intrinsic to the tumor. Rarely, functioning fascicles can run into and through the tumor, a situation that can be quite difficult to recognize (and that is more frequent in neurofibromas). Frequently, dissection and enucleation of the tumor can be done bluntly using dissectors without harming the intact, displaced fascicles. Intermittent irrigation facilitates tissue visualisation and dissection. Typically, the tumor mass can be delivered intact as a single piece. Staying external to the tumor capsule and avoiding encroachment into the substance of the tumor prevents bleeding. Nevertheless, for large masses or plexiform tumors, piecemeal removal may be necessary. After complete dissection of the tumor and isolation of the input and output fascicles, the tumor-bearing fascicles are coagulated and cut within their healthy aspect under magnification. This is the decisive step to minimize the risk of recurrence. The use of electrocautery should be avoided and kept at an absolute minimum. When necessary, a low power setting should be used and the intact portion of the nerve should be protected with cotton patties. After the tumor is resected, the wound is copiously irrigated and is closed in layers. Usually, drains are unnecessary. For details of the surgical procedure, see Figure 18.3.

Oral Boards Review—Management Pearls

1. Microsurgical, function-sparing, complete enucleation of the tumor utilizing intraoperative stimulation is the goal of surgery.
2. Starting dissection at the poles of the tumor facilitates discerning tumor-affected nerve from healthy nerve portions in large tumors.
3. Schwannomas usually arise from one nonfunctioning fascicle.
4. Neurofibromas may involve more than one fascicle, which may still be functional.

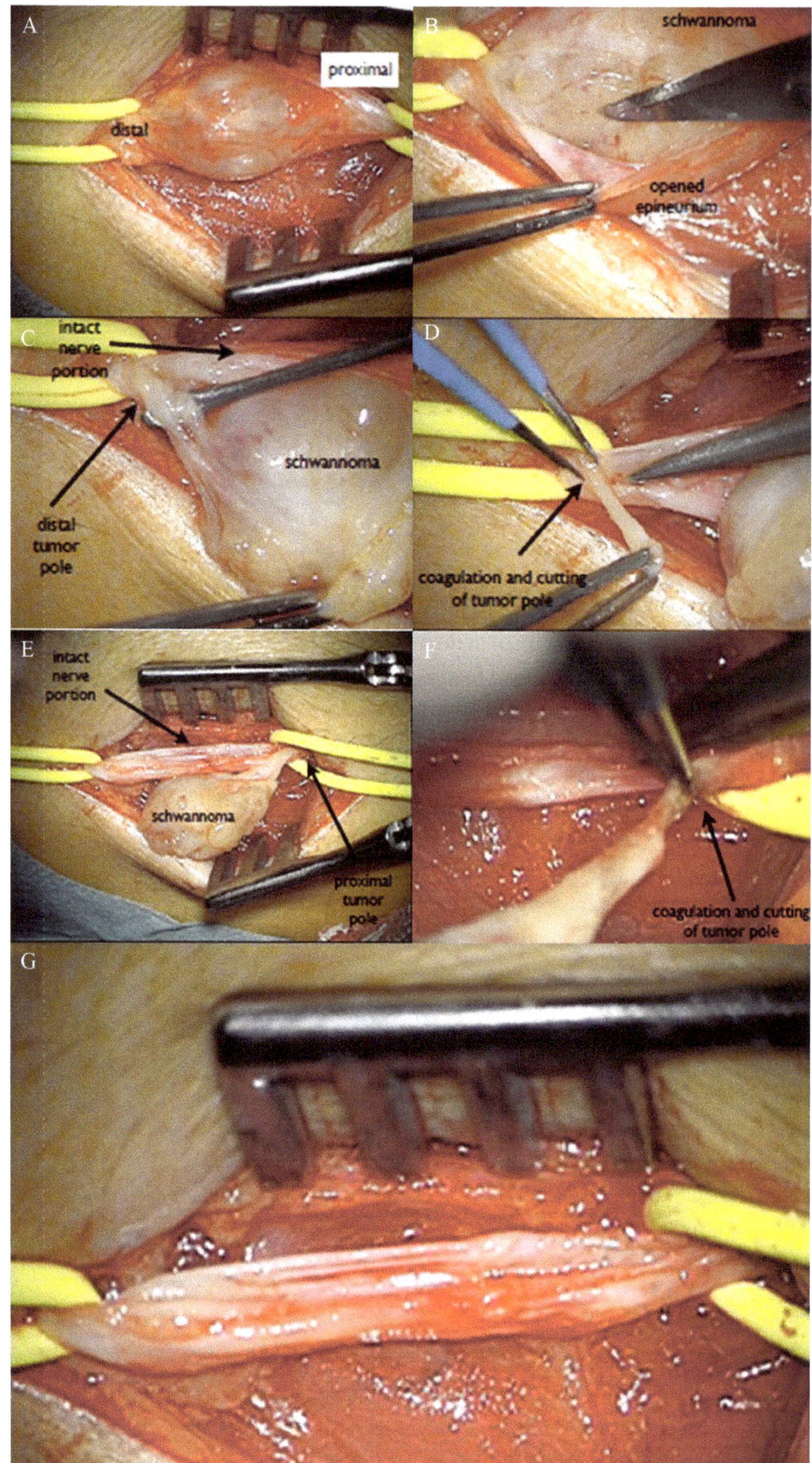

Figure 18.3. Intraoperative photographs showing the steps for resection of a schwannoma. A, The full length of the tumor is exposed, and proximal and distal control is gained by looping the normal nerve proximal and distal to the tumor. B, An epineuriotomy is made in a safe corridor and the tumor capsule is identified. C, Tumor-bearing fascicles are identified and are separated from normal fascicles at the pole of the tumor. D, Tumor-bearing fascicles are coagulated and cut. E, The tumor is dissected free from the normal fascicles as the surgeon works toward the opposite pole of the tumor. F, Tumor-bearing fascicles are isolated at the opposite pole of the tumor and then are coagulated and cut. G, The tumor is completely removed, leaving behind intact, normal nerve fascicles.

Pivot Points

1. Intraoperative signs of infiltration of the intact nerve portion or surrounding tissue may indicate a malignant nerve sheath tumor.
2. Detailed discussion of all possibilities with the patient beforehand is essential.

Aftercare

Patients should be mobilized immediately after surgery. Clinical and MR imaging follow-up is scheduled 3 and 12 months after surgery. In cases of neurofibromatosis or schwannomatosis, while there is no consensus regarding evaluation, consideration should be given to whole-body MR imaging or at least whole-spine and cranial scans. Neurofibromatosis can cause a variety of symptoms, such as learning problems, epilepsy, osteoporosis, scoliosis, brain tumors, etc. To offer adequate treatment beyond nerve tumor surgery, an interdisciplinary team is necessary.

Complications and Management

With proper strategy and microsurgical technique, complication rates can be kept low. After tumor enucleation, a layer of splayed epineurium and intact fascicles remains. This is not tumor capsule, and therefore it is not a potential origin of recurrence and should not be resected in order to avoid severe iatrogenic nerve damage. In case of intraoperative iatrogenic lesion of an intact fascicle, direct microsurgical repair should be done within the same session. Microsurgical nerve repair according to general principles using 10-0 sutures is recommended. Careful intraneural hemostasis is imperative. If possible, electrocautery should be limited and used with low power only. The intact nerve portion can be covered with cotton patties to protect it from the cautery. Frequently, using cotton patties combined with mild pressure suffices to stop the bleeding. Recurrence is rare, but if a nerve sheath tumor regrows or was inadequately removed, redo surgery is more demanding, as it is difficult to discern scar from tumor.[7] Dissecting within the scarred nerve without clearly defined layers leading the way bears a higher risk, increasing the risk of both loss of function and neuropathic pain. Once again, microscopic technique, flushing, intraoperative electrophysiologic monitoring, and high-frequency ultrasound may enhance patient safety. Often, blunt and therefore tissue-sparing dissection is not possible. Instead, careful preparation with micro-knives or micro-scissors has to be performed. Thus, patients have to be informed thoroughly prior to surgery about possible complications and the need for grafting and nerve harvesting. Referral of these patients to experienced nerve surgeons should be considered.

Oral Boards Review—Complication Pearls

1. Transected healthy fascicles should be microsurgically repaired within the same session.
2. Redo resection of nerve sheath tumors is more challenging and has a higher complication rate.

Evidence and Outcomes

In general, results are favorable with benign nerve sheath tumors, with both a low complication rate and high rate of symptomatic improvement. Most studies report a similar complication rate for resection of schwannomas and neurofibromas. Knight et al. reported a 2.5% complication rate in 198 tumors, with complications including postoperative hematoma, neurologic injury, and major vascular injury.[1] Tumor location seems to influence the complication rate, with higher rates in patients with brachial plexus involvement.[8] Preoperative symptoms usually disappear completely or improve significantly postoperatively.[9,10] Recurrence is rare. In a series of 69 schwannomas treated from 2012 to 2016, the authors observed no recurrence (data not published). Hung et al. and Oberle et al. also did not encounter any recurrence in two additional series.[11,12] As mentioned, redo surgery for recurrent tumor is challenging and is associated with higher complication rates. However, there are no reliable data on outcomes after surgery for recurrent nerve tumors.

References

1. Knight DM, Birch R, Pringle J. Benign solitary schwannomas: a review of 234 cases. *J Bone Joint Surg Br.* 2007;89:382–387.
2. Sandberg AA, Stone JF. *The Genetics and Molecular Biology of Neural Tumors*. Humana Press;2008.
3. Baehring JM, Betensky RA, Batchelor TT. Malignant peripheral nerve sheath tumor: the clinical spectrum and outcome of treatment. *Neurology.* 2003;61:696–698.
4. Donner TR, Voorhies RM, Kline DG. Neural sheath tumors of major nerves. *J Neurosurg.* 1994;81:362–373.
5. Tsai WC, Chiou HJ, Chou YH, Wang HK, Chiou SY, Chang CY. Differentiation between schwannomas and neurofibromas in the extremities and superficial body: the role of high-resolution and color Doppler ultrasonography. *J Ultrasound Med.* 2008;27:161–166; quiz 168–169.
6. Gachiani J, Kim D, Nelson A, Kline D. Surgical management of malignant peripheral nerve sheath tumors. *Neurosurg Focus.* 2007;22:E13.
7. Kretschmer T, Antoniadis G, Heinen C, et al. Nerve sheath tumor surgery: case-guided discussion of ambiguous findings, appropriateness of removal, repeated surgery, and nerve repairs. *Neurosurg Focus.* 2007;22:E19.
8. Kim DH, Murovic JA, Tiel RL, Kline DG. Operative outcomes of 546 Louisiana State University Health Sciences Center peripheral nerve tumors. *Neurosurg Clin N Am.* 2004;15:177–192.
9. Artico M, Cervoni L, Wierzbicki V, D'Andrea V, Nucci F. Benign neural sheath tumours of major nerves: characteristics in 119 surgical cases. *Acta Neurochir (Wien).* 1997;139:1108–1116.
10. Huang JH, Samadani U, Zager EL. Brachial plexus region tumors: a review of their history, classification, surgical management, and outcomes. *Neurosurgery Q.* 2003;13:151–161.

11. Hung YW, Tse WL, Cheng HS, Ho PC. Surgical excision for challenging upper limb nerve sheath tumours: a single centre retrospective review of treatment results. *Hong Kong Med J*. 2010;16:287–291.
12. Oberle J, Kahamba J, Richter HP. Peripheral nerve schwannomas—an analysis of 16 patients. *Acta Neurochir (Wien)*. 1997;139:949–953.

Dumbbell Nerve Sheath Tumors

Hussam Abou-Al-Shaar and Mark A. Mahan

19

Case Presentation

A 22-year-old, otherwise healthy woman presents with a 3-month history of progressive gait difficulty, right-sided neck pain, and progressive right upper and lower extremity weakness. She describes weakness involving the entire right side of her body, including her hand, forearm, arm, and leg. She describes pain extending from the lateral neck to the lateral shoulder and down to the lateral portion of the midbrachium. Manual motor examination demonstrates diffuse 4/5 strength in the right upper extremity and 5/5 in the right lower extremity with sustained clonus. The rest of her examination is unremarkable.

The patient does not report any urinary or bowel incontinence. Her past medical and surgical history are unremarkable. She denies history of neck trauma, weight loss, fevers, or generalized fatigue. Detailed assessments of her risks for neuropathies and myelopathies are negative, including vitamin deficiencies, cancer, chemotherapy or radiation exposure, chemical exposure, chronic infections (such as human immunodeficiency virus or hepatitis C), and metabolic diseases (such as diabetes mellitus). Family history is negative for known neurofibromatosis type 1 or 2 (NF1 or NF2), brain tumors, and unexplained early-onset hearing loss.

She reports that she has tried physical therapy, with some improvement in her right-side strength, but she continues to have neck pain.

MR imaging of her spine reveals a large cervical lesion consisting of a C4 nerve root mass extending into the intradural space and severely compressing the spinal cord (Figure 19.1).

Questions

1. What is the likely diagnosis?
2. What key information in the history is essential to obtain?
3. What is the most appropriate imaging modality?
4. What are the characteristic imaging features of these lesions?
5. What other tests can you request?

Assessment and Planning

On the basis of the patient's history, examination, and imaging findings, the neurosurgeon should suspect a nerve sheath tumor of the C4 nerve root with a "dumbbell"

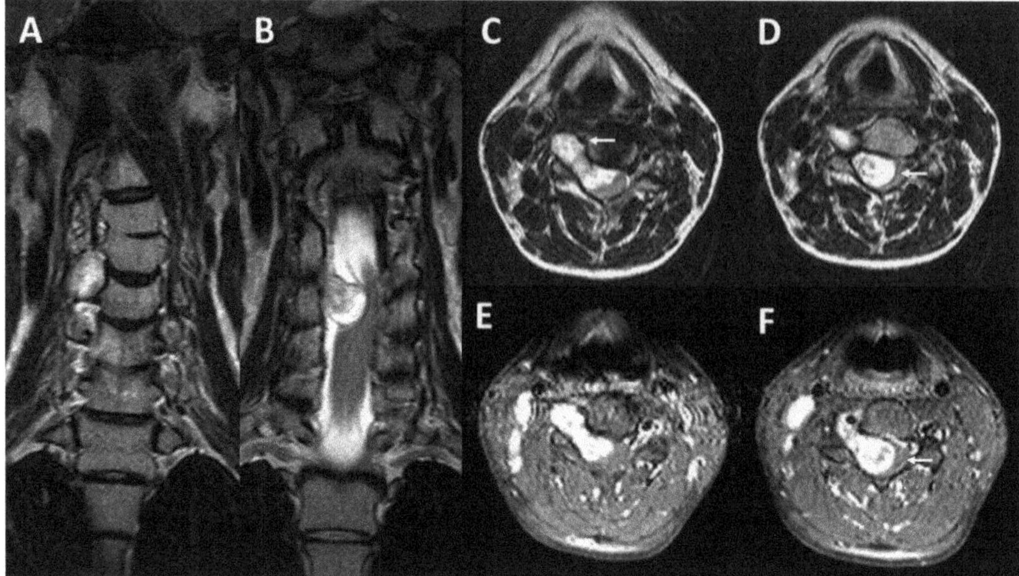

Figure 19.1. Preoperative MR imaging of a dumbbell schwannoma: coronal T2-weighted (A, B), axial T2-weighted (C, D), and axial T1-weighted fat-saturated post-gadolinium (E, F) images. Note the anterior displacement of the vertebral artery (arrow in C) and severe compression of the spinal cord (arrow in D and F).

shape. Approximately 10% of nerve sheath tumors arise from a spinal nerve in the neural foramen and develop a dumbbell-shaped mass. The differential diagnosis of dumbbell tumors is broad. Schwannoma is the most commonly encountered type of dumbbell-shaped tumor, followed by neurofibroma. The differential diagnosis should also take into consideration other neoplastic and nonneoplastic causes, including malignant peripheral nerve sheath tumor (PNST), solitary bone plasmacytoma, chordoma, superior sulcus tumor, spinal metastases, tuberculous spondylitis, vertebral hydatid disease, aneurysmal bone cyst, intraforaminal synovial cyst, traumatic pseudomeningocele, and extradural arachnoid cyst.[1]

Oral Boards Review—Diagnostic Pearls

1. History and examination are crucial—particularly family and infectious history.
2. MR imaging is the gold standard for delineating the lesion and guiding the surgical plan.
3. Schwannomas and neurofibromas account for the majority of dumbbell tumors and can be associated with underlying syndromes. These lesions demonstrate similar imaging features and are hard to differentiate on imaging alone.

4. Cervical dumbbell tumors call for assessment of vertebral artery involvement and the artery's relation to the tumor.
5. Malignant PNSTs are characterized by intense neuropathic pain, larger size, rapid growth, and evidence of necrosis on MR imaging. They are more frequent in patients with NF1 and show uncompensated denervation that is visible on MR imaging as T2 muscle edema or is demonstrable on electromyography (EMG). Malignant PNSTs are sarcomas and require more in-depth, multidisciplinary treatment planning.

Although neoplastic etiologies are the most commonly encountered for dumbbell-shaped lesions, the neurosurgeon should always be vigilant about nonneoplastic etiologies, especially when the history raises suspicion about such unusual lesions. This is of paramount importance because the management of a nonneoplastic lesion can be completely nonsurgical. Therefore, history is critical in the differential diagnosis of a dumbbell-shaped mass. It is crucial to ask patients about a family history of phakomatosis, especially NF1 and NF2, because phakomatoses are inherited in an autosomal dominant fashion and can increase the tendency for the development of nerve sheath tumors, although sporadic nerve sheath tumors are also common. Thus, in such patients, genetic testing may help establish the diagnosis. Moreover, especially in the case of a young woman of childbearing age, genetic counseling is important. Inquiring about a history of tuberculosis or recent contact with infected patients could lead the neurosurgeon toward such rare etiologies and aid in selection of the appropriate test (i.e., chest X-ray, acid-fast bacilli sputum culture for active infection, and Mantoux tuberculin skin test, as well as interferon-gamma release assay for latent infection).

MR imaging is the gold-standard modality for assessment and diagnosis of dumbbell tumors. It is sensitive and specific and will yield essential information about the size, site, cord status, and characteristics of the lesion. It is extremely important to correlate the physical examination with the imaging findings. Because nerve sheath schwannomas and neurofibromas are most commonly encountered in clinical practice, it is essential to know the relevant imaging findings, although nerve sheath schwannomas and neurofibromas usually present with similar imaging features and cannot be distinguished solely by imaging. Both lesions are seen as hypo/isointense lesions on T1-weighted images, with avid contrast enhancement on post-gadolinium images. On T2-weighted images, they are homogeneously hyperintense or show an area of central hypointensity (the target sign). A rim of fat surrounding the tumor may be evident (the split fat sign). Some key features can assist the neurosurgeon in differentiating between the two lesions, but not completely reliably. For example, if the lesion is eccentrically positioned in relation to the parent nerve, this is highly suggestive of a schwannoma, whereas a neurofibroma is typically centrally located. Schwannomas tend to have a more heterogeneous appearance, with degeneration and cystic cavitations, than neurofibromas.[2] If the lesion is located in the cervical segment, it is important to assess the vertebral artery's course, patency, and relation to the tumor for optimal operative planning. A CT scan of the spine can assist in understanding the osseous anatomy, because dumbbell tumors tend to grow slowly and exhibit adjacent bone remodeling. This may facilitate diagnosis as well as operative planning, if an instrumented fusion were to be necessary to facilitate tumor removal. Positron emission tomography (PET)-CT or apparent diffusion coefficient (ADC) mapping may be valuable when there is concern about a malignant PNST. PET scans may demonstrate increased uptake in both benign and malignant PNSTs, which may confuse the differentiation between benign and malignant. Most benign nerve sheath tumors demonstrate a standardized uptake value (SUV) of < 4.9 g/mL, while most malignant PNSTs have an SUV > 7.9 g/mL, while values between 4.9 and 7.9 constitute a gray area where the test is not definitive.[3,4]

Finally, electrodiagnostic studies may be a valuable addition, especially when there is increased concern about a malignant nerve sheath tumor. Electrodiagnostic studies provide evidence of acute and chronic changes within the dermatomes and myotomes of the spinal roots. Thus, whereas large but slowly growing tumors may demonstrate chronic remodeling of motor units, aggressive lesions tend to show uncompensated, acute evidence of denervation (e.g., fibrillations, sharp waves, insertional activity).

The hallmarks of a malignant nerve sheath tumor include pain at rest (particularly nocturnal pain), severe neuropathic pain (commonly described as burning or crushing), size greater than 5 cm, heterogeneous enhancement, history of NF1, and evidence of atrophy.[2] An image-guided biopsy should be performed, particularly when either ADC mapping or PET-CT suggests higher likelihood of malignancy. Management of malignant PNSTs is highly involved and is discussed elsewhere in this volume (Chapter 20).

Questions

1. What are the surgical approaches that could be utilized for this lesion?
2. What are the advantages and disadvantages of each?
3. How would you deal with a cervical dumbbell tumor encasing the vertebral artery?
4. What intraoperative tools will you request for the surgery?

Decision-Making

The first step in decision-making is studying and analyzing each individual patient's case to understand the size, site, and characteristics of the dumbbell tumor and its relation to the adjacent structures. Many classification systems for dumbbell tumors (e.g., Eden's classification, Asazuma's classification, Toyama's classification) have been developed for optimal tumor assessment and surgical planning.[5–7]

The approach for addressing a dumbbell tumor of the cervical region should be tailored to the individual patient's case. The standard anterior cervical approach, the anterolateral approach, the midline posterior approach, or a combination of approaches are most widely used for these lesions. In the posterior approach, it is important that the bony exposure is adequate for complete visualization of the tumor and may require multilevel laminectomies and facetectomies. In cases where the vertebral artery is encased by the tumor, the cephalad and caudal portions entering and leaving the tumor must be

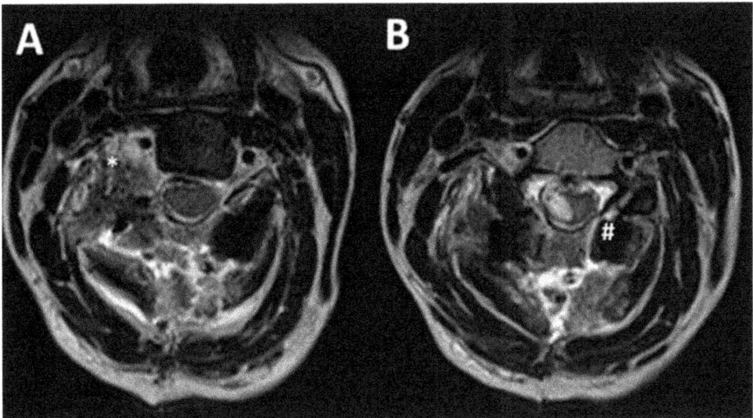

Figure 19.2. Postoperative axial T2-weighted MR imaging depicting complete resection of a dumbbell schwannoma. Note the restored anatomic position of the vertebral artery (indicated by asterisk in A) and partial expansion of the spinal cord (pound sign in B) after complete tumor removal.

exposed for control, and the vertebral artery should be freed by meticulous dissection. In addition, if the vertebral artery is iatrogenically injured during tumor dissection and resection, the artery may be ligated if there is adequate collateral circulation, or it may be directly repaired. If preoperative planning suggests that the vertebral artery may be at risk intraoperatively, a balloon test occlusion should be considered preoperatively to provide information on the safety of vertebral artery sacrifice in the case of an iatrogenic injury. Finally, if spinal stabilization is needed, instrumentation should be placed on the contralateral side prior to destabilization, so that intraoperative settling after osseous removal does not limit surgical resection or create iatrogenic deformity (Figure 19.2).

Approaches to the thoracic spine include the standard midline posterior approach, posterior subscapular approach, trans-sternal–transthoracic approach, mini-thoracotomy, thoracoscopic approach, costotransversectomy for a posterolateral approach, or a combination of anterior and posterior approaches. In such approaches, it is crucial to identify the artery of Adamkiewicz and its subcostal and/or lumbar branches for optimal surgical planning. Moreover, identification and securing of the great vessels is important early on during the procedure. Lumbar spinal dumbbell tumors can be accessed through retroperitoneal approaches with a paramedian or flank incision or via posterior/posterolateral approaches, depending on the extraforaminal extent (Figure 19.3).

Intraoperative neurophysiologic monitoring is an important adjunct. It is the authors' practice to utilize EMG monitoring along with somatosensory and motor evoked potentials in all cases.

Radiosurgery may be considered in cases of salvage or recurrent dumbbell tumors, but there is a paucity of literature that formally reviews results. While the results are not specific to dumbbell tumors, radiosurgery for intradural, extramedullary benign nerve sheath tumors has been shown to provide a high rate of local control. Radiosurgery has been demonstrated to relieve pain but is typically not associated with improvement in other neurologic symptoms. The reported rate of radiation-induced myelopathy ranges from 1% to 4% after treatment of these lesions.[8–12]

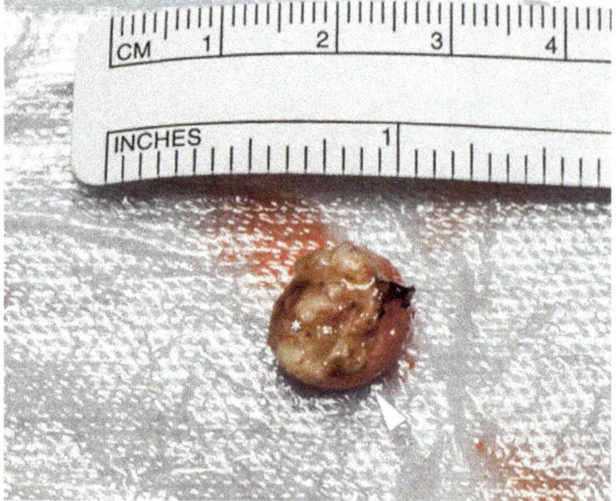

Figure 19.3. Pathologic specimen of the extraforaminal portion of the tumor, resected away from the nerve sheath. Note the typical bland tan-white texture of the interior of the tumor (asterisk) and the smooth border of the capsule (arrowhead). The cauterized portion is the distal end of the fascicle from which the tumor arose.

Questions

1. What are the complications associated with dumbbell tumor resection?
2. What could you do to decrease the rate of intraoperative nerve injury?

Surgical Procedure

The procedure is carried out under general anesthesia with appropriate hemodynamic monitoring, including intra-arterial pressure monitoring if the vertebral artery is to be in the surgical field. Triggered and free-running EMG monitoring along with somatosensory and motor evoked potentials are established prior to patient positioning, especially if there is critical narrowing around the spinal cord. A 10-mg dose of dexamethasone is used to control airway swelling and neural inflammation. In the case presented, the patient was placed in a Mayfield head holder and then was positioned prone on gel rolls. The patient should be gently padded in position. Once the patient is stably placed on the operating table, somatosensory and motor evoked potentials should be recorded again to document any changes from the baseline. The authors utilize long-acting local anesthetics to minimize postoperative narcotic requirements.

For our patient, the lateral portions of the facet joints were exposed bilaterally, with a wider exposure on the side of the tumor, including exposure of the insertions of the posterior and middle scalene muscles. Because we had determined that resection of the entire lateral mass posterior to the tumor was necessary, hardware was placed contralaterally and trajectories for placement of cervical lateral mass screws were drilled on the ipsilateral side. Full laminectomies were performed to allow complete decompression of the spinal cord. The caudal aspect of the C3 lateral mass, the complete C4 lateral mass, and the rostral aspect of the C5 lateral mass were drilled out for an osteotomy of the spine to allow complete mobilization and resection of the C4 nerve sheath tumor. Once clear visualization of the nerve sleeve is achieved, the venous plexus around the nerve sheath can be coagulated using the bipolar cautery. Thus, the entire tumor is visualized prior to the beginning of resection, and no further drilling is necessary after the thecal sac is opened.

The tumor adjacent to the spinal cord is removed first, so that manipulation does not translate to the compressed spinal cord. In the case presented, the C4 and C5 rootlets were mobilized around the tumor to allow gentle retraction, and the dentate ligaments were sectioned rostrally and caudally to allow rotation of the spinal cord, as the tumor arose from a C4 ventral rootlet. Dumbbell tumors are exophytic and can often be gently tugged from underneath the spinal cord (after sectioning of arachnoid membranes) and then divided, which allows for immediate decompression of the spinal cord. Ultrasonic aspiration can also be used to remove tumor adjacent to or underneath the cord.

Attention is then turned laterally to the nerve sleeve to debulk/resect the tumor. Once the tumor capsule is identified, the tumor can be removed by intracapsular dissection to avoid contact with the vertebral artery. The venous plexus is circumferential around the spinal nerve, so it is often easier to manage the venous plexus early with definitive coagulation and division, rather than repeatedly interrupting the procedure for hemostasis. When the dumbbell tumor is a schwannoma, the remainder of the spinal nerve is in a separate sleeve. When it is a neurofibroma, the tumor is adjacent to the fascicles, and careful inspection and stimulation are useful for achieving safe removal of the tumor.

Watertight dural closure should be achieved. A Valsalva maneuver can be used to check for any evidence of cerebrospinal fluid leak. For spinal stabilization following complete facetectomy, after dural closure, screws are placed in an acceptable trajectory on the ipsilateral side. Bone grafting material may be used to augment fusion, if it is performed.

Oral Boards Review—Management Pearls

1. A plan for managing the vertebral artery through direct exposure, preoperative embolization, or other techniques should be established prior to surgical resection.
2. Intracapsular dissection of the tumor is important to avoid injury to the viable and functioning nerve fibers.
3. Stabilization might be necessary to avoid the risk of spinal instability, as full resection of a facet joint is frequently necessary to remove the entirety of the nerve.
4. Continuous neurophysiologic monitoring is vital throughout the procedure. Intraoperative stimulation is necessary to facilitate preservation of motor fibers. If the nerve root must be sacrificed, nerve transfers can frequently be performed to minimize denervation morbidity.

Pivot Points

1. Complete removal of dumbbell tumors should be achieved whenever possible to avoid the risk of recurrence, as revision surgery is complex and is associated with more complications.
2. Preservation of the rootlets/fascicles embedded within the tumor should always be attempted, and the rootlets/fascicles should be resected only after the functionality is checked with intraoperative stimulation and neurophysiologic monitoring.

Aftercare

Corticosteroids and antibiotics are generally not necessary or indicated after the preoperative doses. The neurologic status of the patient must be checked frequently. If a drain is placed, monitoring of the drain output and color is important. Pain can be controlled with appropriate regimens.

Physical therapy is generally started on the first day after the operation and is tailored to the patient's needs.

Complications and Management

As with any procedure, there are some inherent risks unique to each approach. Injury to the esophagus can occur with anterior approaches to the cervical region, whereas in the thoracic region, the most feared complication is injury to the great vessels. Despite these risks, the major concern is the risk for neurologic deficit resulting from resection of roots/rootlets/fascicles embedded within the tumor. The risk of neurologic deficit ranges from 2.3% to 63%, including both temporary and permanent deficits; however, it is not uncommon that the involved nerve is nonfunctional by the time of surgery and complete removal of the nerve leads to no discernible functional deficits (as the adjacent nerves have provided collateral reinnervation).[13–18] This issue can be optimally addressed intraoperatively by the use of root stimulation and neurophysiologic monitoring to assess the functionality of the root and whether it can be divided without incurring postoperative deficit, in case the root cannot be separated from the tumor. If the nerve root must be sacrificed and a deficit is incurred, the distal nerve can frequently be transferred to minimize denervation morbidity.

Vertebral artery injury is another feared complication of cervical dumbbell tumor surgery. It can be adequately addressed starting preoperatively by analyzing the vertebral artery's course and relation to the tumor. In addition, intraoperatively, the proximal and distal portions of the vertebral artery should be identified and secured for control prior to proceeding with tumor resection. Finally, meticulous intracapsular dissection should be carried out to avoid iatrogenic injury during the procedure.

The risk of spinal instability can be minimized by performing facetectomies of less than 25% of each facet joint; however, if stabilization is necessary, instrumentation can be utilized to avoid postoperative spinal instability. Other reported complications include cerebrospinal fluid leakage, intraoperative blood loss, Horner syndrome, dyspnea, deep venous thrombosis, pulmonary embolism, arachnoiditis, vertebral deformities, hematoma, infection, pseudomeningocele formation, and fusion-related complications, such as hardware failure, pseudarthrosis, and adjacent-segment disease.[17,19]

Oral Boards Review—Complications Pearls

1. Nerve roots can be preserved during surgical resection by using intraoperative root stimulation and neurophysiologic monitoring to assess the functionality of the involved root. New postoperative deficits can be addressed with distal nerve transfers.
2. Risk of vertebral artery injury can be minimized by extensive preoperative analysis of its course and relation to the tumor as well as meticulous intraoperative intracapsular dissection and proximal and distal control.
3. Facetectomy of less than 25% of each facet joint can reduce the risk of spinal instability and the need for stabilization.

Evidence and Outcomes

Prospective controlled studies on the management of dumbbell tumors are generally lacking. Because of the long-term risk of tumor recurrence, complete removal of dumbbell tumors should be the goal whenever possible. In one series, the recurrence rate of spinal nerve sheath tumors was 10.7% at 5 years and 28.2% after 10 to 15 years.[20] In addition, revision surgery is usually more complex and is associated with more complications.

Preservation of the roots embedded within the tumor should always be attempted. Sometimes, radical resection may be achieved only by jeopardizing the root(s) from which the tumor is arising, which may result in a neurologic deficit after the resection of tumor-involved nerve root(s). The reported risk is extremely variable among studies, ranging from 2.3% to 63%, including both temporary and permanent deficits.[13–18] Regardless, complete tumor resection is usually achieved in the majority of patients. Various studies show total resection rates of 51% to 97% for dumbbell tumors, with a higher rate of complete resection for schwannomas than for neurofibromas.[13,15,21–24] Cervical tumors have been shown to have the lowest rate of complete resection.[23] While intraoperative electrophysiologic monitoring has not been shown to reduce complications, its use has been associated with an increased rate of gross total resection.[17] Moreover, most patients do well postoperatively, and the majority of patients who have mild postoperative neurologic deficits regain function over a 6- to 12-month period.[13,15] New and profound deficits after tumor removal may require treatment with distal nerve transfers. Generally, in the authors' experience, patients who have severe neurologic deficits preoperatively are less likely to experience improvement, whereas those with mild deficits tend to demonstrate a more pronounced improvement. For example, severe weakness associated with muscle atrophy is not commonly reversed over time, due to the duration of atrophy and the proximal location of the nerve lesion. Similarly, individuals with syndromic dumbbell tumors (e.g., patients with NF2) are much less likely to experience improvement and have a higher tendency for recurrent disease and complex reoperation.[23]

References

1. Kivrak AS, Koc O, Emlik D, Kiresi D, Odev K, Kalkan E. Differential diagnosis of dumbbell lesions associated with spinal neural foraminal widening: imaging features. *Eur J Radiol.* 2009;71:29–41.
2. Karsy M, Guan J, Ravindra VM, Stilwill S, Mahan MA. Diagnostic quality of magnetic resonance imaging interpretation for peripheral nerve sheath tumors: can malignancy be determined? *J Neurol Surg A Cent Eur Neurosurg.* 2016;77:495–504.
3. Ahlawat S, Blakeley J, Montgomery E, Subramaniam RM, Belzberg A, Fayad LM. Schwannoma in neurofibromatosis type 1: a pitfall for detecting malignancy by metabolic imaging. *Skeletal Radiol.* 2013;42:1317–1322.
4. Benz MR, Czernin J, Dry SM, et al. Quantitative F18-fluorodeoxyglucose positron emission tomography accurately characterizes peripheral nerve sheath tumors as malignant or benign. *Cancer.* 2010;116:451–458.
5. Asazuma T, Toyama Y, Maruiwa H, Fujimura Y, Hirabayashi K. Surgical strategy for cervical dumbbell tumors based on a three-dimensional classification. *Spine (Phila Pa 1976).* 2004;29:E10–14.
6. Eden K. The dumb-bell tumours of the spine. *Br J Surg.* 1941;28:549–570.
7. Fujimura Y, Takahata T, Toyama Y. Clinical analysis of 83 cases of the dumbbell tumors in the spine: morphological classification and surgical management. *J Jap Med Soc Paraplegia.* 1992;5:86–87.
8. Dodd RL, Ryu MR, Kamnerdsupaphon P, Gibbs IC, Chang SD Jr, Adler JR Jr. CyberKnife radiosurgery for benign intradural extramedullary spinal tumors. *Neurosurgery.* 2006;58:674–685.
9. Gerszten PC, Burton SA, Ozhasoglu C, McCue KJ, Quinn AE. Radiosurgery for benign intradural spinal tumors. *Neurosurgery.* 2008;62:887–895; discussion 895–896.
10. Sachdev S, Dodd RL, Chang SD, et al. Stereotactic radiosurgery yields long-term control for benign intradural, extramedullary spinal tumors. *Neurosurgery.* 2011;69:533–539; discussion 539.
11. Selch MT, Lin K, Agazaryan N, et al. Initial clinical experience with image-guided linear accelerator-based spinal radiosurgery for treatment of benign nerve sheath tumors. *Surg Neurol.* 2009;72:668–674; discussion 674–675.
12. Shin DW, Sohn MJ, Kim HS, et al. Clinical analysis of spinal stereotactic radiosurgery in the treatment of neurogenic tumors. *J Neurosurg Spine.* 2015;23:429–437.
13. Cherqui A, Kim DH, Kim SH, Park HK, Kline DG. Surgical approaches to paraspinal nerve sheath tumors. *Neurosurg Focus.* 2007;22:E9.
14. Kim P, Ebersold MJ, Onofrio BM, Quast LM. Surgery of spinal nerve schwannoma. Risk of neurological deficit after resection of involved root. *J Neurosurg.* 1989;71:810–814.
15. Nakamura M, Iwanami A, Tsuji O, et al. Long-term surgical outcomes of cervical dumbbell neurinomas. *J Orthop Sci.* 2013;18:8–13.
16. Nanda A, Kukreja S, Ambekar S, Bollam P, Sin AH. Surgical strategies in the management of spinal nerve sheath tumors. *World Neurosurg.* 2015;83:886–899.
17. Safaee MM, Lyon R, Barbaro NM, et al. Neurological outcomes and surgical complications in 221 spinal nerve sheath tumors. *J Neurosurg Spine.* 2017;106(1): 103–111.
18. Seppala MT, Haltia MJ, Sankila RJ, Jaaskelainen JE, Heiskanen O. Long-term outcome after removal of spinal schwannoma: a clinicopathological study of 187 cases. *J Neurosurg.* 1995;83:621–626.

19. Safaee M, Oh T, Barbaro NM, et al. Results of spinal fusion after spinal nerve sheath tumor resection. *World Neurosurg*. 2016;90:6–13.
20. Klekamp J, Samii M. Surgery of spinal nerve sheath tumors with special reference to neurofibromatosis. *Neurosurgery*. 1998;42:279–289; discussion 289–290.
21. Abe J, Takami T, Naito K, Yamagata T, Arima H, Ohata K. Surgical management of solitary nerve sheath tumors of the cervical spine: a retrospective case analysis based on tumor location and extension. *Neurol Med Chir (Tokyo)*. 2014;54:924–929.
22. Conti P, Pansini G, Mouchaty H, Capuano C, Conti R. Spinal neurinomas: retrospective analysis and long-term outcome of 179 consecutively operated cases and review of the literature. *Surg Neurol*. 2004;61:34–43; discussion 44.
23. Safaee M, Parsa AT, Barbaro NM, et al. Association of tumor location, extent of resection, and neurofibromatosis status with clinical outcomes for 221 spinal nerve sheath tumors. *Neurosurg Focus*. 2015;39:E5.
24. Safavi-Abbasi S, Senoglu M, Theodore N, et al. Microsurgical management of spinal schwannomas: evaluation of 128 cases. *J Neurosurg Spine*. 2008;9:40–47.

Malignant Peripheral Nerve Sheath Tumors

Marie-Noëlle Hébert-Blouin

20

Case Presentation

A 66-year-old woman presents to her neurosurgeon with left foot weakness and left leg pain. Over the preceding 6 months, she developed progressive weakness of her left foot associated with electrical sensations and hypesthesia in the sole of her foot. She also noted an enlarging mass in her left posterior thigh. The mass is painful, and the pain disturbs her sleep. The pain has been progressively worsening. She has difficulty sitting on a chair or lying flat because pressure on the mass increases her pain. Over the last year, she sustained an unintentional 30-pound weight loss. Of note, at age 33 she was diagnosed with neurofibromatosis type 1 (NF1), based on multiple skin neurofibromas, a left femoral neurofibroma, and a daughter with NF1. On physical examination, she has weakness of left plantar flexion and toe flexion, hypesthesia of the sole of the foot, and a large fixed painful mass in the left posterior thigh. The remainder of the neurologic examination is normal.

Questions

1. What is the likely diagnosis?
2. What are the most appropriate imaging modalities?
3. What is the appropriate timing of the diagnostic workup?

Assessment and Planning

The neurosurgeon suspects the presence of a nerve sheath tumor involving the tibial portion of the patient's left sciatic nerve. The differential diagnosis includes a benign peripheral nerve sheath tumor (PNST), likely a neurofibroma or atypical neurofibroma in this patient given the context of NF1, a malignant PNST, or another musculoskeletal malignancy. Given the patient's history of NF1, the large size and rapid growth of the lesion, the pain, and the neurologic deficits (motor and sensory), a malignant PNST is the most likely diagnosis.

Malignant PNSTs are soft tissue sarcomas arising from a peripheral nerve or a pre-existing benign nerve sheath tumor (usually neurofibroma) or are sarcomas with features of Schwann-cell differentiation. The exact cellular origin of malignant PNSTs remains unclear, although they are thought to originate from Schwann cells or pluripotent neural crest cells.[1] Malignant PNSTs constitute 5% to 10% of soft tissue sarcomas and can arise sporadically (in approximately 50% of cases), can be associated with NF1 (in 22% to 50% of cases), or can be a consequence of radiation therapy (in approximately 10% of cases, on average 15 years after radiation).[2–6] In the general population, malignant PNSTs are rare (incidence of 0.001%).[6] However, patients with NF1, a hereditary autosomal dominant disorder that involves the NF1 tumor suppressor gene, have a lifetime risk of developing a malignant PNST between 6% and 13%.[6,7] These patients have an even higher risk (up to 18 times) if they have an internal plexiform neurofibroma; plexiform neurofibromas have a 10% risk of malignant transformation.[8] Most malignant PNSTs occur in patients between the ages of 20 and 50 years, with median onset in the fifth decade in the general population and in the third decade in patients with NF1.[9]

The molecular events contributing to the development of a malignant PNST are unclear, but many different genetic aberrations have been demonstrated. No difference has been shown between NF1-associated and sporadic malignant PNSTs. The genetic changes affect signaling pathways that modulate cellular proliferation, growth, and apoptosis. Proteins that have been implicated in the pathogenesis of malignant PNSTs include neurofibromin 1, phosphatase and tensin homolog (PTEN), insulin-like growth factor 1 receptor (IGF1R), epidermal growth factor receptor (EGFR), and mitogen-activated protein kinases (MAPKs).[6]

Differentiating between benign and malignant PNSTs clinically is challenging and may not always be possible. Clinical features suggestive of a malignant PNST include pain (particularly constant, spontaneous pain and night pain), neurologic deficits (paresthesias, sensory loss, weakness), rapid growth, and association with NF1 and radiation, but there is considerable overlap with the clinical features of benign PNSTs. Regardless, when these features are present, suspicion for malignancy should be raised. Imaging, including ultrasound, CT, MR imaging, and fluorodeoxyglucose-positron emission tomography (FDG-PET), can provide useful information and help in evaluation and diagnosis of malignant PNSTs. However, while the findings on imaging can be suggestive, particularly in the right clinical context, they are not completely diagnostic for malignant PNSTs.

Ultrasound, CT, and MR imaging can determine the tumor size, location, involved nerve(s), and local invasiveness with variable resolution. MR imaging provides better definition of the tumor characteristics and relationship to the nerve, especially if a high-resolution MR scanner, such as a 3-Tesla scanner, is used. On MR imaging, malignant PNSTs are typically larger tumors (> 5 cm) and may have ill-defined margins with associated peritumoral edema and infiltration of adjacent tissue. Intratumoral lobulation, heterogeneity, or cystic changes and irregular or peripheral contrast enhancement are more frequently observed in malignant PNSTs than in benign PNSTs.[10–15] However, there is considerable overlap in the appearance of both benign and malignant PNSTs, making their distinction challenging and unreliable.[16] One study found that the statistically predictive factors for malignancy included tumor size > 5 cm, peripheral enhancement, perilesional edema, and intratumoral cystic change. However, the presence of two or more of these factors was only 61% sensitive but 90% specific.[15] The presence of these features should raise suspicion of malignancy and prompt further workup, but, in the right clinical context, the absence of these features should not eliminate consideration of malignancy.

FDG-PET can help identify malignant PNSTs in patients with a concerning lesion or in patients with multiple tumors, such as in some NF1 patients. Tumor glucose utilization is measured with the maximum standardized uptake value (SUV_{max}); a lower tumor SUV_{max} suggests a benign PNST, whereas a higher tumor SUV_{max} suggests a malignant PNST. An SUV_{max} greater than 6.1 has a sensitivity of 94% and a specificity of 91% for malignant PNST.[10] However, overlap exists between the SUV_{max} of malignant PNSTs and that of neurofibromas, and an even greater overlap exists between the SUV_{max} of malignant PNSTs and that of schwannomas. Some authors suggest that tumor-to-liver ratio (> 1.5) may be superior to an SUV_{max} threshold, and that metabolically active whole-body tumor volume and whole-body total lesion glycolysis may better identify malignant changes in patients with NF1.[17–19] Currently, the combination of FDG-PET with CT or MR imaging offers the best ability to distinguish benign and malignant PNSTs.

In the present case, the neurosurgeon requests MR imaging of the left thigh and sciatic nerve and an FDG-PET scan. Given the concern for malignant PNST, the imaging is requested on an urgent basis. MR imaging (Figure 20.1) shows a 15-cm very heterogeneous mass in the posterior midthigh that involves the tibial nerve, with heterogeneous enhancement and a central non-enhancing portion suggestive of necrosis. Peritumoral edema and some ill-defined margins are seen. The FDG-PET (Figure 20.2) shows increased FDG uptake in the periphery (SUV_{max} of 6.7) with photopenia centrally, likely consistent with tumor necrosis.

Questions

1. When a malignant PNST is suspected, what is the next diagnostic step?
2. Which preoperative workup is essential to plan for appropriate treatment?
3. Why is the correct pathologic diagnosis of malignant PNST challenging?

Oral Boards Review—Diagnostic Pearls

1. Malignant PNSTs, the sixth most common soft tissue sarcoma, arise in three contexts:
   a. Sporadically (approximately half of cases)
   b. In patients with NF1 (approximately half of cases)
   c. After radiation therapy (approximately 10% of cases)
2. Clinical symptoms that raise suspicion for malignant PNST (red flags) are:
   Large mass (> 5 cm)
   Fixed mass
   Pain (spontaneous, severe, night pain)
   Neurologic deficit (motor or sensory)
   Rapid growth
   New-onset pain in a known neurofibroma (especially in patients with NF1)
3. The most useful imaging in the evaluation of a malignant PNST is MR imaging in conjunction with FDG-PET.

4. MR imaging findings associated with malignant PNSTs are:
   Large tumors (> 5 cm)
   Ill-defined margins
   Peritumoral edema
   Infiltration of adjacent tissue
   Intratumoral lobulation, heterogeneity, or cystic changes
   Irregular or peripheral contrast enhancement
5. FDG-PET with a SUV_{max} > 6.1 has a high sensitivity and specificity for the diagnosis of a malignant PNST.

Decision-Making

Although clinical history and imaging can be suggestive of malignant PNST, they do not confirm the diagnosis. A pathologic diagnosis is required. A variety of approaches are acceptable, including biopsy prior to definitive surgery. Given that the treatment, similar to the treatment of other soft tissue sarcomas, is radical surgical resection with adjuvant radiation, a diagnosis is required before planning the definitive surgery. The biopsy can be performed via a percutaneous route or an open, multiple quadrant biopsy. Depending on the accessibility of the lesion, a CT-guided or PET/CT-guided biopsy can also be an option.[17] Occasionally, a nondiagnostic biopsy or a sampling error can occur, especially in cases of neurofibromas. Caution is necessary, especially in cases of negative (nonmalignant PNST) biopsy results, which can be misleading. Another option is a staged approach, with first a gross total resection, taking care not to violate the tumor capsule, followed by definitive surgery (second stage) after a full pathologic examination confirming a malignant PNST as the diagnosis.

There are no guidelines for how to proceed and which approach to take; the process is often guided by the surgeon's preference. In our institution, if a malignant PNST is suspected, a biopsy is usually performed. If the tumor is large and accessible, a percutaneous biopsy is performed, with CT or ultrasound guidance if necessary. The biopsy track is determined in conjunction with the oncologic surgeon, to plan for its resection during definitive surgery. If a percutaneous biopsy cannot be performed, an open biopsy is usually performed. In our institution, a two-stage approach (gross total resection followed by definitive surgery) is done in cases in which the biopsy is negative or inconclusive or in cases in which malignant PNST is considered unlikely.

The diagnosis of a malignant PNST requires a histologically malignant tumor arising either from a peripheral nerve or from a pre-existing benign nerve sheath tumor (usually a neurofibroma) or a tumor arising in a patient with NF1. In other cases, the diagnosis can be made when features of Schwann-cell differentiation are seen on histologic, immunohistochemical, and ultrastructural examination. However, the diagnosis of a malignant PNST can be challenging because its histologic appearance is variable, and there are no definitive markers or widely accepted diagnostic criteria. Moreover, other sarcomas, benign soft tissue tumors, and non-epithelial tumors (especially melanoma) can mimic a malignant PNST. Another difficulty is to distinguish

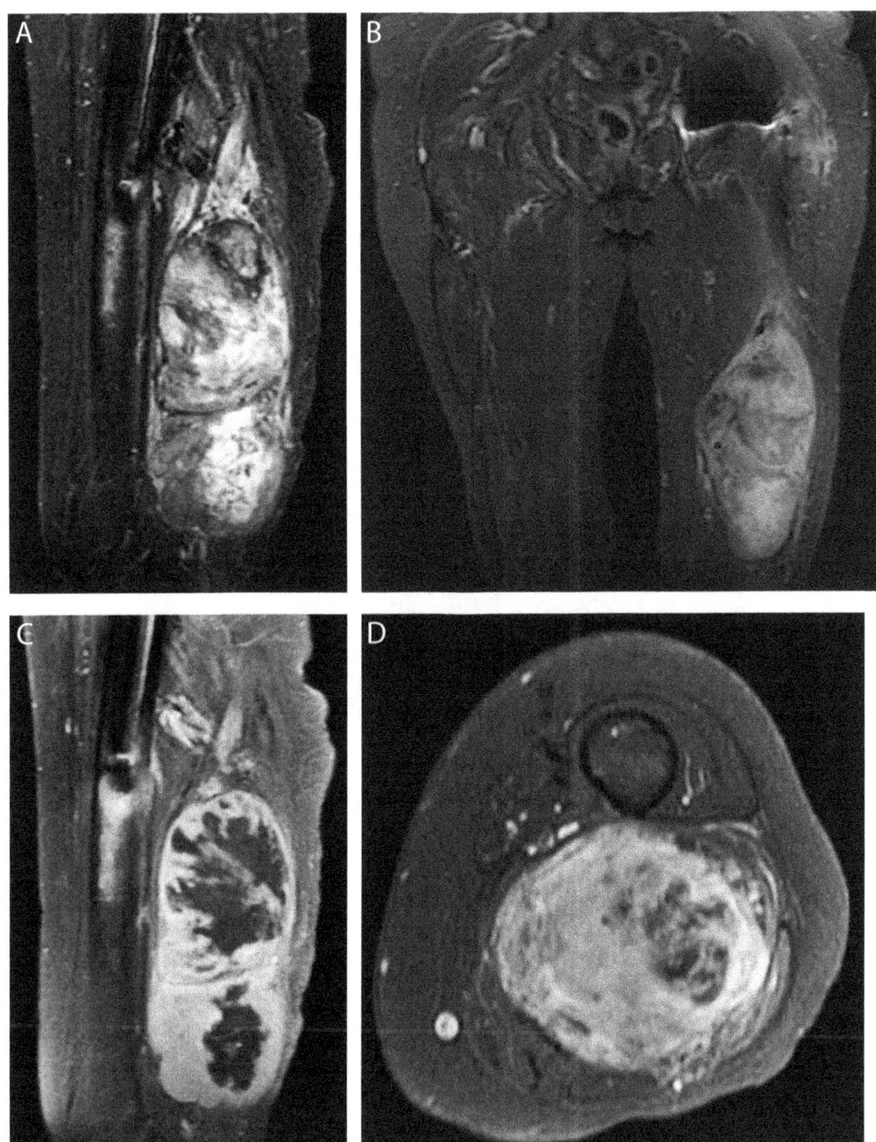

Figure 20.1. A, Sagittal fast STIR (**short-tau inversion-recovery**) MR image showing the heterogeneity of a large midthigh lesion involving the tibial division of the sciatic nerve. Note the perilesional edema at the superior pole of the lesion. B, Coronal fast STIR MR image of the lesion, again showing its large size and heterogeneity. C, Sagittal T1-weighted, fat-saturated, post-gadolinium MR image at the same level as A, showing peripheral heterogeneous enhancement. D, Axial T1-weighted, fat-saturated, post-gadolinium MR image approximately at the midlesion level, showing heterogeneous enhancement. Note the irregular margins of the lesion.

low-grade malignant PNSTs from neurofibromas and neurofibromas with atypical features, because these lesions likely represent a histologic continuum.[1,6] Because the diagnosis is challenging, it is important to make definitive treatment decisions based on final permanent sections and not based on frozen sections.

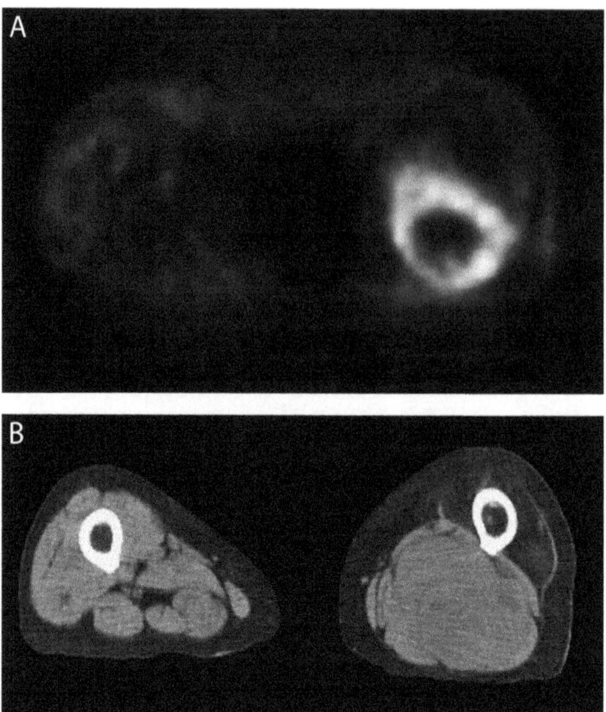

Figure 20.2. A, Axial ^{18}F-FDG-PET image at the midthigh level showing increased heterogeneous FDG uptake in the periphery (SUV_{max} of 6.7) and photopenia centrally, likely consistent with tumor necrosis. B, Corresponding axial CT image at the same level showing the mass at the midthigh level.

After confirming the diagnosis, a preoperative metastatic workup is important, as it will influence the subsequent treatment plan. It is important to note that, at presentation, 10% to 16% of patients already have distant metastatic disease.[20] The most common sites for metastasis are the lungs, followed by the bones, liver, brain, and adrenal glands; regional lymph node involvement is uncommon.[6,21,22] If the workup reveals metastatic disease, palliative surgery and adjuvant radiation and chemotherapy are suggested.

Due to the complexity of the diagnosis and treatment of malignant PNSTs, patients should be treated by an experienced multidisciplinary team of physicians, including surgical oncologists, radiation oncologists, and medical oncologists, as well as radiologists and pathologists with specialization in sarcoma.

In the present case, percutaneous biopsy confirms a malignant PNST and the patient's chest CT shows multiple lung metastases. The patient is discussed and treated by a multidisciplinary sarcoma treatment team. She undergoes palliative radiation therapy and resection.

Questions

1. What is the main goal of surgery?
2. What are the surgical principles of malignant PNST resection?

Surgical Procedure

During surgery for malignant PNSTs, the goal is complete removal of the tumor with wide histologically negative margins of resection. Local control is thought to decrease the risk of systemic metastasis and is a strong predictor of survival. Surgery for malignant PNSTs often requires en-bloc resection of major nerves, accepting the potential significant functional losses. Adjacent contaminated soft tissues should also be removed. Resectability varies depending on tumor location; for example, resectability is approximately 20% in the paraspinal region and 95% in extremities.[22,23] In most patients with a malignant PNST in an extremity, the limb can be preserved, with amputation required in a small proportion of primary and recurrent tumors to achieve complete tumor resection. The surgical principles of malignant PNST resection are: no violation of the tumor capsule, nerve sacrifice, removal of adjacent potentially contaminated soft tissue (2-cm margins), and limb preservation when feasible. Full pathologic examination is performed on permanent sections. Nerve reconstruction is generally not advocated, given that radiation and chemotherapy will compromise regeneration and that the natural history is often not long enough for the patient to benefit from the reconstruction.

The surgical management of low-grade malignant PNSTs may be different from the management of high-grade malignant PNSTs. A study has shown that negative surgical margins did not have a significant effect on the clinical outcome of patients with low-grade malignant PNSTs or atypical neurofibromas.[24]

Oral Boards Review—Management Pearls

1. Biopsy (percutaneous, fine-needle, or open) is important to confirm the diagnosis of malignant PNST and to plan for surgery.
2. One approach is staged surgery: The first stage aims at gross total resection without violating the capsule, and the second stage is definitive surgery to obtain wide negative margins once pathology is confirmed.
3. The main goal of surgery is complete en-bloc resection with wide negative margins.
4. Management of malignant PNSTs should be performed by a specialized multidisciplinary sarcoma team that includes a surgical oncologist, radiation oncologist, medical oncologist, and specialized radiologist and pathologist.
5. If malignant PNST is suspected, a metastatic workup should be performed.
6. The surgical principles for malignant PNST resection include:
   a. No violation of the tumor capsule
   b. Nerve sacrifice
   c. Removal of adjacent potentially contaminated soft tissue (2-cm margins)
   d. Limb preservation (when feasible)

Pivot Points

1. If malignant PNST is suspected clinically and on imaging, a biopsy should be performed to plan for further treatment, including radical en-bloc resection.

2. If malignant PNST is suspected and the biopsy is negative, sampling error should be considered.
3. If the metastatic workup is positive, palliative surgery and adjuvant radiation and chemotherapy are suggested.
4. If pathology shows a neurofibroma with atypical features or a low-grade malignant PNST, obtaining negative surgical margins may not be as critical, as it appears not to have a significant impact on the clinical outcome of patients.

Aftercare

There are no definitive follow-up guidelines for management of a malignant PNST after surgical resection. Both neoadjuvant and postoperative adjuvant radiation therapy are thought to provide local control and may delay the onset of recurrence. Despite radiation therapy's small effect on long-term survival rates, the Oncology Consensus Group recommends it as a uniform treatment policy for malignant PNST, even when the surgical margins are clean.[25] The typical dose, 6,000 to 7,000 cGy, includes the tumor or operative field with a 5-cm field margin. Postoperative radiation therapy is most commonly given, but some centers, including ours, use preoperative radiation therapy.[22] The rationale for preoperative radiation therapy is that it may provide better success in obtaining a tumor-free margin and may kill tumor cells more effectively because of undisturbed vascularity. It should be considered especially when it will be difficult to provide optimal radiotherapy after excision due to location, size, and distribution, if dissection is anticipated along a major neurovascular bundle, with the possibility of leaving microscopic disease in critical structures, if remote tissue flaps or skin grafts are required, or if wound management issues are anticipated.[26–28] Other options include brachytherapy or intraoperative electron irradiation, which have been shown to possibly improve local control in small series.

Chemotherapy is usually given to patients with metastatic malignant PNST, with unresectable tumors, or with high-risk tumors (> 5 cm). Currently available recommendations are based on case reports, small case series, and on regimens proven to be successful for other sarcomas. In general, malignant PNSTs are relatively resistant to chemotherapy. In 20% to 25% of patients, there is a partial response to a regimen of doxorubicin with or without ifosfamide.[29] A meta-analysis showed that this regimen conferred a benefit at 10 years for progression-free survival and reduction of both local and distant relapse, but no significant overall survival benefit.[30] Currently, targeting of various molecular pathways implicated in malignant PNSTs, such as the RAS-MAPK, Hsp90, PI3K/AKT/mTOR, and EGFR signaling cascades, is being explored.

Complications and Management

The major complications of malignant PNSTs, because they are high-grade sarcomas, are local recurrence and the development of distant metastases. Local recurrences are found in 40% to 65% of patients, with most (75%) developing within 24 months of the first resection (median 22 months).[6,23,31–33] Local recurrence can be treated with repeat resection. Risk factors for local recurrence include positive margins of resection and head and neck tumors. Distant metastases develop in 30% to 60% of patients and are a frequent cause of mortality.[6,23,32] The most common metastasis sites are the lungs, followed by the soft tissues, bones, liver, brain, and adrenal glands; regional lymph node involvement is uncommon. Between 10% and 16% of patients already have distant metastatic disease at presentation.[20] The median time to metastasis is 13 months, with 75% of distant recurrence occurring within 24 months.[20,33] Risk factors for metastatic disease include the size of the primary tumor, the tumor grade, and local recurrence. Although systemic chemotherapy is administered to manage metastatic malignant PNSTs, survival remains low.

In the present case, after initial palliative resection and radiation therapy, the patient developed a local recurrence 10 months later and died 4 months after that.

Oral Boards Review—Complications Pearls

1. Local recurrence occurs in 40% to 65% of patients.
    a. Repeat resection can be performed.
    b. Local recurrence increases the risk of metastasis and is a risk factor for poor survival.
2. Distant metastasis occurs in 30% to 60% of patients, with 10% to 16% having metastasis at presentation.
    a. Chemotherapy is usually administered, but survival remains low.

Evidence and Outcomes

Malignant PNSTs are aggressive sarcomas and their prognosis is generally poor. In fact, in a survival nomogram for sarcoma, malignant PNST histology had the highest sarcoma-related mortality.[34] Patients with high-grade malignant PNSTs have a 5-year survival between 23% and 69% and a mortality rate of up to 75%.[6,35,36] Risk factors for poor survival include tumors larger than 5 cm, local recurrence, tumor site (head, neck, and trunk having poorer prognosis), high-grade tumors with advanced histology, heterologous rhabdomyoblastic differentiation, and positive surgical margins.[26] The most consistently reported risk factors are size > 5 cm followed by incomplete resection with positive margins.[37–39] Wide negative margins are a strong predictor of survival.[3,25,40] In fact, in one study 3- and 5-year survival with positive versus negative margins were 47% and 22% versus 74% and 67%, respectively.[23] Paraspinal disease in particular has been associated with reduced survival, likely owing to the difficulty of achieving negative margins. The 2-year survival for paraspinal disease is approximately 35%, while the 5-year survival is only 16%, with the median survival being 8.5 months.[3,41,42]

Although patients with NF1 were thought to have a worse prognosis, no consensus has been reached about whether NF1 constitutes an independent risk factor for poor prognosis or not. A recent meta-analysis showed that NF1-related malignant PNSTs had a poorer prognosis than sporadic malignant PNSTs, but the prognosis for the two groups converged over the last decade, so that there likely is no difference.[43] Recent data, however, do suggest that radiation-induced malignant PNSTs likely have a poorer prognosis than sporadic malignant PNSTs (47% versus 67% 5-year survival).[44]

The best prognosis is conferred by gross total resection with negative margins prior to metastasis.[31,42,45] Both the local recurrence and distant metastatic rates are increased with positive margins.[20,46,47] Radiation is a key component of the treatment regimen. Brachytherapy or intraoperative electron irradiation significantly increases survival, with 3- and 5-year survival rates without therapy of 61% and 50% versus with therapy of 84% and 72%.[23] Postoperative radiation also improves local disease control and 5-year overall survival (5-year survival is 65% with radiation and 38% without it).[40]

Malignant PNST remains a diagnostic and therapeutic challenge, for which surgery is the mainstay of effective treatment, with multimodal therapy used to optimize tumor control. A better understanding of the molecular biology of malignant PNSTs may lead to biologic targets and change or improve treatments.

References

1. Thway K, Fisher C. Malignant peripheral nerve sheath tumor: pathology and genetics. *Ann Diagn Pathol.* 2014;18:109–116.
2. Ducatman BS, Scheithauer BW. Postirradiation neurofibrosarcoma. *Cancer.* 1983;51:1028–1033.
3. Ducatman BS, Scheithauer BW, Piepgras DG, Reiman HM, Ilstrup DM. Malignant peripheral nerve sheath tumors. A clinicopathologic study of 120 cases. *Cancer.* 1986;57:2006–2021.
4. Fuchs B, Spinner RJ, Rock MG. Malignant peripheral nerve sheath tumors: an update. *J Surg Orthop Adv.* 2005;14:168–174.
5. Grobmyer SR, Reith JD, Shahlaee A, Bush CH, Hochwald SN. Malignant peripheral nerve sheath tumor: molecular pathogenesis and current management considerations. *J Surg Oncol.* 2008;97:340–349.
6. James AW, Shurell E, Singh A, Dry SM, Eilber FC. Malignant peripheral nerve sheath tumor. *Surg Oncol Clin N Am.* 2016;25:789–802.
7. Evans DG, Baser ME, McGaughran J, Sharif S, Howard E, Moran A. Malignant peripheral nerve sheath tumours in neurofibromatosis 1. *J Med Genet.* 2002;39:311–314.
8. McGaughran JM, Harris DI, Donnai D, et al. A clinical study of type 1 neurofibromatosis in north west England. *J Med Genet.* 1999;36:197–203.
9. Shurell E, Tran LM, Nakashima J, et al. Gender dimorphism and age of onset in malignant peripheral nerve sheath tumor preclinical models and human patients. *BMC Cancer.* 2014;14:827.
10. Benz MR, Czernin J, Dry SM, et al. Quantitative F18-fluorodeoxyglucose positron emission tomography accurately characterizes peripheral nerve sheath tumors as malignant or benign. *Cancer.* 2010;116:451–458.
11. Demehri S, Belzberg A, Blakeley J, Fayad LM. Conventional and functional MR imaging of peripheral nerve sheath tumors: initial experience. *AJNR Am J Neuroradiol.* 2014;35:1615–1620.
12. Derlin T, Tornquist K, Munster S, et al. Comparative effectiveness of ^{18}F-FDG PET/CT versus whole-body MRI for detection of malignant peripheral nerve sheath tumors in neurofibromatosis type 1. *Clin Nucl Med.* 2013;38:e19–25.
13. Matsumine A, Kusuzaki K, Nakamura T, et al. Differentiation between neurofibromas and malignant peripheral nerve sheath tumors in neurofibromatosis 1 evaluated by MRI. *J Cancer Res Clin Oncol.* 2009;135:891–900.

14. Salamon J, Mautner VF, Adam G, Derlin T. Multimodal imaging in neurofibromatosis type 1-associated nerve sheath tumors. *Rofo*. 2015;187:1084–1092.
15. Wasa J, Nishida Y, Tsukushi S, et al. MRI features in the differentiation of malignant peripheral nerve sheath tumors and neurofibromas. *AJR Am J Roentgenol*. 2010;194:1568–1574.
16. Mautner VF, Friedrich RE, von Deimling A, et al. Malignant peripheral nerve sheath tumours in neurofibromatosis type 1: MRI supports the diagnosis of malignant plexiform neurofibroma. *Neuroradiology*. 2003;45:618–625.
17. Brahmi M, Thiesse P, Ranchere D, et al. Diagnostic accuracy of PET/CT-guided percutaneous biopsies for malignant peripheral nerve sheath tumors in neurofibromatosis type 1 patients. *PLOS ONE*. 2015;10:e0138386.
18. Combemale P, Valeyrie-Allanore L, Giammarile F, et al. Utility of 18F-FDG PET with a semi-quantitative index in the detection of sarcomatous transformation in patients with neurofibromatosis type 1. *PLOS ONE*. 2014;9:e85954.
19. Salamon J, Papp L, Toth Z, et al. Nerve sheath tumors in neurofibromatosis type 1: assessment of whole-body metabolic tumor burden using F-18-FDG PET/CT. *PLOS ONE*. 2015;10:e0143305.
20. Anghileri M, Miceli R, Fiore M, et al. Malignant peripheral nerve sheath tumors: prognostic factors and survival in a series of patients treated at a single institution. *Cancer*. 2006;107:1065–1074.
21. Farid M, Demicco EG, Garcia R, et al. Malignant peripheral nerve sheath tumors. *Oncologist*. 2014;19:193–201.
22. Gupta G, Mammis A, Maniker A. Malignant peripheral nerve sheath tumors. *Neurosurg Clin N Am*. 2008;19:533–543, v.
23. Wong WW, Hirose T, Scheithauer BW, Schild SE, Gunderson LL. Malignant peripheral nerve sheath tumor: analysis of treatment outcome. *Int J Radiat Oncol Biol Phys*. 1998;42:351–360.
24. Bernthal NM, Putnam A, Jones KB, Viskochil D, Randall RL. The effect of surgical margins on outcomes for low grade MPNSTs and atypical neurofibroma. *J Surg Oncol*. 2014;110:813–816.
25. Ferner RE, Gutmann DH. International consensus statement on malignant peripheral nerve sheath tumors in neurofibromatosis. *Cancer Res*. 2002;62:1573–1577.
26. Angelov L, Davis A, O'Sullivan B, Bell R, Guha A. Neurogenic sarcomas: experience at the University of Toronto. *Neurosurgery*. 1998;43:56–64; discussion 64–65.
27. Nielsen OS, Cummings B, O'Sullivan B, Catton C, Bell RS, Fornasier VL. Preoperative and postoperative irradiation of soft tissue sarcomas: effect of radiation field size. *Int J Radiat Oncol Biol Phys*. 1991;21:1595–1599.
28. Peat BG, Bell RS, Davis A, et al. Wound-healing complications after soft-tissue sarcoma surgery. *Plast Reconstr Surg*. 1994;93:980–987.
29. Santoro A, Tursz T, Mouridsen H, et al. Doxorubicin versus CYVADIC versus doxorubicin plus ifosfamide in first-line treatment of advanced soft tissue sarcomas: a randomized study of the European Organization for Research and Treatment of Cancer Soft Tissue and Bone Sarcoma Group. *J Clin Oncol*. 1995;13:1537–1545.
30. Sarcoma Meta-analysis Collaboration. Adjuvant chemotherapy for localised resectable soft-tissue sarcoma of adults: meta-analysis of individual data. *Lancet*. 1997;350:1647–1654.
31. Baehring JM, Betensky RA, Batchelor TT. Malignant peripheral nerve sheath tumor: the clinical spectrum and outcome of treatment. *Neurology*. 2003;61:696–698.

32. Goertz O, Langer S, Uthoff D, et al. Diagnosis, treatment and survival of 65 patients with malignant peripheral nerve sheath tumors. *Anticancer Res.* 2014;34:777–783.
33. Ramanathan RC, Thomas JM. Malignant peripheral nerve sheath tumours associated with von Recklinghausen's neurofibromatosis. *Eur J Surg Oncol.* 1999;25:190–193.
34. Kattan MW, Leung DH, Brennan MF. Postoperative nomogram for 12-year sarcoma-specific death. *J Clin Oncol.* 2002;20:791–796.
35. Eilber FC, Brennan MF, Eilber FR, Dry SM, Singer S, Kattan MW. Validation of the post-operative nomogram for 12-year sarcoma-specific mortality. *Cancer.* 2004;101:2270–2275.
36. Lin CT, Huang TW, Nieh S, Lee SC. Treatment of a malignant peripheral nerve sheath tumor. *Onkologie.* 2009;32:503–505.
37. LaFemina J, Qin LX, Moraco NH, et al. Oncologic outcomes of sporadic, neurofibromatosis-associated, and radiation-induced malignant peripheral nerve sheath tumors. *Ann Surg Oncol.* 2013;20:66–72.
38. Stucky CC, Johnson KN, Gray RJ, et al. Malignant peripheral nerve sheath tumors (MPNST): the Mayo Clinic experience. *Ann Surg Oncol.* 2012;19:878–885.
39. Zou C, Smith KD, Liu J, et al. Clinical, pathological, and molecular variables predictive of malignant peripheral nerve sheath tumor outcome. *Ann Surg.* 2009;249:1014–1022.
40. Kar M, Deo SV, Shukla NK, et al. Malignant peripheral nerve sheath tumors (MPNST)—clinicopathological study and treatment outcome of twenty-four cases. *World J Surg Oncol.* 2006;4:55.
41. Jandali S, Diluna ML, Storm PB, Low DW. Use of the vascularized free fibula graft with an arteriovenous loop for fusion of cervical and thoracic spinal defects in previously irradiated pediatric patients. *Plast Reconstr Surg.* 2011;127:1932–1938.
42. Kourea HP, Bilsky MH, Leung DH, Lewis JJ, Woodruff JM. Subdiaphragmatic and intrathoracic paraspinal malignant peripheral nerve sheath tumors: a clinicopathologic study of 25 patients and 26 tumors. *Cancer.* 1998;82:2191–2203.
43. Kolberg M, Holand M, Agesen TH, et al. Survival meta-analyses for >1800 malignant peripheral nerve sheath tumor patients with and without neurofibromatosis type 1. *Neuro Oncol.* 2013;15:135–147.
44. Watson KL, Al Sannaa GA, Kivlin CM, et al. Patterns of recurrence and survival in sporadic, neurofibromatosis type 1-associated, and radiation-associated malignant peripheral nerve sheath tumors. *J Neurosurg.* 2017;126:319–329.
45. Wanebo JE, Malik JM, VandenBerg SR, Wanebo HJ, Driesen N, Persing JA. Malignant peripheral nerve sheath tumors. A clinicopathologic study of 28 cases. *Cancer.* 1993;71:1247–1253.
46. Gronchi A, Casali PG, Mariani L, et al. Status of surgical margins and prognosis in adult soft tissue sarcomas of the extremities: a series of patients treated at a single institution. *J Clin Oncol.* 2005;23:96–104.
47. Porter DE, Prasad V, Foster L, Dall GF, Birch R, Grimer RJ. Survival in malignant peripheral nerve sheath tumours: a comparison between sporadic and neurofibromatosis type 1-associated tumours. *Sarcoma.* 2009;2009:756395.

Section 4

Peripheral Nerve Trauma

Adult Total Brachial Plexus Injury

Mustafa Nadi and Rajiv Midha

21

Case Presentation

A 46-year-old, right-handed female was involved in a motor vehicle accident as a restrained driver and was transferred to a level I trauma facility. Initial physical exam showed minimal disturbance in level of consciousness, multiple scalp lacerations, a deep abrasion on the left side of the patient's neck just above the clavicle, and difficulty breathing. Before intubation, the patient was noted to be in moderate to severe pain and was unable to move her left arm. CT scans and X-rays showed mild traumatic subarachnoid hemorrhage, bilateral elbow fracture-dislocations, a stable fracture of the T2 lamina, a pulmonary contusion, multiple bilateral rib fractures, and a right pneumothorax. A chest tube was inserted and both elbows were fixated by the orthopedic team. Follow-up examination revealed that the patient was awake and very responsive to verbal stimuli. She was extubated after 2 days. She was able to move all other limbs with normal strength (the right upper extremity could not be fully assessed due to orthopedic fixation), but no movement was elicited in her left upper extremity, even with painful stimulation. In addition, the left upper extremity was flaccid and no reflexes could be elicited. The palpebral fissure and pupil on the left side were smaller than on the right side.

Questions

1. What is the next step?
2. What is the differential diagnosis?
3. What is the most appropriate imaging modality?
4. What are the most appropriate anatomic areas to image, and why?
5. What is the appropriate timing of the diagnostic workup?

Assessment and Planning

The differential diagnosis in this case includes total (pan-) brachial plexus injury (BPI), cervical spinal cord injury, contralateral cerebral contusion, and severe musculoskeletal injury. Given complete loss of motor function in all muscle groups of the left arm, sensory loss from C5 to T1, a flaccid limb without reflexes, and the local wound at the left side of neck, the most likely diagnosis is pan-plexus injury. Cervical spine injury usually results in quadriparesis rather than monoplegia. Contralateral high cortical contusions due to head trauma or a depressed skull fracture can manifest

Table 21.1.
Nerve Root Injured and Respective Motor Deficits

Neural Structure	Muscles Affected—Neurologic Deficit
C5	Supraspinatus, infraspinatus, deltoid—shoulder abduction, forward flexion, external rotation
C6	Biceps, brachialis, brachioradialis, supinator—elbow flexion and supination
C7	Triceps, pronator teres, latissimus dorsi—elbow extension and pronation
C8	Wrist and finger flexors, finger and thumb extensors, some hand intrinsics
T1	Hand intrinsics

as hemiparesis, but motor tone is typically preserved. Furthermore, these injuries were excluded early on by the head CT scan. Although severe local musculoskeletal injury, including injury to the rotator cuff and upper extremity bones, can be in the differential, these injuries may affect shoulder and arm movement but not hand function or sensation. X-rays can help rule out extensive fractures. Given the most likely diagnosis, MR imaging of the left brachial plexus was requested.

It is mandatory to perform a thorough clinical exam to determine the extent, site, and severity (nature) of BPI (Table 21.1). Proper physical examination and a high index of suspicion are required to recognize the presence of BPI. The diagnosis is often delayed, particularly when concomitant injuries are present. Individual muscle power, sensation, reflexes, and motor tone should be evaluated. Many times this is not possible in the acute phase of trauma because of other life-threatening injuries and/or a disturbed level of consciousness. When the patient is hemodynamically and neurologically stable, a second clinical assessment should be conducted. The goal of clinical assessment is to localize the lesion to the supra- or infraclavicular plexus and to classify the injury as preganglionic or postganglionic. For supraclavicular injuries, clinical assessment helps identify the portion of the plexus that is injured: upper (C5-C6 ± C7), lower (C8-T1), or pan (C5-T1).

Oral Boards Review—Diagnostic Pearls

1. The clinical evaluation is crucial for the accurate diagnosis of BPI. Proper physical examination and a high index of suspicion are required to recognize the presence of BPI. The diagnosis is often delayed, particularly when concomitant injuries are present.
2. Inspection of the position of the upper extremity can give a hint about the portion of the plexus that is injured. An adducted and internally rotated arm, extended elbow, and pronated forearm (waiter's tip posture) indicates injury to the upper plexus (C5-C6). A claw hand with an extended wrist can result from injury to the lower plexus (C7, C8, and T1). A completely flail, insensate upper extremity signals a pan-plexus injury (C5-T1).

3. X-rays of the cervical spine and chest can reveal associated injuries or findings, such as cervical transverse process fractures, which correlate with spinal nerve root avulsions, or an elevated hemidiaphragm, indicating phrenic nerve (C4, C5 spinal roots) damage. MR imaging can reveal a pseudomeningocele (indirect sign of root avulsion) as well as the details of brachial plexus anatomy and involvement.
4. Electrodiagnostic tests can confirm the clinical picture, determine the injury level and severity, and help predict recovery in some cases. Nerve conduction studies (NCS) and electromyography (EMG) should first be performed 3 to 4 weeks after the injury and should be performed serially to document any recovery. In preganglionic injuries, sensory nerve action potentials (SNAPs) are normal and compound muscle action potentials (CMAPs) are absent, with clinically complete weakness and sensory loss. In postganglionic injuries, SNAPs will be affected as well.
5. The function of the spinal accessory nerve (SAN; an extra-plexal nerve) should be assessed by evaluating trapezius muscle strength, because the SAN can be an important donor for nerve transfer procedures.
6. Interval follow-up examination is important to observe for signs of spontaneous recovery. A Tinel sign can indicate the front of recovery, which can be followed over time. Typically, as recovery occurs, the location of the Tinel sign will progress more distally. If the location of the Tinel sign remains fixed at a given location, it may localize a neuroma.

MR imaging should be deferred until the patient is clinically stable. In the patient presented, the brachial plexus MR imaging included the cervical area and demonstrated severe soft tissue disruption in the left lower neck and supraclavicular region of the brachial plexus. Currently, MR imaging is the gold standard for evaluating the levels of spinal nerve root injury. The direct signs of spinal nerve root injury are complete or partial rootlet avulsions from the spinal cord, whereas pseudomeningocele, lateral cord displacement, and spinal cord edema and hemorrhage are indirect findings that may suggest nerve root avulsion (Figure 21.1). MR imaging can therefore help differentiate between pre- and postganglionic BPI, but it is not always diagnostic. Some centers prefer CT myelography over MR myelography in the evaluation for nerve root avulsion.

Electrodiagnostic studies in the case presented were planned for 3 weeks after trauma. NCS and EMG showed no motor response in the upper limb and normal sensory (SNAP) responses. This was consistent with preganglionic avulsion of the brachial plexus. Six weeks after the injury, the patient was re-evaluated, at which time she complained of severe pain throughout her left upper extremity. Physical examination revealed a flail left upper limb, normal trapezius function (innervated by the SAN), anesthesia in the C5-T1 dermatomes, a moist hand, and partial drooping of her left eyelid (partial Horner syndrome, which is a clue to the proximal nature of the injury at T1). An inspiration/expiration chest X-ray showed preserved diaphragmatic excursion, confirming the functionality of the left phrenic nerve (which can potentially be used for nerve transfer). Real-time ultrasound is another modality that can be utilized to assess movement of the diaphragm.

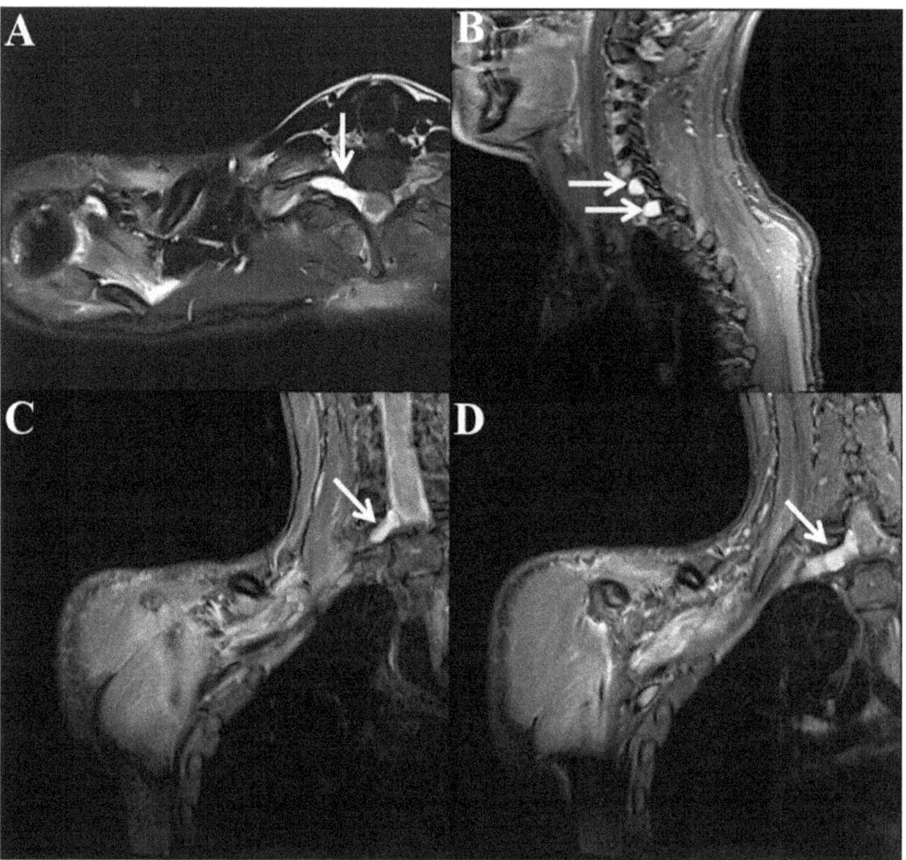

Figure 21.1. A, Axial, T2-weighted MR image showing a pseudomeningocele (arrow). B, Sagittal, T2-weighted MR image showing pseudomeningoceles in the neural foramina at C7-T1 and T1-T2 (C8 and T1 roots). C, Coronal, T2-weighted MR image showing a pseudomeningocele at the level of the C8 nerve root. D, Coronal, T2-weighted MR image showing a pseudomeningocele at the level of the T1 nerve root.

Questions

1. How do the clinical and radiologic findings influence surgical planning?
2. What is the most appropriate timing for surgical intervention in this patient?
3. How should surgery be approached in a patient with pan-plexus injury?
4. What is the major goal of surgery in patients with pan-plexus injury? What are the priorities for reconstruction?

Decision-Making

The patient showed features of preganglionic avulsions, including severe pain in an insensate arm and Horner syndrome, with the clinical features supported by radiologic and electrodiagnostic results. The patient also had moist skin on her hand, another clue that the injury was preganglionic. A moist hand occurs from a sympathectomy effect, whereas postganglionic lesion leads to dry skin because of a lack of sweating. In preganglionic injuries, the central nervous system is disconnected from the peripheral nervous system, as the nerve rootlets have been disconnected from the spinal cord. Consequently, there is no or little hope for spontaneous recovery and reconstruction should be planned as early as possible, typically 2 to 3 months after trauma. Moreover, in cases of preganglionic injury, nerve graft repair is not an option; surgical options include nerve transfers (in the case of pan-plexus injury, using only extra-plexal donors), free muscle transfer, and secondary reconstruction. In cases where the injury is thought to be postganglionic or it is unclear, the patient should be observed for 3 to 6 months for signs of spontaneous recovery. Surgical decision-making and planning should be undertaken at that time.

The goal of brachial plexus surgery is primarily to reanimate motor function and secondarily to provide some protective sensation to the hand. In adult pan-plexus injury, the first priority is to regain elbow flexion and the second priority is dynamic shoulder stabilization, because abduction, external rotation, and shoulder stability are required for optimal elbow flexion. Elbow extension and wrist and finger extension and flexion are lower priorities. Intrinsic hand function has the lowest priority because of its distance from the donor nerves and poor prognosis for recovery in adults. Sensory reinnervation has been gaining increased attention, and the goal is to obtain protective sensation of the hand via the median nerve distribution.

In the present case and similar cases, despite clinical and electrodiagnostic evidence of preganglionic injury of C5 and C6, the authors usually incorporate supraclavicular exploration of the brachial plexus into any surgical plan. If C5 and/or C6 is found to be viable, then a nerve graft is typically performed. The precise nerve targets depend on whether only one or both of C5 and C6 are viable. Regardless of whether C5 and C6 are viable, nerve transfers are typically required to achieve the goals of reconstruction. Given that the entire brachial plexus has been injured, extra-plexal donors are required. Potential extra-plexal donors in these cases include the SAN, intercostal nerves, phrenic nerve, and contralateral C7. The authors have abandoned use of the contralateral C7 due to poor outcomes and the potential significant complications. In addition, a decision must be made whether to reinnervate only the patient's native upper extremity muscles or to include a free gracilis muscle transfer. In the case presented, a plan was made to explore the supraclavicular plexus to assess C5 and C6 and otherwise to perform nerve transfers using the phrenic nerve and SAN as donors. The patient was very sedentary; otherwise, the use of the phrenic nerve as a donor would have been controversial. The SAN is a good donor but its use in pan-plexus injuries is somewhat controversial because it takes away the potential for a trapezius tendon transfer. Given the patient's multiple rib fractures, the ipsilateral intercostal nerves were not considered as donors for transfers. Although rib fractures increase the risk of finding nonviable intercostal nerves intraoperatively, usually a sufficient number of viable intercostal nerves can still be found, even in the context of rib fractures.[1] Caution should also be exercised in using intercostal nerves for transfer in cases of ipsilateral phrenic nerve injury with hemidiaphragm paralysis, particularly if preoperative pulmonary function tests are abnormal.[1,2] An advantage of utilizing intercostal nerve transfers is the potential for sensory reinnervation. The sensory portion of the intercostal nerves can be transferred to the lateral cord contribution of the median nerve in order to attempt to restore protective sensation in the hand.

Questions

1. What is the most common surgical approach for BPI reconstruction?
2. What are the potential donor nerves for nerve transfer in adult pan-plexus injury?
3. What are the potential sources of nerve graft material?

Surgical Procedure

The surgery is performed under general anesthesia without the use of neuromuscular blockade to allow intraoperative nerve stimulation. The patient is positioned supine with the head rotated 30° to 60° to the contralateral side. The affected shoulder is slightly lifted off the table by an interscapular gel pad. This enables the shoulder to drop down, increasing the neck-shoulder angle and providing a wider supraclavicular view and working access. The ipsilateral neck, ipsilateral chest, and full upper extremity are prepped and draped to allow a combined supra- and infraclavicular approach (Figure 21.2). Both legs from the knee distally are also prepped and draped for potential sural nerve harvest.

The supraclavicular exposure is performed first, using a transverse skin incision about 1.5 to 2 cm rostral to the clavicle. The incision originates slightly medial to the lateral border of the sternocleidomastoid (SCM) muscle, parallels the clavicle, and stops at the midportion of the trapezius muscle, with a length of approximately 8 cm. This enables access to both the SAN and the phrenic nerve through the same incision, in addition to access to the brachial plexus. The incision is deepened through the subcutaneous tissue to dissect the platysma, to create subplatysmal flaps, and to expose the lateral border of the SCM. The lateral 1 cm of the clavicular head of the SCM can be taken off the clavicle to increase exposure.

Next, the supraclavicular fat pad is mobilized inferomedially to superolaterally. The external jugular vein and transverse cervical artery and vein are ligated and secured with hemoclips. A key landmark in accessing the brachial plexus is the omohyoid

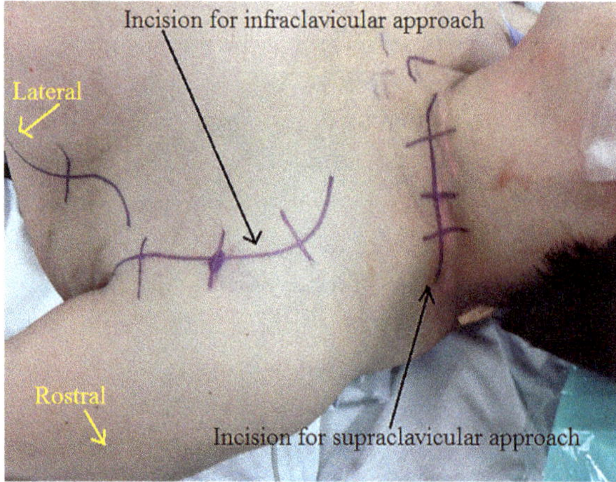

Figure 21.2. Intraoperative view of the incision marking for supra- and infraclavicular approaches for brachial plexus exploration.

muscle. Throughout the dissection superficial to the omohyoid, supraclavicular nerves may be encountered. These nerves can be preserved in order to trace them proximally to identify the cervical plexus and C4, and they can also be utilized in some cases as nerve graft material. The omohyoid should be identified as it crosses posterolaterally over the superior trunk. The tendinous portion of the omohyoid can be identified and tagged with tendon stitches, and the omohyoid can be divided. Retraction of the two ends of the omohyoid provides great access to the deeper brachial plexus structures. The suprascapular nerve (SSN) follows the same lateral course as the omohyoid, and both head toward the suprascapular notch. After dissection of the lateral border of the SCM, it is turned medially to enable careful examination of the fascia overlying the anterior scalene muscle that covers the phrenic nerve. After trauma, this area can be scarred, and often no discernible anatomic planes can be identified. The phrenic nerve can be found just deep to the fascia overlying the anterior scalene; its identification can be facilitated by direct electrical stimulation, which results in hemidiaphragm contraction and noticeable chest wall movement.

Once the phrenic nerve is dissected and isolated over a length, the anterior scalene can be incised to access the supraclavicular plexus elements, the first element being the superior trunk. After that, the anterior and posterior divisions of superior trunk can be identified, along with the SSN (Figure 21.3A). In cases of severe injury, the superior trunk and its trifurcation may be retracted significantly, at times even into the infraclavicular space. Once the superior trunk is identified, C7 and the middle trunk can be located deep to the anterior scalene. The inferior trunk can be located medial to the omohyoid and beneath the anterior scalene in contact with the subclavian artery.

The next step is dissection along the nerve roots to the level of the neural foramina. When intact roots appear to be present, somatosensory evoked potentials (SSEP) and motor evoked potentials (MEP) can be monitored to confirm continuity of the root with the central nervous system. In cases where a viable C5 or C6 root is found, the neuromatous end can be resected back to healthy nerve and the root can be used in reconstruction. Once exploration of the C5 and C6 nerve roots is completed and the superior trunk trifurcation into the anterior division, posterior division, and SSN has been identified, attention is turned to the infraclavicular exposure.

When required, the infraclavicular exposure is made via an oblique incision in the deltopectoral groove. While it is not always necessary, this incision can be T'd into the supraclavicular incision. After the skin and subcutaneous tissue are opened and dissection is made along the cephalic vein, the superficial fascia of the pectoralis major muscle can be identified and incised. This allows the muscle fibers to be split and retracted in order expose the deep fascia. Incising the deep fascia allows identification of the pectoralis minor muscle. The pectoralis minor should be isolated circumferentially and then, while the deeper elements are protected, the tendinous insertion onto the coracoid process can be divided. Once it is divided, the axillary fat pad and infraclavicular plexus elements can be visualized. The cords of the brachial plexus can be identified in this location and are named for their relations to the axillary artery. The uppermost structure on the lateral side of the pectoralis minor is the lateral cord. It should be properly identified by dissecting its course to find the lateral contribution to the median nerve, the musculocutaneous nerve (Figure 21.3B), and its branch to the coracobrachialis. After

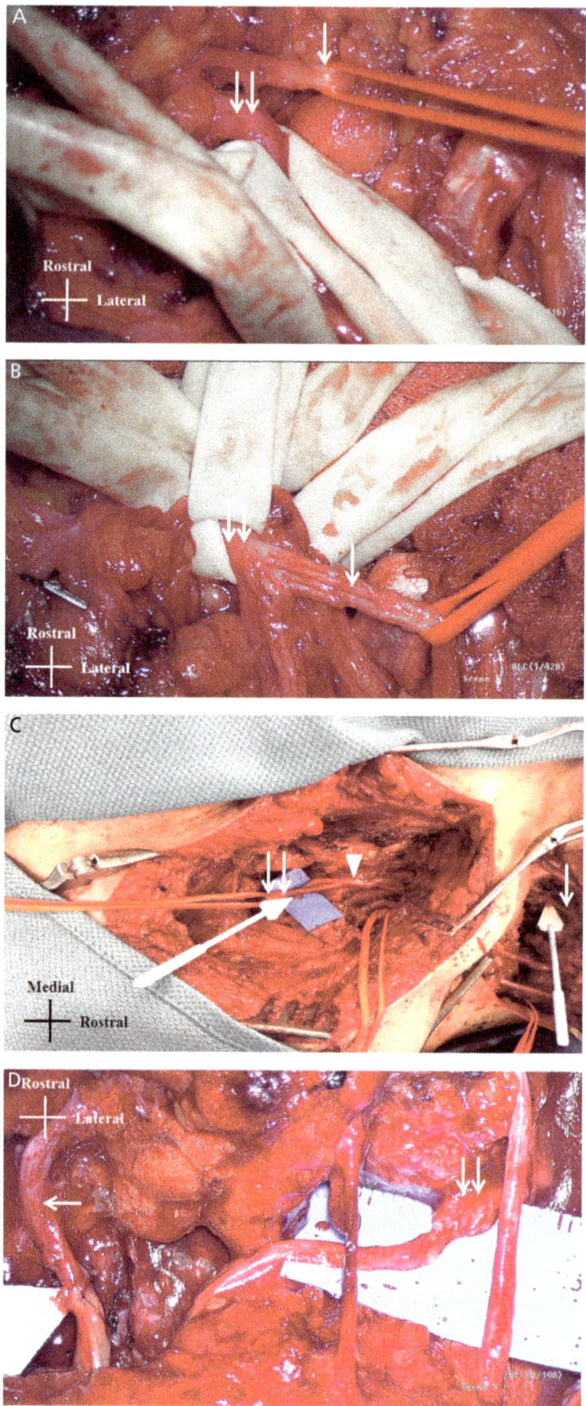

Figure 21.3. Intraoperative images of brachial plexus injury repair. A, Identification of the suprascapular nerve (arrow) and posterior division of the superior trunk (double arrow). B, The lateral cord (double arrow) and musculocutaneous nerve (arrow) lengthening after internal neurolysis. C, Coaptation sites of cabled sural nerve graft (arrowhead) from the supraclavicular phrenic nerve (arrow) to infraclavicular musculocutaneous nerve (double arrow). D, Proximal (supraclavicular) sites of coaptation for the two major donor nerves, the phrenic nerve (arrow, transferred to the musculocutaneous nerve) and the spinal accessory nerve (double arrow, transferred to the suprascapular nerve).

that, the axillary artery can be identified and secured. It is the landmark for finding the posterior and medial cords. The posterior cord is lateral and deep to the artery. The posterior cord can then be traced distally to identify the axillary nerve and the radial nerve. Because of scarred and anatomically distorted tissue planes, it is mandatory to use several landmarks to identify the brachial plexus elements. Intraoperative nerve stimulation is of great help in this respect, although in the case of pan-plexus injury, stimulation may not elicit any response.

At this point, the typical targets for reinnervation, which may include the anterior division of the superior trunk, the SSN, the axillary nerve, the lateral cord contribution to the median nerve, and/or the musculocutaneous nerve, have all been identified and exposed. The next step is to find the donor nerves and to isolate a reasonable length to allow nerve transfer. Phrenic nerve isolation is discussed above. The other donor nerve used in the case presented was the SAN. The trapezius muscle should be retracted laterally and dissected along its medial and deeper surface to reveal the SAN. Considerable length of the nerve should be isolated and the nerve transected as distally as possible.

In the present case, brachial plexus exploration revealed complete avulsion of all spinal nerve roots, including C5 and C6, rendering them nonviable. The superior trunk and its trifurcation were retracted into the infraclavicular space. The reconstructive strategy in this case utilized a phrenic to musculocutaneous nerve transfer and a SAN to SSN transfer. The phrenic to musculocutaneous nerve transfer was performed using two 10-cm sural nerve grafts (Figure 21.3C). Due to the significant retraction of the SSN, the SAN to SSN nerve transfer (Figure 21.3D) required a cabled interposed nerve graft, with one sural nerve cable and one supraclavicular nerve cable, each 9 cm long. The microscope was used for internal neurolysis and coaptation (9-0 nylon was used in an epineurial fashion at each coaptation site), and the coaptations were reinforced with fibrin glue. Once the coaptations were completed, the wound was copiously irrigated, hemostasis was achieved, and the wounds were closed in layers.

Oral Boards Review—Management Pearls

1. In adult pan-plexus injury, the first priority is to regain elbow flexion and the second priority is dynamic shoulder stabilization, because abduction, external rotation, and shoulder stability are required for optimal elbow flexion.
2. Adult pan-plexus injury without viable nerve roots requires the use of extra-plexal donors. Potential nerve donors include the phrenic nerve, SAN, and intercostal nerves.

Pivot Points

1. Brachial plexus surgery is challenging both mentally and manually. Thorough preoperative assessment and planning and intraoperative re-evaluation are pivotal to implementing a successful reconstruction strategy.

2. Intraoperative anatomic and electrophysiologic assessments of nerve integrity are key to successful surgical decision-making and execution.

Aftercare

No immediate recovery is expected after BPI repair. It is a slow process and requires education of patients and their families or caregivers. Targeted physiotherapy is crucial to maintain joint range of motion. Physiotherapy is typically instituted 3 weeks postoperatively. The arm is typically maintained in a sling or shoulder immobilizer for the first 3 weeks in order to not disrupt the coaptation sites and to allow them to heal. Patients should be followed in the outpatient setting for a prolonged period of time, as regeneration and neural recovery time is lengthy (1 inch/month). Long-term physiotherapy is particularly important with nerve transfers, given the relearning that must occur in order to make the transfers successful. Pain management with appropriate pharmacotherapy is also crucial.

Tendon and/or muscle transfer in addition to arthrodesis can be secondarily considered and can improve function. Psychological support is critically important to patients with this kind of permanent deficit. Most patients require family and community support along with medical remedies to avoid long-term depression and suicidal ideation.

Complications and Management

Devastating complications of brachial plexus reconstruction are uncommon. Nonetheless, both intraoperative and postoperative complications have been encountered and are important to be aware of.

Potential significant intraoperative complications include thoracic duct injury, injury to major blood vessels, and pneumothorax. Injury to the thoracic duct can occur during left-sided brachial plexus exploration (right-sided dissection can result in lymphatic leakage from smaller lymphatics). Chylous fistula can lead to electrolyte, fluid, and protein abnormalities, and its treatment may require hospitalization. Chylothorax can occur and may carry high mortality. Therefore, once thoracic duct injury is identified, it should be repaired or the duct should be ligated. The vessels that are vulnerable are the vertebral artery (throughout foraminal dissection), the subclavian artery and vein (during proximal subclavicular dissection), and the axillary artery and circumflex humeral artery (in quadrangular space dissection). Significant injuries may require consultation with vascular surgery colleagues. Injury to the apical lung pleura may cause a pneumothorax. This can occur especially in the dissection of the lower trunk. Pleural or pericardial transgression can also occur during the harvest of intercostal nerves for transfer. A chest X-ray should be performed postoperatively when intercostal nerves are harvested. A chest tube may be required in the case of a pneumothorax.

Potential postoperative complications include hematoma or seroma, wound infection, and deafferentation pain. When the nerve roots are avulsed in preganglionic lesions, the sensory neurons in the deafferented dorsal column start to generate spontaneous signals that are felt to be the basis for the (often) intractable deafferentation pain syndrome. Patients often report a severe burning or crushing sensation in the limbs. The pain is usually severe and episodic. Treatment of deafferentation pain should start early and with a multidisciplinary approach. Antidepressants, anticonvulsants, and narcotics may play a role. The treatment must be customized to the nature of the pain and to the patient. Gabapentin is useful and has a good safety margin. Acupuncture, hypnosis, biofeedback, and various desensitization protocols can be used. In cases of refractory pain, surgical intervention to disrupt the signals generated in the dorsal root entry zone (DREZ) of the dorsal columns is the last resort when conservative measures fail. This invasive procedure is called DREZ lesioning. The patient in the case presented developed persistent pain in her arm that she described as "pouring hot water on it"; the pain was managed reasonably well with a combination of duloxetine, gabapentin, and hydromorphone.

Oral Boards Review—Complications Pearls

1. Injury to the phrenic nerve, which is adjacent to the upper trunk of the brachial plexus, can cause hemidiaphragm paralysis.
2. The thoracic duct can be injured during left-sided brachial plexus exploration.
3. A postoperative chest X-ray should be obtained when intercostal nerves are harvested to rule out pneumothorax.
4. Deafferentation pain associated with nerve root avulsion injuries can be severe and requires a multidisciplinary approach to management.

Evidence and Outcomes

Several factors may influence the final outcome. The nature of the injury, its severity and extent, other neurologic deficits, associated spinal cord injury, the patient's age, nearby skeletal fractures, and joint deformities and contractures, as well as vascular injuries are all important to consider. In the present case, the patient had multiple factors leading to a poor prognosis: total BPI with five nerve root avulsions, nearby structures with limited functionality (elbow and shoulder), and age of 46 years (older than most patients with BPI). In general, the prognosis for patients with pan-plexus injury is poor. When C5 is found to be preserved and can be used as a donor, there is somewhat better hope for shoulder and elbow function recovery.[3]

SAN to SSN transfer in pan-plexus injury patients has had mild success. In one large study, the mean recovery of shoulder abduction was 58.5°. Only approximately 40% of patients achieved any active external rotation, and in those patients, recovery was modest.[4] The modest success of this procedure has led some to consider preservation of the SAN and trapezius function for later tendon transfer. More recently, better results have been achieved with dual nerve transfer utilizing intercostal nerve to anterior branch of the axillary nerve transfer and SAN to SSN transfer. This was studied in a smaller number of patients, but mean abduction was 93.83° and mean external rotation was 54°.[5]

Both the phrenic nerve and intercostal nerves have been studied as donors for reanimation of elbow flexion in patients with pan-plexus injury. Intercostal nerve transfer to the biceps branch of the musculocutaneous nerve has shown moderate success, with two thirds of patients recovering at least antigravity elbow flexion and approximately one quarter recovering M4 or better elbow flexion in one study.[6] In another study that directly compared the phrenic nerve to the intercostal nerves as donors for elbow flexion, average elbow flexion strength was similar between the two, but the phrenic nerve had a slightly higher percentage of good outcomes (83%) than the intercostal nerves (70%).[7] In young, otherwise healthy patients with good preoperative lung function, phrenic nerve sacrifice typically results in a small decrease in lung function postoperatively that recovers over the following year.[8] The simultaneous use of intercostal nerves and the phrenic nerve significantly increases the risk of complications, and this practice is not recommended.[1,2]

Free functioning gracilis muscle transfer has been increasingly utilized in patients with pan-plexus injury.[9–12] The group at the Mayo Clinic has shown that approximately 70% of patients undergoing free functioning gracilis muscle transfer achieve at least M3 strength.[9,11] In their hands, this procedure outperformed intercostal to musculocutaneous nerve transfer, with only 42% achieving at least M3 elbow flexion in the latter group.[11] Overall, these results are encouraging.

Sensory reconstruction using intercostal nerve transfer has also shown some success. In one study, 50% to 75% of patients were able to perceive warm and/or cold and all patients in the study regained at least some useful sensation in the hand.[13] This technique shows promise in providing protective sensation to the affected hand.

The limited recovery potential of BPI has led researchers to investigate, propose, and implement several novel directions. These advances include dual free muscle transfers, nerve root reimplantation, and amputation with reanimation of myoelectric prostheses.[14–16] Ideally, future research will build on these exciting discoveries to further improve the outlook for patients with total BPI.

References

1. Kovachevich R, Kircher MF, Wood CM, Spinner RJ, Bishop AT, Shin AY. Complications of intercostal nerve transfer for brachial plexus reconstruction. *J Hand Surg Am.* 2010;35:1995–2000.
2. Kita Y, Tajiri Y, Hoshikawa S, Hara Y, Iijima J. Impact of phrenic nerve paralysis on the surgical outcome of intercostal nerve transfer. *Hand Surg.* 2015;20:47–52.
3. Kim DH, Cho YJ, Tiel RL, Kline DG. Outcomes of surgery in 1019 brachial plexus lesions treated at Louisiana State University Health Sciences Center. *J Neurosurg.* 2003;98:1005–1016.
4. Bertelli JA, Ghizoni MF. Results of spinal accessory to suprascapular nerve transfer in 110 patients with complete palsy of the brachial plexus. *J Neurosurg Spine.* 2016;24:990–995.
5. Chu B, Wang H, Chen L, Gu Y, Hu S. Dual nerve transfers for restoration of shoulder function after brachial plexus avulsion injury. *Ann Plast Surg.* 2016;76:668–673.
6. Cho AB, Iamaguchi RB, Silva GB, et al. Intercostal nerve transfer to the biceps motor branch in complete traumatic brachial plexus injuries. *Microsurgery.* 2015;35:428–431.
7. Liu Y, Lao J, Zhao X. Comparative study of phrenic and intercostal nerve transfers for elbow flexion after global brachial plexus injury. *Injury.* 2015;46:671–675.

8. Xu WD, Gu YD, Lu JB, Yu C, Zhang CG, Xu JG. Pulmonary function after complete unilateral phrenic nerve transection. *J Neurosurg*. 2005;103:464–467.
9. Barrie KA, Steinmann SP, Shin AY, Spinner RJ, Bishop AT. Gracilis free muscle transfer for restoration of function after complete brachial plexus avulsion. *Neurosurg Focus*. 2004;16:E8.
10. Krauss EM, Tung TH, Moore AM. Free functional muscle transfers to restore upper extremity function. *Hand Clin*. 2016;32:243–256.
11. Maldonado AA, Kircher MF, Spinner RJ, Bishop AT, Shin AY. Free functioning gracilis muscle transfer versus intercostal nerve transfer to musculocutaneous nerve for restoration of elbow flexion after traumatic adult brachial pan-plexus injury. *Plast Reconstr Surg*. 2016;138:483e–488e.
12. Nicoson MC, Franco MJ, Tung TH. Donor nerve sources in free functional gracilis muscle transfer for elbow flexion in adult brachial plexus injury. *Microsurgery*. 2017;37(5):377–382.
13. Hattori Y, Doi K, Sakamoto S, Yukata K. Sensory recovery of the hand with intercostal nerve transfer following complete avulsion of the brachial plexus. *Plast Reconstr Surg*. 2009;123:276–283.
14. Aszmann OC, Roche AD, Salminger S, et al. Bionic reconstruction to restore hand function after brachial plexus injury: a case series of three patients. *Lancet*. 2015;385:2183–2189.
15. Carlstedt T, Anand P, Hallin R, Misra PV, Noren G, Seferlis T. Spinal nerve root repair and reimplantation of avulsed ventral roots into the spinal cord after brachial plexus injury. *J Neurosurg*. 2000;93:237–247.
16. Doi K, Muramatsu K, Hattori Y, et al. Restoration of prehension with the double free muscle technique following complete avulsion of the brachial plexus. Indications and long-term results. *J Bone Joint Surg Am*. 2000;82:652–666.

22

Adult Upper Trunk Brachial Plexus Injury

Jared M. Pisapia, Zarina S. Ali, Gregory G. Heuer, and Eric L. Zager

Case Presentation

A 33-year-old painter presented after sustaining an injury at work when multiple cans of paint fell from an elevated shelf onto his right shoulder. He immediately experienced sharp shoulder pain and was unable to abduct the shoulder or flex the elbow. He had preserved movement of his hand and forearm. He was initially evaluated in the emergency department, where plain X-rays of the shoulder confirmed the presence of a nondisplaced clavicular fracture. The patient was managed nonoperatively with a sling. Upon follow-up 6 weeks later, the patient continued to notice impairment of shoulder movement and elbow flexion, and he had developed atrophy of the right shoulder muscles. On physical examination, there was no evidence of Horner syndrome. Visual inspection revealed atrophy of the right deltoid, infraspinatus, and biceps muscles, with glenohumeral subluxation. Motor strength testing was normal in the trapezius, rhomboids, serratus anterior, pectoralis, latissimus dorsi, triceps, pronator teres and quadratus, forearm flexor and extensor muscle groups, and hand intrinsic muscles. The patient had 1/5 strength in the deltoid, supraspinatus, infraspinatus, and biceps muscles. He had partial loss of supination. He had decreased sensation to light touch and pinprick along the lateral arm and forearm extending to the thumb. Reflexes were normal except at the right biceps, where the reflex was absent. Percussion over the supraclavicular region yielded pain and paresthesias along the lateral arm.

Questions

1. What is the most likely diagnosis?
2. What is the most likely site of injury/compression?
3. What are the next steps in the diagnostic evaluation?
4. When in relation to the time of injury should the next diagnostic steps be performed?

Assessment and Planning

A diagnosis of brachial plexus injury is suspected. Specifically, blunt injury to the upper trunk is likely, based on the mechanism of injury, pattern of muscle weakness, and pattern of sensory deficits. Stretch/contusion injuries make up approximately

50% of brachial plexus lesions, with over 35% of injuries specifically affecting the C5, C6, and/or C7 roots.[1] Caudal displacement of the shoulder in relation to the cranium places excessive traction on the upper plexus, leading to injury. Since the upper trunk is formed by the C5 and C6 spinal nerves, a lesion at this level produces weakness of the deltoid and supraspinatus muscles, resulting in loss of shoulder abduction. Atrophy of the deltoid muscle is often prominent and is easily appreciated when the affected side is compared to the contralateral side. In addition, weakness of the infraspinatus muscle results in loss of shoulder external rotation. Biceps, brachialis, and brachioradialis muscle weakness results in a lack of elbow flexion. In addition, supination is partially compromised due to biceps paralysis, although the supinator, which receives radial innervation, may be intact. Additional C7 involvement is associated with variable loss of triceps and forearm musculature. The injury pattern associated with an upper trunk injury is termed Erb's palsy, and it is characterized clinically by the waiter's tip posture—adduction and internal rotation at the shoulder and pronation and extension at the elbow. Sensory loss is commonly seen over the C5 and C6 dermatomes and may be incomplete.

When patients present with a brachial plexus injury, it is important to determine the portion of the brachial plexus that is injured and also to differentiate between pre- and postganglionic injuries, as both have important treatment implications. Preganglionic lesions typically represent root avulsions from the spinal cord. The neurologic examination can provide clues regarding pre- versus postganglionic injury. The dorsal scapular nerve innervating the levator scapulae and rhomboids arises very proximally from C5. The long thoracic nerve innervating the serratus anterior receives contributions from C5, C6, and C7, with these contributions arising very proximally. Thus, assessing the rhomboids and serratus anterior clinically and electrophysiologically is important in determining how proximal the injury is. Weakness of the rhomboid and serratus anterior muscles suggests a proximal injury, likely preganglionic. Horner syndrome, due to disruption of the sympathetic chain, suggests a preganglionic injury, specifically at the C8-T1 levels. Preganglionic injuries are often accompanied by fractures of the transverse process or first rib and generally require a high-impact mechanism of injury.

Additional electrodiagnostic and imaging studies may support the presence of a preganglionic injury. For instance, electromyography (EMG) shows loss of innervation to the cervical paraspinal muscles in a preganglionic injury. Similarly, a sensory nerve action potential (SNAP) obtained from an anesthetic finger suggests a preganglionic injury (the sensory nerve cell body in the dorsal root ganglion is intact). EMG is commonly performed 3 to 4 weeks after the injury to allow time for Wallerian degeneration to occur in case of axonotmesis or neurotmesis, so that these injury types can be differentiated from neurapraxia. CT or MR myelography can help define the level of nerve root injury and may show pseudomeningocele formation, which is suggestive of a preganglionic injury. This study should not be performed in the acute setting, as clotted blood may occlude expansion of a pseudomeningocele and yield a false-negative result. The brachial plexus may be visualized by MR imaging. Imaging findings of a pseudomeningocele or empty nerve root sleeves suggest a preganglionic injury, whereas the presence of a traumatic neuroma or widespread plexus edema suggests a postganglionic injury. Finally, an elevated hemidiaphragm may be evident on radiographic imaging due to phrenic nerve damage, which suggests a proximal, likely preganglionic, injury.

Mimics of upper trunk injury that should be considered in the differential diagnosis include rotator cuff injury, cervical disc disease at C4-C5 and C5-C6, infraclavicular plexus injury (e.g., lateral and posterior cord injury), and cervical spinal cord injury. Bilateral upper extremity symptoms should prompt consideration of a central cervical pathology. Disc herniations are commonly accompanied by neck pain and radiation of pain in a specific dermatomal distribution. Cervical spine MR imaging may demonstrate cervical cord signal change, disc herniation, or foraminal narrowing. Motor strength testing and EMG can help to differentiate the affected muscles. Ultimately, an understanding of brachial plexus anatomy will narrow the differential diagnosis.

Oral Boards Review—Diagnostic Pearls

1. Upper trunk injury is suggested by weakness in the following muscles (and corresponding movements): supraspinatus and deltoid (shoulder abduction), infraspinatus (external rotation), and biceps (elbow flexion, forearm supination).
2. Preganglionic injury is suggested by the following physical exam and imaging findings: weakness in rhomboid and serratus anterior muscles, winged scapula, lack of Tinel sign in the supraclavicular fossa, pseudomeningocele formation, elevated hemidiaphragm, Horner syndrome, and first rib and/or transverse process fractures.
3. EMG is commonly performed 3 to 4 weeks after the injury.
4. The differential diagnosis of upper trunk injury includes cervical disc disease at C4-C5 and C5-C6, rotator cuff injury, infraclavicular plexus injury, and cervical spinal cord injury.

Questions

1. What are the options for nerve reconstruction in upper trunk brachial plexus injuries and what are the advantages and disadvantages of each strategy?
2. How does evidence of pre- versus postganglionic injury influence treatment strategy?
3. How does time from injury influence the decision to operate?
4. What are the surgical objectives for restoring function in upper trunk injury?

Decision-Making

Nerve reconstruction strategies for upper trunk brachial plexus injuries include nerve graft, nerve transfer, or a combination, and each approach has advantages and disadvantages. Nerve grafting, in which one or more of the non-avulsed roots is coapted distally to a trunk, division, cord, or peripheral nerve with an interposed autologous nerve graft, has the benefit of simulating the native branching pattern of the brachial plexus. With nerve grafting, multiple distal muscles are targets for reinnervation.[2]

However, an increased number of target muscles corresponds to a reduced number of regenerating axons available to each individual muscle. Furthermore, a nerve graft requires that regenerating axons cross two coaptation sites, which may further decrease the number of axons reaching a target muscle. Time to reinnervation may be prolonged, depending on the distance from the proximal nerve stump to the target muscle. Nerve regeneration occurs at approximately 1 inch per month or 1 mm per day. Nerve grafting is only an option for postganglionic injuries with a viable nerve stump remaining.

For preganglionic injuries where nerve root stumps are not available to serve as sites for grafting, nerve transfers may be used. Fascicles from an uninjured nerve are microsurgically transferred to the distal peripheral nerve supplied by injured roots at a location proximal to the target muscle.[3] Multiple nerve transfers may be combined in a single patient to restore multiple movements. Although nerve transfers do not necessarily simulate the native branching pattern of the brachial plexus, reinnervation of the target muscle is maximized, as all regenerating axonal input is targeted to a single, smaller denervated target. Additional benefits include reduced distance and, therefore, reduced time to reinnervation of target muscle, crossing of a single suture junction, and reduced fibrosis at the operative site, as compared to the injury site.[4]

In addition to the selection of a surgical repair strategy, the timing of potential surgical intervention is a key consideration in the decision-making process. Upper trunk injuries range from neurapraxic or stretch injuries, which resolve spontaneously over time, to nerve root avulsions, which do not spontaneously recover. Surgical intervention is not warranted in neurapraxic injuries, whereas nerve reconstruction is required for the treatment of avulsion injuries. Axonotmetic injuries, in which variable axonal injury is present but with maintained epineurium, are monitored for evidence of reinnervation. In general, the optimal timing of surgery is reported to be 3 to 6 months after injury in patients who have not shown clinical reinnervation.[5] This time frame allows for spontaneous regeneration to occur after a neurapraxic injury, while not allowing too much time to pass before changes in the distal nerve stump, neuromuscular junction, and muscle preclude reinnervation following surgical repair. After 12 to 18 months of denervation, a target muscle may not be able to recover strength, even with robust nerve regeneration. Accordingly, for patients with late presentation (6 to 12 months after injury), even in the setting of a postganglionic injury with viable nerve stumps, nerve grafting may not be an option. Because nerve transfer reduces the time to reinnervation, nerve transfer is a viable option for patients with a late presentation. Some authors advocate for early surgical intervention within 3 to 6 weeks for near-total plexus involvement with a high-energy mechanism of injury in which spontaneous regeneration is highly unlikely due to severe injury.[6,7] For partial upper plexus involvement, surgery is recommended within 3 to 6 months if there is either no recovery or a plateau in neurologic recovery. If more than 1 year has passed between the time of injury and presentation, so that there is concern for muscle atrophy or failure of nerve reinnervation, orthopedic procedures, such as shoulder arthrodesis to stabilize the humeroscapular joint, lower trapezius to infraspinatus tendon transfer to restore external rotation, and single or double free gracilis muscle transfer (Doi procedure), especially in cases of pan-plexus injury, should be considered.[8–10] These secondary reconstructive options do not have the same time constraints as nerve graft repair or nerve transfer and can be performed at any time after injury. Furthermore, they remain options in the setting of primary nerve reconstruction failure.

The objective of surgical intervention is to restore upper extremity function, as loss of shoulder abduction, external rotation, elbow flexion, and forearm supination associated with C5-C6 root and upper trunk injuries results in significant disability. Although prioritization differs by surgeon, the top functional priorities of nerve reconstruction are restoration of elbow flexion, shoulder abduction, and external rotation.[11] A multinational survey of peripheral nerve surgeons supported these surgical objectives.[3]

Questions

1. What are the intraoperative options for assessing the suitability of nerve roots for grafting versus transfer?
2. What nerve repair strategies may be used in the case of C5 and C6 avulsions (preganglionic injury)?
3. What is the branching pattern of the upper trunk from cranial and posterior to caudal and anterior?
4. What are the potential complications specific to operating in the region of the upper trunk?

Surgical Procedure

For suspected upper trunk injury, the traditional approach is supraclavicular brachial plexus exploration to define the lesion, which is the basis for the repair strategy. Under general anesthesia without neuromuscular blockade, the patient is positioned supine with a folded towel between the shoulder blades to elevate the chest. The head is turned to the contralateral side and is slightly extended on a donut roll. The supraclavicular and infraclavicular regions are widely prepped (Figure 22.1A). In addition, sites of harvest for potential nerve grafts, such as the lower extremity in the case of the sural nerve, and sites of potential donor or recipient nerve, such as the upper extremity or chest, are exposed as well. Needle EMG electrodes are placed in the appropriate muscle groups for intraoperative neuromonitoring. For the supraclavicular approach, the authors perform a transverse incision approximately 1.5 cm above the clavicle and extending across the posterior triangle of the neck from the posterior edge of the sternocleidomastoid to the trapezius muscle (Figure 22.1B). The incision may be placed in a skin crease for cosmesis. The platysma is incised and a subplatysmal dissection is performed for improved superior-inferior exposure. Dissection along the posterior border of the sternocleidomastoid is performed, and the underlying fat pad is mobilized, beginning inferomedially to allow retraction superolaterally (Figure 22.2). The lateral edge of the SCM may be divided at the clavicle if necessary to optimize the exposure. Attempts are made to preserve the supraclavicular sensory nerves, posterior belly of the omohyoid muscle, and transverse cervical vessels, although these structures may be divided if needed to improve exposure. Bipolar cautery is used for hemostasis and cauterization of lymphatic

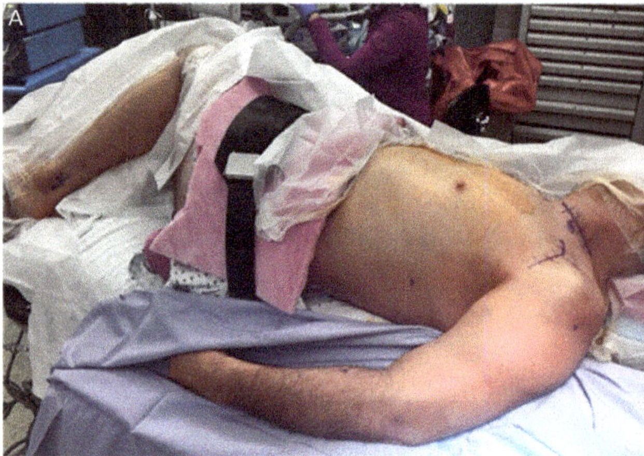

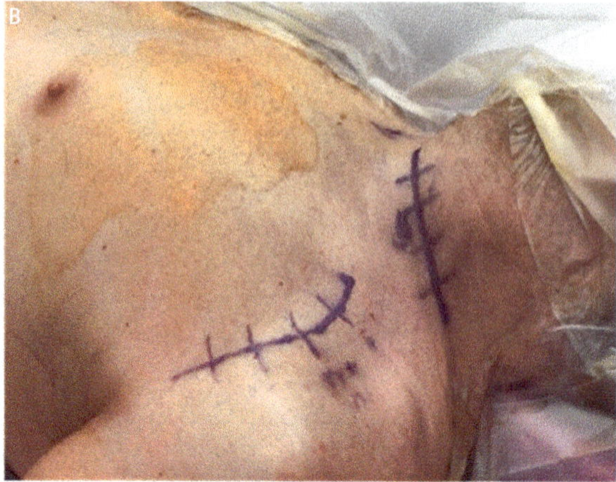

Figure 22.1. Positioning and incision for repair of upper trunk injury. A, The patient is positioned supine with the head turned to the right for a left supraclavicular brachial plexus exploration. The chest, arm, and lower leg are prepped for possible nerve graft or nerve transfer. B, An incision is marked in the supraclavicular region 1.5 cm above the clavicle and extending to the posterior edge of the trapezius muscle. The deltopectoral groove is marked for possible infraclavicular dissection, if needed.

channels. On the left side, the thoracic duct is identified if possible and is either preserved or securely ligated. An intraoperative nerve stimulator is used to confirm the identification of the phrenic nerve, which descends in a lateral to medial direction overlying the anterior scalene muscle. The nerve may be traced back to the C5 spinal nerve. The contribution of C5 to the phrenic nerve typically occurs as the phrenic nerve crosses the lateral border of the anterior scalene. Once C5 is identified, the remaining nerve roots contributing to the brachial plexus can be identified passing

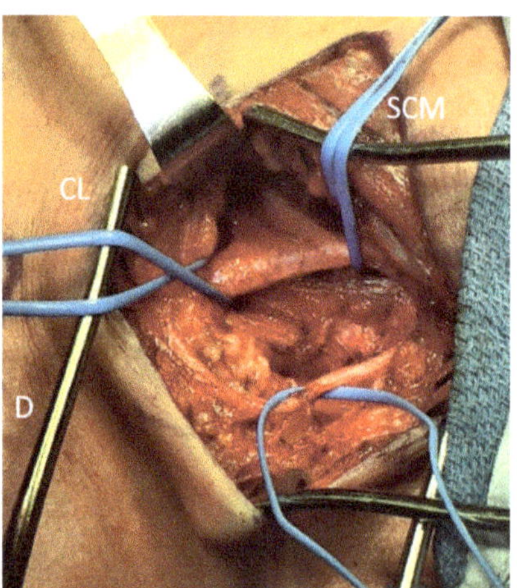

Figure 22.2. Intraoperative photograph of supraclavicular brachial plexus exploration. The phrenic nerve (blue loop, 2 o'clock position) may be traced back to the injured and enlarged upper trunk (blue loop, 9 o'clock position). A large supraclavicular sensory nerve is identified (blue loop, 6 o'clock position). CL = clavicle; D = deltoid; SCM = sternocleidomastoid muscle.

between the anterior and middle scalene muscles, along with the subclavian artery inferiorly. Once the spinal nerves are identified, circumferential dissection and external neurolysis are performed.

Nerve Grafting

Intraoperative neural stimulation and monitoring involving stimulation of spinal nerves with needle EMG in corresponding muscles are used to differentiate the exposed nerves and to identify the level of injury. If no compound motor action potential or motor responses are observed, scar tissue is resected and the nerve is sectioned sharply proximal to the site of stimulation. If healthy fascicles are observed, then the root is considered amenable to direct nerve grafting.[12] If the appearance of healthy fascicles is questionable, a frozen section of the proximal stump is examined; the presence of ganglion cells indicates nerve root avulsion and grafting from that level is not pursued. A healthy root contains greater than 50% myelinated axons.[13] If a healthy root is identified, the proximal stump is then sutured to a nerve graft (often autologous sural nerve) in an end-to-end, epineurial fashion using one or two 8-0 or 10-0 nylon sutures and reinforced with fibrin glue (Figure 22.3). Common grafts include C5 to the posterior division of the upper trunk or posterior cord.[5] Others include C5 and/or C6 to the suprascapular nerve, anterior division of the upper trunk, axillary nerve, or musculocutaneous nerve (MCN).[14] Contrary to prior anatomic diagrams in which the anterior division is more cranial than the posterior division of the upper trunk, a recent cadaveric study showed that the branching pattern of the upper trunk from cranial and posterior to caudal and anterior follows the sequence of suprascapular nerve, posterior division, and then anterior division (acronym SPA), which has important implications in both nerve grafting and nerve transfer procedures.[15] Following repair, the supraclavicular fat pad is reflected medially. Hemostasis is obtained. The wound is irrigated and is closed in anatomic layers.

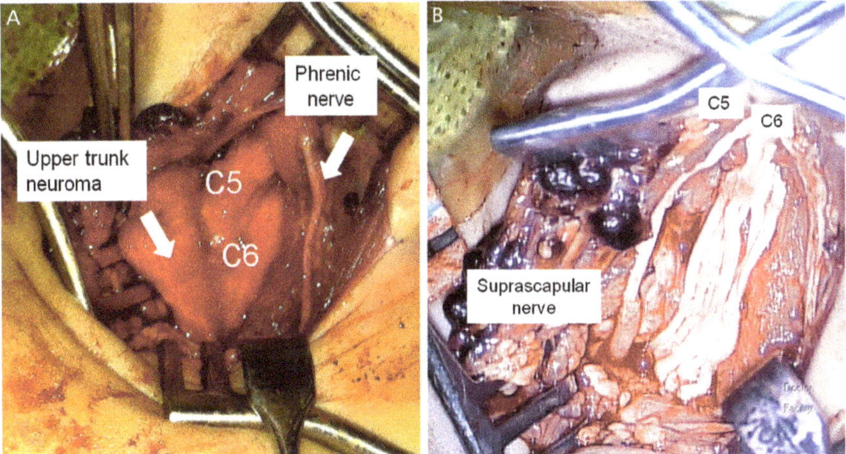

Figure 22.3. A, Supraclavicular exposure showing the phrenic nerve, C5 and C6 spinal roots, and an upper trunk neuroma. B, The neuroma is excised and multiple interpositional sural nerve grafts are placed for repair.

Nerve Transfers

If viable nerve roots are not available, as in the case of preganglionic injury, a combination of distal nerve transfers may be used for restoring upper extremity function after upper trunk injury. For instance, the Oberlin procedure involves transfer of an ulnar nerve fascicle to the biceps branch of the MCN for restoration of elbow flexion.[16] An incision is made in the medial biceps-triceps groove overlying the neurovascular bundle (Figure 22.4). The MCN is found between the biceps and brachialis muscles. The nerve is followed proximally until a prominent biceps branch is identified. The ulnar nerve is located and the epineurium is opened using microsurgical technique and the operating microscope. Gentle internal neurolysis allows separation of the fascicles (Figure 22.5A). Stimulation is applied to each fascicle and motor/EMG response is assessed. The fascicle serving the flexor carpi ulnaris with little or no hand intrinsic function is selected and is sharply divided distally (the mnemonic is "donor distal"). The biceps branch of the MCN is sectioned proximally, and the nerve stumps are brought together for coaptation (Figure 22.5B). Advantages of the nerve transfer include the short distance to denervated motor endplates, the single suture line, and the good size match between donor and recipient nerves.[17] The transfer is also done in a virgin, unscarred surgical site. A double fascicle transfer may be performed in which a fascicle of the median nerve is transferred to the brachialis branch of the MCN;

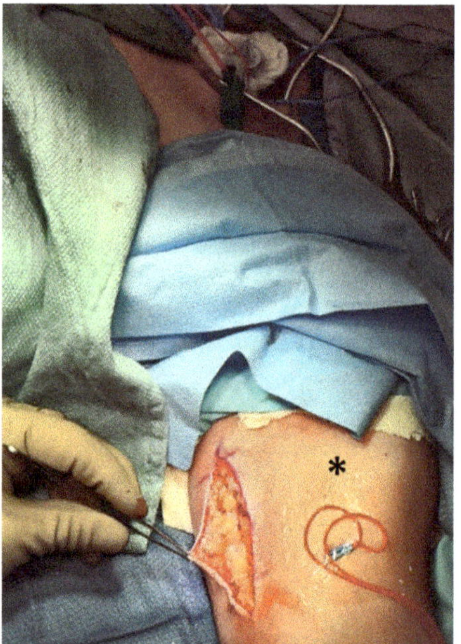

Figure 22.4. Oberlin nerve transfer. An incision is made in the medial biceps-triceps groove overlying the neurovascular bundle for transfer of an ulnar nerve fascicle to the biceps branch of the musculocutaneous nerve for restoration of elbow flexion. Asterisk (*) marks an intraoperative monitoring needle placed in the left biceps.

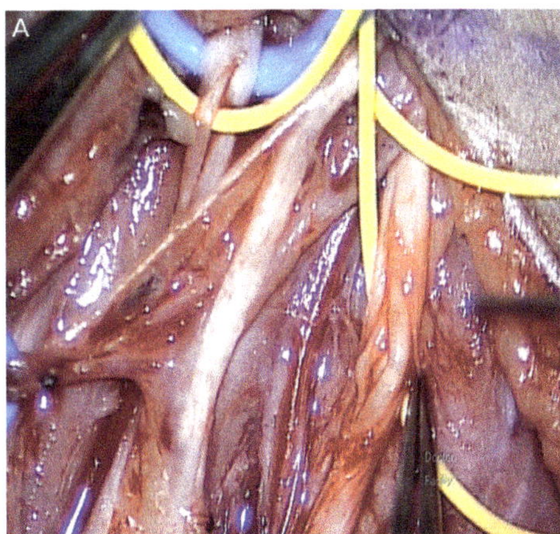

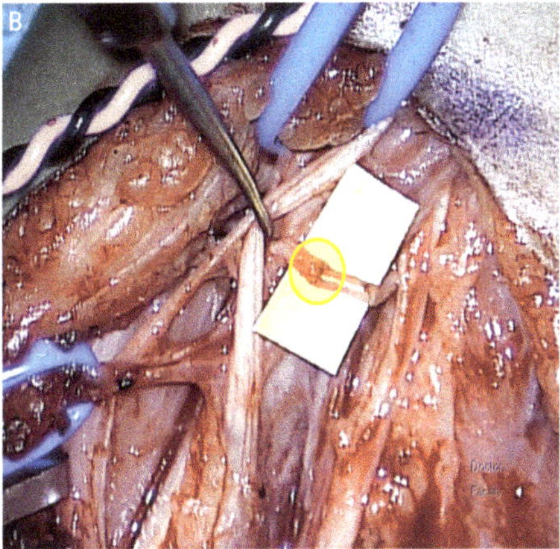

Figure 22.5. A, In the Oberlin procedure, the biceps branch (yellow loop, top left) of the musculocutaneous nerve (blue loop) is incised proximally, and internal neurolysis of the ulnar nerve (yellow loop, right) is performed. B, An ulnar fascicle is incised distally and coapted to the biceps branch (yellow circle).

however, somewhat surprisingly, a randomized study did not show a difference in outcome between the Oberlin (single transfer) and double fascicular transfer.[18–20] To restore shoulder abduction, stabilization, and external rotation, a posterior approach for double nerve transfer may be used in which the distal spinal accessory nerve is transferred to the suprascapular nerve and the medial triceps branch of the radial nerve is transferred to the axillary nerve.[21,22] Although the above three nerve transfers are commonly used in the management of upper trunk injury, many other transfers exist, with donors including the phrenic nerve, intercostal nerves, and contralateral C7 spinal nerve or middle trunk.[17] Also, combinations of nerve graft and nerve transfer may be used in select cases.

Oral Boards Review—Management Pearls

1. If a postganglionic injury is suggested by preoperative evaluation and neuromonitoring, serial sectioning of the spinal nerve may be performed to determine if healthy fascicles are present for nerve grafting.
2. Common grafts used in upper trunk injury include C5 and C6 spinal nerves to anterior and/or posterior divisions of the upper trunk, suprascapular nerve, axillary nerve, or MCN.
3. The branching pattern of the upper trunk from cranial and posterior to caudal and anterior follows the sequence of suprascapular nerve, posterior division, and then anterior division (acronym SPA).
4. Three common nerve transfers for upper trunk injury include ulnar nerve fascicle to biceps branch of the MCN, distal spinal accessory nerve to suprascapular nerve, and triceps branch of the radial nerve to axillary nerve.

Pivot Point

1. If no motor potential or motor response is observed with intraoperative nerve stimulation, then perform serial sectioning of the nerve to assess for viable fascicles.
2. If healthy fascicles are noted proximally in the C5 and C6 root, then perform nerve grafting.
3. If no healthy fascicles are noted or the C5 and C6 roots are avulsed, then perform nerve transfer.

Aftercare

To avoid tension on the coaptation sites following nerve grafting or transfer, the upper extremity is immobilized in a sling for 3 weeks postoperatively, after which time the patient can begin passive range-of-motion exercises with physical therapy. Patients are kept in the hospital for observation overnight. A chest X-ray is obtained if the patient experiences any respiratory distress. Potential diagnoses include paralyzed hemidiaphragm due to phrenic nerve injury, pneumothorax, and chylothorax. Many patients experience severe neuropathic pain, especially following root avulsion injury, and multidisciplinary management with pain specialists is recommended.

Complications and Management

Potential complications include failure of the nerve graft or transfer and injury to structures surrounding the brachial plexus trunks. Iatrogenic injury to the brachial plexus or phrenic nerve may occur during exposure. Laceration of the phrenic nerve may be treated with primary repair. All open lymph channels should be ligated, clipped, or coagulated. A chylothorax may result from injury to the thoracic duct, which enters the venous system on the left side of the body at the junction of the left internal jugular vein with the subclavian vein. It may be treated with a fat-free diet, open re-exploration, or endovascular embolization of the thoracic duct in select cases.[23] Pneumothorax may occur in exposure of the lower plexus and is treated by a chest tube. Additional complications include subclavian or axillary artery injury, hematoma, and infection.

Oral Boards Review—Complication Pearls

1. Sharp laceration of the phrenic nerve should be repaired primarily at the time of injury.
2. The thoracic duct is located at the junction of the left internal jugular vein and left subclavian artery.
3. Chylothorax and pneumothorax are possible complications of brachial plexus surgery.
4. All open lymph channels should be ligated, clipped, or coagulated.
5. Secondary reconstructive strategies, such as free muscle transfer, joint fusion, and tendon transfer, should be considered when primary nerve reconstruction fails.

Evidence and Outcomes

There is ongoing debate in the literature about the optimal surgical approach for repair of brachial plexus injuries. Supraclavicular exploration followed by nerve grafting when feasible is the traditional approach for upper trunk injuries. In a large series of supraclavicular stretch lesions, among 34 cases where nerve grafting was performed from C5 and C6 to the anterior and posterior divisions of the upper trunk, 19 patients recovered to Medical Research Council (MRC) grade 3, eight patients to grade 4, and seven patients to grade 3 to 4.[14] More recently, some authors have proposed nerve transfer as the initial and primary strategy due to the favorable outcomes associated with certain transfers. For instance, over 90% of patients achieved grade 4 elbow flexion following the Oberlin procedure.[24] For the double transfer to restore shoulder function, 78% achieved better than grade 3 and 46% achieved grade 4 or higher.[2] Furthermore, in a comparative effectiveness study, the Oberlin procedure and nerve transfers were more effective in restoring elbow flexion and shoulder abduction than nerve grafting or a combination of nerve grafting and transfer.[4] Supraclavicular exploration with nerve grafting is still widely accepted as the gold standard for upper trunk repair because it permits the surgeon to define the pathoanatomy and to subsequently devise an individualized treatment plan.[2] However, several authors make an exception in the case of isolated elbow flexion weakness, due to the reliability of the Oberlin procedure.[2,4,25] As experience with nerve transfers continues to increase, further research is required to continually refine the indications for each treatment approach.

References

1. Kim DH, Murovic JA, Tiel RL, Kline DG. Mechanisms of injury in operative brachial plexus lesions. *Neurosurg Focus*. 2004;16:E2.
2. Yang LJ, Chang KW, Chung KC. A systematic review of nerve transfer and nerve repair for the treatment of adult upper brachial plexus injury. *Neurosurgery*. 2012;71:417–429, discussion 429.
3. Belzberg AJ, Dorsi MJ, Storm PB, Moriarity JL. Surgical repair of brachial plexus injury: a multinational survey of experienced peripheral nerve surgeons. *J Neurosurg*. 2004;101:365–376.
4. Ali ZS, Heuer GG, Faught RW, et al. Upper brachial plexus injury in adults: comparative effectiveness of different repair techniques. *J Neurosurg*. 2015;122:195–201.
5. Giuffre JL, Kakar S, Bishop AT, Spinner RJ, Shin AY. Current concepts of the treatment of adult brachial plexus injuries. *J Hand Surg Am*. 2010;35:678–688.
6. Jivan S, Kumar N, Wiberg M, Kay S. The influence of pre-surgical delay on functional outcome after reconstruction of brachial plexus injuries. *J Plast Reconstr Aesthetic Surg*. 2009;62:472–479.
7. Kay SP, Wiberg M, Thornton DJ. Nerves are living structures whose injury requires urgent repair. *J Plast Reconstr Aesthetic Surg*. 2010;63:1939–1940.
8. Barrie KA, Steinmann SP, Shin AY, Spinner RJ, Bishop AT. Gracilis free muscle transfer for restoration of function after complete brachial plexus avulsion. *Neurosurg Focus*. 2004;16:E8.
9. Doi K, Kuwata N, Muramatsu K, Hottori Y, Kawai S. Double muscle transfer for upper extremity reconstruction following complete avulsion of the brachial plexus. *Hand Clin*. 1999;15:757–767.
10. Elhassan B, Bishop A, Shin A, Spinner R. Shoulder tendon transfer options for adult patients with brachial plexus injury. *J Hand Surg Am*. 2010;35:1211–1219.

11. Songcharoen P, Wongtrakul S, Spinner RJ. Brachial plexus injuries in the adult. nerve transfers: the Siriraj Hospital experience. *Hand Clin.* 2005;21:83–89.
12. Kline DG, Hudson AR. Diagnosis of root avulsions. *J Neurosurg.* 1997;87:483–484.
13. Malessy MJ, van Duinen SG, Feirabend HK, Thomeer RT. Correlation between histopathological findings in C-5 and C-6 nerve stumps and motor recovery following nerve grafting for repair of brachial plexus injury. *J Neurosurg.* 1999;91:636–644.
14. Kim DH, Cho YJ, Tiel RL, Kline DG. Outcomes of surgery in 1019 brachial plexus lesions treated at Louisiana State University Health Sciences Center. *J Neurosurg.* 2003;98:1005–1016.
15. Hanna A. The SPA arrangement of the branches of the upper trunk of the brachial plexus: a correction of a longstanding misconception and a new diagram of the brachial plexus. *J Neurosurg.* 2016;125:350–354.
16. Oberlin C, Beal D, Leechavengvongs S, Salon A, Dauge MC, Sarcy JJ. Nerve transfer to biceps muscle using a part of ulnar nerve for C5-C6 avulsion of the brachial plexus: anatomical study and report of four cases. *J Hand Surg Am.* 1994;19:232–237.
17. Ray WZ, Chang J, Hawasli A, Wilson TJ, Yang L. Motor nerve transfers: a comprehensive review. *Neurosurgery.* 2016;78:1–26.
18. Carlsen BT, Kircher MF, Spinner RJ, Bishop AT, Shin AY. Comparison of single versus double nerve transfers for elbow flexion after brachial plexus injury. *Plast Reconstr Surg.* 2011;127:269–276.
19. Mackinnon SE, Novak CB, Myckatyn TM, Tung TH. Results of reinnervation of the biceps and brachialis muscles with a double fascicular transfer for elbow flexion. *J Hand Surg Am.* 2005;30:978–985.
20. Martins RS, Siqueira MG, Heise CO, Foroni L, Teixeira MJ. A prospective study comparing single and double fascicular transfer to restore elbow flexion after brachial plexus injury. *Neurosurgery.* 2013;72:709–714, discussion 714–715.
21. Bertelli JA, Ghizoni MF. Results of spinal accessory to suprascapular nerve transfer in 110 patients with complete palsy of the brachial plexus. *J Neurosurg Spine.* 2016;24:990–995.
22. Colbert SH, Mackinnon S. Posterior approach for double nerve transfer for restoration of shoulder function in upper brachial plexus palsy. *Hand (N Y).* 2006;1:71–77.
23. Nadolski GJ, Itkin M. Thoracic duct embolization for nontraumatic chylous effusion: experience in 34 patients. *Chest.* 2013;143:158–163.
24. Leechavengvongs S, Witoonchart K, Uerpairojkit C, Thuvasethakul P, Ketmalasiri W. Nerve transfer to biceps muscle using a part of the ulnar nerve in brachial plexus injury (upper arm type): a report of 32 cases. *J Hand Surg Am.* 1998;23:711–716.
25. Garg R, Merrell GA, Hillstrom HJ, Wolfe SW. Comparison of nerve transfers and nerve grafting for traumatic upper plexus palsy: a systematic review and analysis. *J Bone Joint Surg Am.* 2011;93:819–829.

Neonatal Brachial Plexus Palsy

Raymond Tse and Angelo B. Lipira

23

Case Presentation

A 3-week-old boy presents to the multidisciplinary brachial plexus clinic because his parents are concerned about the function of his right upper extremity. The parents state that, since birth, he has not seemed to move the arm, and he holds it to his side. He is otherwise healthy. Pregnancy was significant for gestational diabetes, and the child is at the 95th percentile for weight. Labor was prolonged and difficult. Detailed examination reveals an absence of shoulder abduction, external rotation, elbow flexion, and forearm supination (Figure 23.1). The infant is observed to open and close his right hand, as well as flex and extend the wrist. There are no signs of Horner syndrome.

Questions

1. What is the most likely diagnosis and what structures are involved?
2. What are the appropriate next steps to establish the diagnosis?
3. What is the appropriate timing for the diagnostic workup?

Assessment and Planning

The brachial plexus surgeon suspects a birth-related brachial plexus injury involving the upper trunk (C5 and C6 roots). The differential diagnosis includes "pseudoparalysis," meaning lack of movement due to pain related to a non-neurologic injury or process, such as clavicular fracture or a septic shoulder joint. Congenital limb differences, such as arthrogryposis, and central nervous system lesions may also be confused with plexus injury. The diagnoses can usually be distinguished on the basis of physical exam and plain X-rays, if musculoskeletal injuries are suspected. In the case of a fracture or infection, lack of movement is due to pain and resolves with bony healing or resolution of infection.

Neonatal brachial plexus palsy occurs in 0.5 to 3 out of 1000 live births.[1] The majority of infants recover spontaneously, but 10% to 30% do not, and they will benefit from surgical intervention.[2,3] Despite this, for unclear reasons, surgery appears to be underutilized in this patient population.[4] Establishing care early with an experienced multidisciplinary brachial plexus team is critical, as proper diagnosis and management require close follow-up with serial examinations.

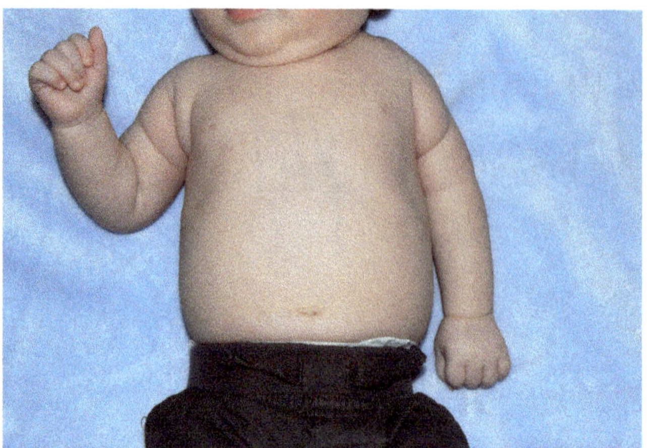

Figure 23.1. Patient presentation. Exam reveals absence of shoulder abduction, external rotation, elbow flexion, and forearm supination.

Multiple root levels of the brachial plexus (C5 through T1) can be involved. The upper trunk (C5 and C6) is most frequently injured, typically from traction that widens the neck–shoulder angle during birth. With increasing severity of injury, lower roots are progressively affected. Presentations can generally be grouped into four patterns according to the Narakas grading scale. Type I involves C5 and C6 deficits (Erb-Duchenne type) with loss of shoulder abduction, shoulder external rotation, elbow flexion, and forearm supination. The limb assumes the Erb posture due to intact antagonist muscles. Type II involves C5 to C7/ C8 deficits (extended Erb type), resulting in the additional loss of elbow and wrist extension. The limb assumes the waiter's tip posture. Type III involves deficits from C5 to C8-T1, resulting in an arm that is generally flaccid or paralyzed. Type IV involves C5 to T1 plus the sympathetic chain, resulting in a flail arm and Horner syndrome. Horner syndrome, defined by unilateral ptosis, miosis, and anhidrosis, indicates injury to the sympathetic chain, which arises near the root of T1. This suggests a proximal injury to the T1 root, but it does not indicate the degree of injury; resolution by 1 month suggests neurapraxia, while persistence is seen in more severe injury types.

The diagnostic challenge for the brachial plexus surgeon is to determine the severity of injury and the potential for recovery. This can only be accomplished through detailed serial exams documenting the evolution of recovery. The authors reserve MR imaging and electromyography (EMG) for patients in whom the decision to proceed with surgical treatment has been made. Some centers, however, utilize these studies earlier in an effort to dichotomize those likely to recover and those unlikely to recover spontaneously.[5–7] Indications for surgical intervention remain controversial. Traditionally, lack of elbow flexion at 3 months has been used as a surgical indication by many surgeons; however, there is evidence that this may be overly aggressive, as a number of these patients will recover function spontaneously.[3,8,9] Many surgeons have since made their operative indications more conservative, considering surgery only when a child has not recovered elbow flexion by 5 or 6 months of age. Given that a single motor function may not fully represent the status of the entire brachial plexus, the authors tend to follow the Toronto protocol, which

Table 23.1.
The Hospital for Sick Children Active Movement Scale

Observation	Grade
Gravity eliminated	
No contraction	0
Contraction, no motion	1
Motion < ½ range	2
Motion > ½ range	3
Full motion	4
Against gravity	
Motion < ½ range	5
Motion > ½ range	6
Full motion	7

Source: Clarke HM, Curtis CG. An approach to obstetrical brachial plexus injuries. *Hand Clinics.* 1995;11(4):563–580.

involves application of the Active Movement Scale (AMS; Table 23.1) and considers specific clinical scenarios.[10] Surgical exploration is recommended in cases of total flail arm (pan-plexus palsy) with persistent Horner syndrome beyond 1 month, when the composite AMS score for elbow flexion, elbow extension, wrist extension, thumb extension, and finger extension is < 3.5 at 3 months, when there is lack of progressive recovery of elbow flexion at 6 months, and when the child is unable to pass the cookie test (composite movement of getting the hand to the mouth with the arm adducted) at 9 months of age.

Once the decision to proceed with surgery has been made, imaging to assess for nerve root avulsion(s) can help with surgical planning. Nerve root avulsion is a preganglionic injury rendering the root nonfunctional and unavailable as a proximal source of axons for target reinnervation. For imaging, the authors prefer MR myelography, as it does not require lumbar puncture or radiation exposure and is highly sensitive in detecting pseudomeningoceles, which are predictive of root avulsion.[11,12] Despite these potential advantages, some centers continue to prefer CT myelography. If nerve transfers are anticipated, EMG can be useful in identifying potential donor nerves for transfer, given that some donor nerves may be affected by the brachial plexus injury. The authors routinely employ ultrasound to assess the function of the diaphragm, because the phrenic nerve can be intertwined in neuroma and limit respiratory reserve.

Questions

1. Which levels of the brachial plexus are affected in the present case?
2. When is the appropriate time for surgical intervention in the present case? What factors should be considered?
3. When is the appropriate time to intervene for an infant with pan-plexus palsy and persistent Horner syndrome?

Oral Boards Review—Diagnostic Pearls

1. The brachial plexus consists of cervical nerves 5 through 8 (C5-C8) and thoracic nerve 1 (T1), with variable contributions from C4 (pre-fixed) or T2 (post-fixed).
2. Physical examination is the key to accurate diagnosis. All other diagnostic modalities (imaging and EMG) should be considered extensions of the physical examination. Lower regions of the plexus are involved with increasing severity of traction and injury. Narakas classified injury types based on extent of root involvement:[13]
   a. Type I (Erb-Duchenne type)—C5 and C6 are affected and the injury presents with loss of shoulder abduction, shoulder external rotation, elbow flexion, and forearm supination. Type I is the most common type.
   b. Type II (extended Erb type)—C5 to C7 (± C8) are affected. Presents with same deficits as in Type I plus loss of elbow and wrist extension, resulting in waiter's tip posture.
   c. Type III (flail limb)—C5 to C8-T1 are affected. Presents with flaccid, paralyzed arm.
   d. Type IV (flail limb with Horner syndrome)—C5 to T1 and the sympathetic chain are affected. Presents with flail arm and Horner syndrome, suggesting proximal T1 injury.
3. Isolated lower plexus palsy involving C8 and T1 (Klumpke's palsy) is extremely rare in neonatal brachial plexus palsy. It classically presents as a clawed hand from loss of ulnar nerve and intrinsic hand muscle function, but there is intact shoulder and elbow function. This injury pattern results from upward traction on the brachial plexus.
4. Both CT and MR myelography are widely used to assess for root avulsions; however, the authors prefer MR myelography because it avoids both lumbar puncture and radiation.
5. Plain X-rays are useful to rule out rib and clavicular fractures and cervical ribs. Skeletal injuries may present with pseudoparalysis of the extremity, which can be confused with brachial plexus injury.
6. Ultrasound is useful to identify hemidiaphragm paralysis from phrenic nerve involvement. This can be missed on plain chest X-rays depending on the stage of the respiratory cycle.

Decision-Making

Once it is determined that spontaneous recovery will be inadequate, a surgical plan is devised based upon preoperative clinical examination and imaging. Neuroma excision and grafting remains the standard approach for nerve reconstruction (Figure 23.2). Nerve transfers sacrifice a functioning nerve to innervate a nonfunctioning nerve and have gained in popularity for adult brachial plexus reconstruction, but their role in neonatal brachial plexus palsies has yet to be fully defined. Nerve grafts take advantage of the abundant proximal regenerating axons, allow for anatomic

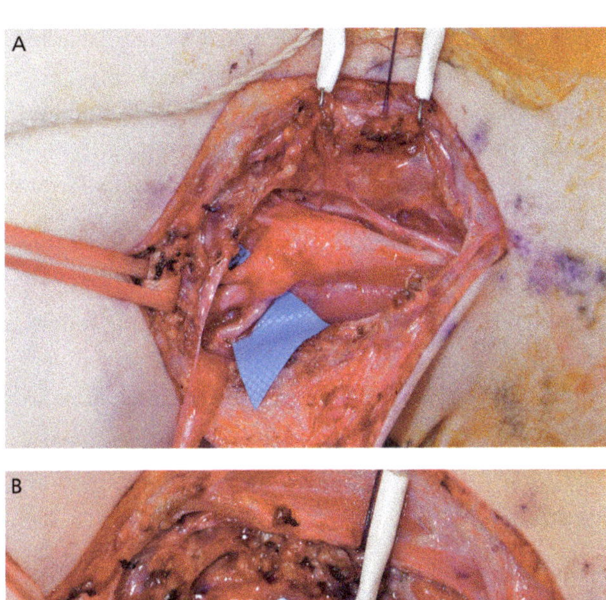

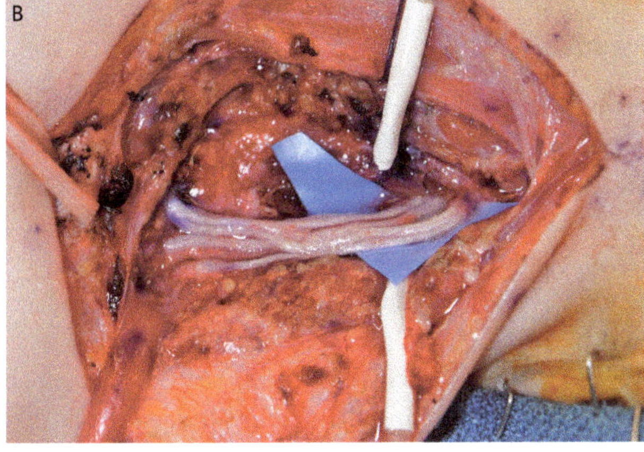

Figure 23.2. A, Surgical exposure of a large neuroma of the upper trunk of the brachial plexus. B, Final result after excision of the neuroma and sural nerve cable grafting of C5 and C6 to the suprascapular nerve, anterior division, and posterior division.

reconstruction, and avoid sacrifice of motor donors. Nerve transfers reduce the distance between regenerating axons and the target, allow for greater motor-to-motor specificity, require fewer sites of coaptation, and can be technically easier to perform. The use of nerve transfers as a primary means of reconstruction in neonatal injuries, when nerve grafting is an option, is controversial, as nerve grafting may provide a greater number of axons, and the effect on growth and development of sacrificing donor nerves for transfers is unknown. Furthermore, in more severe palsies (Narakas Type II or worse), the use of nerve transfers as a primary strategy may leave deficits unaddressed. The use of nerve transfers in addition to grafting when insufficient proximal donors exist is widely accepted. In our practice, we first utilize all available proximal nerve stumps for axon donation through nerve grafting. If distal recipients exceed available proximal donors, as in the case of multiple root avulsions, we employ nerve transfers in addition to grafting. In these situations, we commonly use spinal accessory to suprascapular nerve and intercostal to musculocutaneous nerve transfers.

There is a role for nerve transfers in delayed presentations, isolated deficits, and failed primary reconstructions. It is important to note that, in anything other than a

Narakas Type I palsy, donor nerves for transfer may be unavailable and nerve transfers alone will leave some or many motor deficits unaddressed.[11]

Further intraoperative decision-making will depend on findings of the exploration, direct electrical stimulation of the proximal nerve roots, and histologic examination of cut ends to determine the relative quality of proximal stumps.

> **Questions**
>
> 1. What is the significance of finding evidence of multiple root avulsions on preoperative MR myelography?
> 2. What are the pros and cons of nerve transfer in neonatal brachial plexus reconstruction?

Surgical Procedure

Brachial plexus exploration and reconstruction is a major surgical procedure performed under general anesthesia. The patient is positioned supine with the head turned away from the injured side to allow access to the posterior triangle via an L-shaped incision. The horizontal limb of the incision parallels the clavicle and the vertical limb parallels the posterior sternocleidomastoid (SCM) muscle (Figure 23.3). A superolaterally based subplatysmal flap is elevated, revealing the supraclavicular fat pad, external jugular vein, and cervical plexus. Cervical plexus branches are traced back to the C4 root and phrenic nerve. The supraclavicular fat pad is then divided along the posterior SCM and superior clavicle, revealing the omohyoid muscle, which is typically divided and tagged with suture for repair at the end of the case. The transverse cervical vessels are often encountered at this level as well and may be ligated if necessary. The upper trunk of the brachial plexus is found just deep to the omohyoid and is often

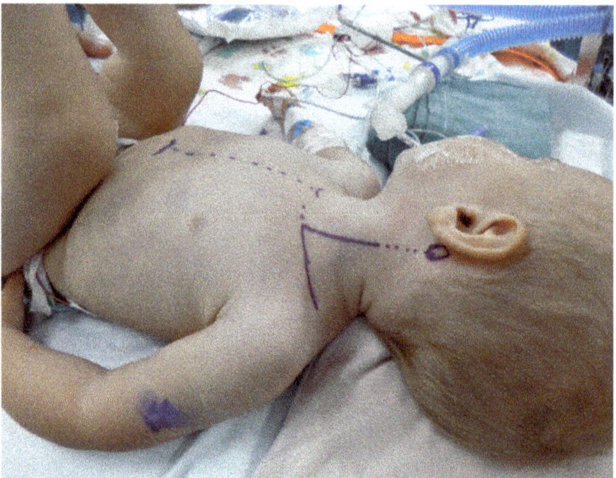

Figure 23.3. The patient is positioned supine with the head turned away from the injured side to allow access the posterior triangle via an L-shaped incision. The horizontal limb of the incision parallels the clavicle and the vertical limb parallels the posterior sternocleidomastoid.

heavily scarred and distorted. The phrenic nerve is carefully mobilized, and it can be followed from C4 to find the upper trunk (C5 and C6). The neuroma is carefully separated from the anterior and middle scalenes. The upper trunk branches are then identified distally under the clavicle and followed proximally toward the trifurcation of the anterior division, posterior division, and suprascapular nerve. The lower roots are then exposed by dissecting further caudally between the anterior and middle scalenes, while heading more posterior with each progressively lower root. In cases of rupture or avulsion, the anatomy may be extremely distorted, and, due to retraction, the structures normally found in the supraclavicular space may be found in the infraclavicular space. Once identified, each nerve root is assessed by direct visualization and possibly by electrical stimulation, but much of the decision to excise a portion of the plexus is based upon preoperative function, because a response to stimulation is not necessarily indicative of useful motor function. In neonates, the utility of intraoperative electrophysiologic testing (nerve conduction and evoked potentials) is controversial. The injured nerve segments are excised to healthy-appearing nerve. It is the authors' practice to send frozen sections to pathology for analysis, although this is not universally done at all centers. The combination of the histologic appearance of the proximal nerve roots and the response to electrical stimulation is used to determine the relative quality of proximal nerve roots for nerve grafting.

Bilateral sural nerves are typically harvested through three small transverse incisions on each leg (Figure 23.4). If visualization is difficult, an endoscope is used. A plan is then made based on preoperative exam, findings of the exploration, direct electrical stimulation of proximal nerve roots, and histologic examination of the cut ends. For upper trunk injuries with available proximal C5 and C6 roots, we typically graft C5 to the suprascapular nerve, anterior division, and posterior division, and C6 to the anterior and posterior divisions (Figure 23.5). For more severe injuries with lower-level root involvement and multiple avulsions, we typically prioritize cable grafts for hand function (C8 and T1) and employ nerve transfers for other functions (e.g., spinal accessory to suprascapular nerve, intercostals to musculocutaneous nerve). Nerve coaptation is performed under an operative microscope, securing grafts with fibrin glue proximally and then distally, working from deep to superficial. Additional supplementation with suture is optional. The grafts are tailored so that they are tension-free in the position of greatest length, with the head rotated and abducted away from the affected side. The omohyoid is repaired, and the supraclavicular fat pad is repaired over the grafted nerves to provide protection and a gliding surface. The skin is closed in layers.

Oral Boards Review—Management Pearls

1. Care must be taken when working deep to the junction of the SCM and the clavicle to avoid injury to the thoracic duct (left side) or the subclavian vessels.
2. Excessive retraction of the SCM may expose the carotid sheath and expose the internal jugular vein and carotid artery to potential injury.
3. Reconstructive priorities are hand function, elbow flexion, and shoulder stability and function.

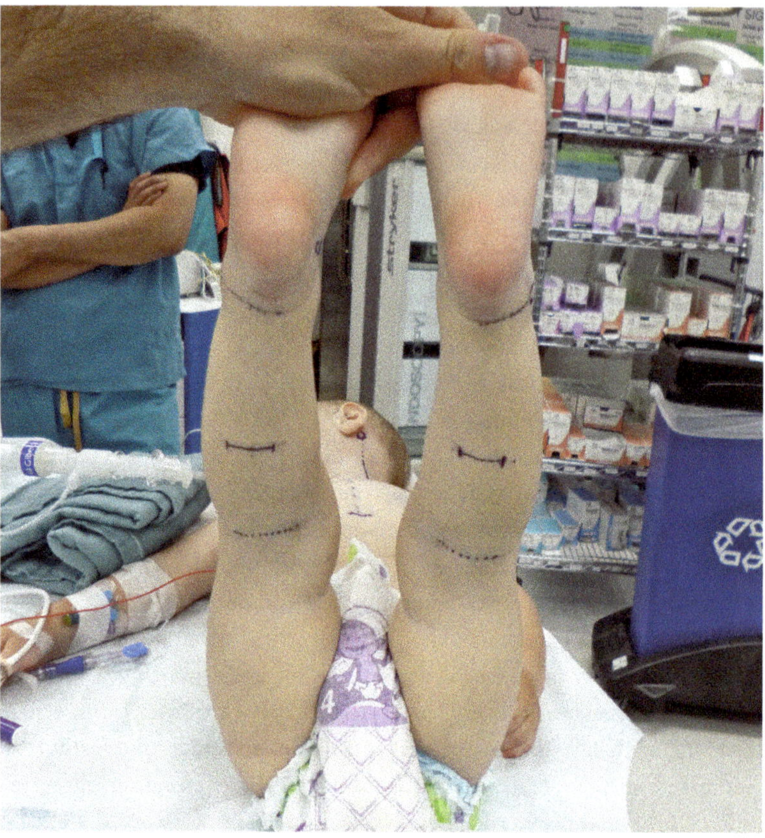

Figure 23.4. Bilateral sural nerves are harvested through three small transverse incisions on each leg. The proximal incision is placed in a natural crease behind the knee, and the distal incision in a natural crease lateral to the Achilles tendon. The middle incision is placed at the musculotendinous junction of the gastrocnemius and Achilles tendon.

Pivot Points

1. Patients with too few proximal donors (e.g., multiple root avulsions, pan-plexus palsy) often require nerve transfers using extra-plexal donors in addition to cable grafting.
2. The availability of proximal donors is ultimately not known until intraoperative exploration, so the surgeon must be prepared for multiple possible scenarios (e.g., nerve transfers in addition to grafting).

Aftercare

Infants are immobilized for 3 to 5 weeks. If the shoulder is supple and there is no significant glenoid dysplasia on preoperative MR imaging, a cuff-and-collar sling is used

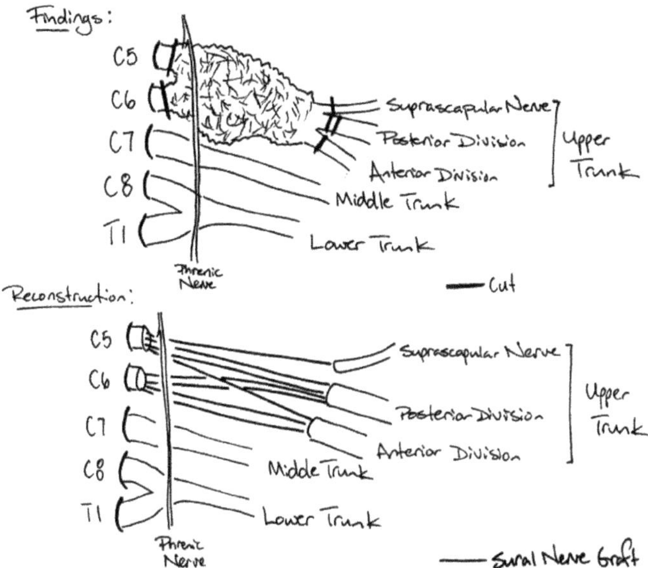

Figure 23.5. Sketch from operative note depicting neuroma of upper trunk and planned cable nerve graft reconstruction of suprascapular nerve, anterior division, and posterior division from C5 and C6 roots.

for 3 weeks, followed by an additional 2 weeks of leaving the arm within the shirt (i.e., the arm is not brought through the sleeve) to avoid significant abduction. If the shoulder is stiff and there is significant glenohumeral dysplasia, the internal rotators are temporarily denervated with botulinum toxin A and the shoulder is stretched into external rotation using a shoulder spica cast for the full 5 weeks. In all cases, range-of-motion stretching is resumed after 5 weeks.

Complications and Management

There are many critical structures in the vicinity of the brachial plexus that the surgeon must be aware of. Overly aggressive traction on the supraclavicular fat pad or excessive retraction of the SCM can pull the carotid sheath into the operative field and place its contents at risk. Phrenic nerve injury with transient or permanent diaphragm dysfunction can occur if the nerve is not handled gently. Bipolar cautery should be used in the division of the fat pad to seal the lymphatics and to avoid postoperative lymph leak and/or lymphocele. On the left side, the thoracic duct is at risk during dissection posterior to the SCM–clavicle junction. During proximal root dissection, the vertebral artery is at risk for injury. In injuries where the lower trunk must be accessed (e.g., pan-plexus injury), the subclavian vessels must be cautiously separated and the lung apex must be avoided.

Musculoskeletal problems, including internal rotation contracture and glenohumeral dysplasia, are common, and treatments include physical therapy, shoulder reduction and casting, botulinum A injection for motor imbalance, and surgeries, including shoulder tendon transfers and humeral osteotomy.

Oral Boards Review—Complication Pearls

1. Structures at risk include the carotid artery, internal jugular vein, phrenic nerve, thoracic duct, subclavian vessels, and nerves of the brachial plexus itself.
2. All neonatal brachial plexus patients require ongoing physical therapy and monitoring for musculoskeletal sequelae.

Evidence and Outcomes

When following the Toronto protocol in the treatment of neonatal brachial plexus palsy, reasonable expectations are for 90% of patients to have improvements, 5% to 10% of patients to have no improvements beyond baseline, and 1% to 5% of patients to experience functional losses related to a complication or failed reinnervation. Following reconstruction, neuromotor function may be initially diminished, but it should return to preoperative levels by 6 months if nerve reconstruction is successful. Improvements continue from there but tend to plateau at 2 to 3 years after surgery.

References

1. Borschel GH, Clarke HM. Obstetrical brachial plexus palsy. *Plast Reconstr Surg.* 2009;124:144e–155e.
2. Pondaag W, Malessy MJ, van Dijk JG, Thomeer RT. Natural history of obstetric brachial plexus palsy: a systematic review. *Dev Med Child Neurol.* 2004;46:138–144.
3. Waters PM. Comparison of the natural history, the outcome of microsurgical repair, and the outcome of operative reconstruction in brachial plexus birth palsy. *J Bone Joint Surg Am.* 1999;81:649–659.
4. Squitieri L, Steggerda J, Yang LJ, Kim HM, Chung KC. A national study to evaluate trends in the utilization of nerve reconstruction for treatment of neonatal brachial plexus palsy [outcomes article]. *Plast Reconstr Surg.* 2011;127:277–283.
5. Malessy MJ, Pondaag W, Yang LJ, Hofstede-Buitenhuis SM, le Cessie S, van Dijk JG. Severe obstetric brachial plexus palsies can be identified at one month of age. *PLOS ONE.* 2011;6:e26193.
6. Van Dijk JG, Pondaag W, Buitenhuis SM, Van Zwet EW, Malessy MJ. Needle electromyography at 1 month predicts paralysis of elbow flexion at 3 months in obstetric brachial plexus lesions. *Dev Med Child Neurol.* 2012;54:753–758.
7. Vanderhave KL, Bovid K, Alpert H, et al. Utility of electrodiagnostic testing and computed tomography myelography in the preoperative evaluation of neonatal brachial plexus palsy. *J Neurosurg Pediatr.* 2012;9:283–289.
8. Gilbert A, Pivato G, Kheiralla T. Long-term results of primary repair of brachial plexus lesions in children. *Microsurgery.* 2006;26:334–342.
9. Michelow BJ, Clarke HM, Curtis CG, Zuker RM, Seifu Y, Andrews DF. The natural history of obstetrical brachial plexus palsy. *Plast Reconstr Surg.* 1994;93:675–680, discussion 681.
10. Clarke HM, Curtis CG. An approach to obstetrical brachial plexus injuries. *Hand Clin.* 1995;11:563–580, discussion 580–561.

11. Somashekar D, Yang LJ, Ibrahim M, Parmar HA. High-resolution MRI evaluation of neonatal brachial plexus palsy: A promising alternative to traditional CT myelography. *AJNR Am J Neuroradiol.* 2014;35:1209–1213.
12. Tse R, Nixon JN, Iyer RS, Kuhlman-Wood KA, Ishak GE. The diagnostic value of CT myelography, MR myelography, and both in neonatal brachial plexus palsy. *AJNR Am J Neuroradiol.* 2014;35:1425–1432.
13. Narakas AO. *The paralysed hand.* Edinburgh: Churchill Livingstone;1987.

Axillary Nerve Injury

Russell A. Payne and Elias B. Rizk

24

Case Presentation

A 43-year-old male presents to the peripheral nerve clinic 6 months after a snow skiing accident. During the accident, he struck a tree, resulting in an anterior dislocation of his right shoulder. His shoulder was reduced after approximately 3 hours. Evaluation at that time was negative for associated fracture or rotator cuff tear. His shoulder was immobilized in a sling for 3 weeks. He then began a course of physical therapy. He initially had difficulty abducting his arm past approximately 30°. However, over the course of 6 months, he has regained nearly normal shoulder abduction. He has noted atrophy of his right deltoid muscle over that time. He complains of a constant, dull ache in his shoulder. He also fatigues easily when engaged in overhead activities or when his right arm is abducted. On examination, all active and passive range of motion is normal, with the exception of forward flexion of the shoulder, which is limited. Deltoid motor examination reveals no muscle activation. External rotation of the right shoulder is 4+/5. The remainder of the motor examination is normal. There is significant atrophy of the deltoid (Figure 24.1). Sensory examination is normal. A nerve conduction study (NCS)/electromyogram (EMG) was obtained and showed normal median and ulnar nerve motor conduction studies, normal amplitudes, and normal latencies. Sensory studies were normal in the median, ulnar, and lateral antebrachial cutaneous distributions. Ulnar and median nerve F-latencies were normal. On EMG examination, there was continuous spontaneous activity (3+ fibrillation potentials/positive sharp waves) in the deltoid. Motor unit action potentials (MUAPs) could not be elicited in the deltoid. The biceps, latissimus dorsi, levator scapulae, and rhomboids were normal.

Questions

1. Which nerves are affected and what are their courses? Which muscles do they innervate?
2. What physical exam findings are consistent with damage to the affected nerves?
3. What is the significance of the NCS/EMG findings?
4. What are the important factors related to timing of NCS/EMG studies?

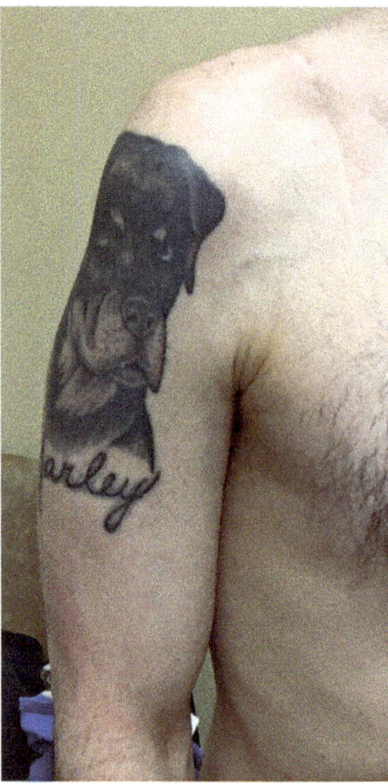

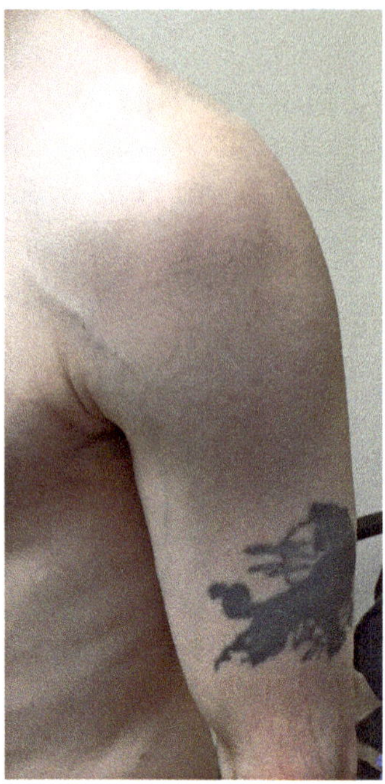

Figure 24.1. Side-by-side comparison of the deltoid muscles demonstrating profound atrophy.

Assessment and Planning

A diagnosis of an isolated axillary nerve injury is made. The axillary nerve carries fibers from C5-C6 and arises from the posterior cord, wraps over the inferior edge of the subscapularis and travels with the posterior humeral circumflex artery through the quadrangular space. It then travels around the surgical neck of the humerus and divides into anterior and posterior branches. The anterior branch primarily provides motor innervation to the anterior and middle deltoid but also gives off several small cutaneous branches. The posterior branch provides innervation to the posterior deltoid and teres minor and then continues on to become the superior lateral brachial cutaneous nerve.

Axillary nerve injury has been associated with a variety of sports, both contact and noncontact.[1] Neurologic injuries are well known to be associated with shoulder trauma, particularly anterior dislocation of the shoulder. The incidence of neuropathy associated with anterior shoulder dislocation is reported to be as high as 65%.[2,3] Among the associated nerve injuries, the axillary nerve is the most commonly injured nerve.[2] A common association is the triad of anterior shoulder dislocation, peripheral nerve injury, and rotator cuff tear.[4,5] Thus, when a patient presents with anterior dislocation of the shoulder, it is important to assess the rotator cuff and to assess for peripheral nerve injury. Patients with the full triad have poorer outcomes than patients with only one or two findings of the triad.[6]

The axillary nerve innervates the deltoid and teres minor muscles. The deltoid is the major abductor of the shoulder, particularly past approximately 30°. The teres minor contributes to external rotation of the arm. Shoulder abduction and external rotation can be remarkably good despite complete loss of axillary nerve function. In addition to the deltoid, the rotator cuff muscles (i.e., supraspinatus, infraspinatus, and subscapularis) also contribute to abduction of the shoulder. While these muscles are optimally oriented to abduct the shoulder over the first 30°, when the axillary nerve is injured, the muscles can take on a compensatory role, making for nearly normal range of motion. With the loss of the rotator cuff either through concomitant nerve injury to the suprascapular nerve or rotator cuff tear, significant disability with loss of shoulder abduction will be apparent.[7,8] While range of motion can appear remarkably normal with an isolated axillary nerve injury, because the rotator cuff muscles are not optimally oriented for abduction beyond 30°, the shoulder will fatigue easily, which often will limit activities.[9] Patients with isolated axillary nerve injuries are often very functional but are highly dependent on the rotator cuff muscles for functionality. Since rotator cuff tears increase with age and since loss of deltoid function may predispose to rotator cuff tears, restoration of axillary nerve function is important for preventing severe disability.[9–12] Teres minor function is also lost in axillary nerve palsies. While the teres minor muscle contributes to external rotation of the arm, the infraspinatus is the major external rotator. Thus, loss of the teres minor will result in only minor weakness of external rotation.

Electrodiagnostic studies are useful in determining the extent of injury and, perhaps more importantly, extent of reinnervation and recovery. It is important both that the clinical examination be followed sequentially and that sequential electrodiagnostic studies be used to extend the clinical examination to determine if reinnervation and recovery are present. The presence of MUAPs on neurophysiologic testing means that there are axons in continuity with the target organ. This may be due to collateral sprouting as early as 12 weeks after injury or due to axonal regeneration later on.

Oral Boards Review—Diagnostic Pearls

1. In isolated axillary nerve injury, shoulder abduction and external rotation can be remarkably normal as long as the rotator cuff is intact. A common finding is fatigability that limits activities due to loss of deltoid function.
2. In general, NCS/EMG should be done 3 to 6 weeks after injury. Prior to this time, fibrillations do not appear on EMG.
3. The presence of MUAPs on neurophysiologic testing means that there are axons in continuity with the target organ. This may be due to collateral sprouting as early as 12 weeks after injury or due to axonal regeneration later on. Either way, this finding excludes nerve grafting or nerve transfer as a treatment option. The absence of MUAPs on testing for several months suggests a lack of recovery.

Questions

1. What factors influence whether surgical intervention should be performed?
2. What is the timing of surgery?
3. Broadly speaking, what are the options for nerve repair?

Decision-Making

The patient in the presented case is 6 months from his injury and has no clinical or electrodiagnostic signs of recovery. Six months is sufficient time to allow for spontaneous recovery in the case of a neurapraxic injury. With no signs of recovery, surgical exploration should be offered. There is no absolute consensus regarding the appropriate observation period before offering surgical exploration. However, most agree that a period of 3 to 6 months is appropriate with sequential clinical examinations and electrodiagnostic studies. It is important not to delay surgery, as denervation atrophy can render muscles useless even in the setting of neurotization. Decision-making is difficult when minor recovery is observed but seems to plateau without a functional level of deltoid activity. Some favor earlier surgical intervention because a shorter delay from injury to surgery has been associated with improved outcomes, but, even with significant delay in surgery (i.e., 12 months or possibly longer), good outcomes can be achieved.[13,14]

In general, nerve repair can be divided into direct nerve repair, nerve grafting, and nerve transfers. At 3 to 6 months after injury, the authors generally favor surgical exploration of the axillary nerve with intraoperative nerve action potential (NAP) monitoring. In cases where there is a neuroma-in-continuity and NAPs are present across the lesion, we favor neurolysis alone. In cases where NAPs are absent across the lesion, we favor resection of the neuroma, with primary repair if possible or graft repair if the gap is too wide for primary repair. We typically use the sural nerve for graft material, but other sources could be utilized, including the superficial radial sensory nerve or the medial antebrachial cutaneous nerve. Outcomes with this approach have generally been favorable.[1,14–16]

In cases of longer delay between injury and surgery, the authors favor nerve transfer. The typical nerve transfer operation that we utilize is transfer of a triceps branch of the radial nerve to the axillary nerve via a posterior approach. In general, nerve transfer for isolated axillary nerve injury has favorable outcomes that are comparable to nerve graft repair.[12,17] How these options relate to time between injury and surgery, however, is unclear.

Many nerve transfers have been described in the literature, and a multitude of donor nerves have been proposed.[18] In general, the donor nerve should be one that has not been affected severely by the injury, it should carry a healthy number of motor fibers, and other muscles should duplicate the action of the muscle it innervates so that there is not significant loss of function. Spatially, the donor and recipient nerves must be closely related.

Orthopedic procedures may be possible in the event of nerve surgery failure or when the delay from injury to evaluation is too long for nerve surgery to be a viable option. The options include tendon transfer and, in some cases, shoulder fusion. While tendon transfer options are not the primary concern when considering options for nerve transfer, the tendon transfer options should at least be considered when selecting the nerve donor.

Questions

1. What is the anatomy of the quadrangular space and the triangular interval?
2. Is there a role for neuromonitoring in this case? What kind?
3. How can one assess for axonal continuity intraoperatively?
4. How is nerve graft length related to recovery?

Surgical Procedure

The patient presented has an isolated axillary nerve palsy and is 6 months from his injury. In a case like this, the authors favor an anterior infraclavicular approach for exploration of the axillary nerve with intraoperative NAP monitoring.

The procedure is performed under general anesthesia without the use of paralytic agents to allow for neuromonitoring. The patient is positioned supine with the arm slightly abducted. An incision is made from the clavicle to the axilla in the deltopectoral groove. As dissection is deepened, the cephalic vein is identified running in the deltopectoral groove. The muscle fibers of the deltoid and pectoralis major are identified and separated. Separating and retracting the deltoid from the pectoralis major allows for identification of the muscle fibers of the pectoralis minor attaching to the coracoid process. Note that, on the lateral portion of the coracoid process, the short head of the biceps and the coracobrachialis originate. The pectoralis minor can then be suture-tagged and divided. Retraction of the divided pectoralis minor reveals the cords of the brachial plexus and the axillary artery. First, the lateral cord is identified and looped. Neurolysis of the lateral cord is then performed as distal as possible and the lateral cord contribution to the median nerve is identified. The median nerve is then dissected free from the axillary artery. Next, the lateral cord is gently retracted to allow identification of the posterior cord. Neurolysis of the posterior cord is then performed, with identification of the thoracodorsal nerve and branches to the subscapularis along its course. The division of the posterior cord into the radial nerve and axillary nerve is then identified. The axillary artery is retracted medially, typically with an encircling Penrose drain, to allow further exposure of the axillary nerve. Neurolysis of the axillary nerve is continued distally until its entrance into the quadrangular space. At this point, intraoperative NAPs are recorded across the identified lesion. If NAPs are present across the lesion, neurolysis alone is performed. In cases where NAPs are absent across the identified neuroma-in-continuity, the neuroma is resected and graft repair is performed. In this case, NAPs were absent. The neuroma was resected and sural nerve was harvested and was used for nerve graft repair. In cases where the lesion is extensive, the anterior infraclavicular approach can be combined with a posterior approach to allow exposure of normal axillary nerve distal to its passage through the quadrangular space, where nerve graft coaptation can be performed. Alternatively, the posterior approach can be utilized to perform transfer of a triceps branch of the radial nerve to the axillary nerve, rather than performing nerve graft repair with a long graft.

Once the nerve graft repair is performed, typically using two 9-0 nylon sutures and Tisseel fibrin sealant at each coaptation site, then the pectoralis minor is reattached to the coracoid process. The wound is copiously irrigated. The incision is closed in layers.

Oral Boards Review—Management Pearls

1. Surgery should not be delayed in patients that have shown no recovery on repeat clinical examination and electrodiagnostic testing. Typically, surgery is undertaken 3 to 6 months after injury, if no improvement is observed. Waiting longer can result in irreversible denervation atrophy and limited recovery.
2. Nerve grafting and nerve transfer are both acceptable options for isolated axillary nerve injury.

Pivot Points

1. If intraoperative stimulation of the nerve in question causes activation of the target muscle, the nerve is in continuity. For best results, the nerve should undergo neurolysis instead of reconstruction.
2. For best results, normal fascicular anatomy should be identified in both the proximal/donor segment and the distal/recipient segment.

Aftercare

All incisions are closed with absorbable sutures and Steri-Strips. The extremity is not immobilized, but a sling is used for comfort. Strenuous activity is restricted until after follow-up; however, use of the extremity is encouraged. After nerve transfer, patients work with a physical therapist in order to increase functionality of the limb. We counsel our patients that recovery will not be immediate because the peripheral nervous system regenerates at about 1 inch per month.

Complications and Management

The complications are the same as the complications of most nerve surgeries. All patients have a risk of infection and difficulty with wound healing, at both the primary operative site and the donor site. Preoperatively, it is important to discuss with the patient the possibility of no improvement or even worsening function after surgery, because the donor nerve or surrounding nerves manipulated during exposure may be injured. Vascular injury, while rare, can be life threatening. In cases of vascular injury, it is important to gain proximal and distal control of the vessel in order to control the bleeding and then to enlist the help of vascular surgery colleagues for definitive management. In cases of unsuccessful nerve surgery, consultation with orthopedic surgery may be beneficial for consideration of orthopedic procedures, such as tendon transfer.

Evidence and Outcomes

There are no randomized controlled trials that compare nerve graft repair versus nerve transfer for reconstruction of the axillary nerve. The superiority of one technique over the other cannot be determined. While nerve grafting has a long history in nerve surgery, the use of nerve transfers is a more recent development, with many favoring nerve transfer over nerve grafting due to its relative ease and low morbidity. Transfers have traditionally been reserved for preganglionic injuries, such as root avulsions, but are now being used in postganglionic injuries as well. Others favor nerve grafting, citing the higher ratio of proximal to distal motor fibers as well as the superiority of the anatomic reconstruction. A review of the literature reveals no consensus on this subject. Regardless, the overall outcomes for isolated axillary nerve palsy are good.

Kline and Kim reported a large series of solitary axillary nerve palsies. They utilized an approach similar to that described in this chapter: exploration of the axillary nerve via an anterior infraclavicular approach and intraoperative NAP monitoring. Among their cohort, 46 patients had complete preoperative loss of axillary nerve function and absent NAPs intraoperatively. Of the 46, three underwent resection of the neuroma with primary repair and 43 required nerve graft repair. Mean postoperative deltoid strength was 3.8 on the LSU scale.[16]

Lee and colleagues[19] reported outcomes of surgical intervention for 26 isolated axillary nerve injuries associated with sports. They also utilized an approach similar to that described in this chapter. When the lesion was regular and NAPs were present across the lesion, neurolysis alone was performed. When the lesion was irregular, regardless of the results of NAP testing, the lesion was resected and repaired primarily or graft repaired. Among nine patients with partial loss of axillary nerve function and positive NAPs in whom neurolysis alone was performed, the mean postoperative deltoid grade was LSU 4.2.

Bonnard and colleagues[13] found that 85% of patients with isolated axillary nerve palsy who underwent nerve graft repair regained useful deltoid function (M3 or better on the Medical Research Council grading scale). They found that the time from injury to surgery and patient age contributed to the likelihood of success. When time from injury to surgery exceeded 5.3 months, the outcome was worse than when the time was less than 5.3 months. Based on these results, Bonnard and colleagues favor surgery at 3 months after injury. They also found that advancing age decreased the likelihood of a successful outcome.[13]

While Bonnard et al. found that delay in repair is associated with worsened outcomes, when evaluation is unavoidably delayed, there are data to support delayed repair with good outcomes. In 12 patients who underwent axillary nerve graft repair an average of 11.25 months after the injury, all 12 regained at least M3 deltoid function.[14] Some consider a significant lag between injury and surgery to be an indication for nerve transfer rather than graft repair. Nerve transfer has also been shown to be successful for isolated axillary nerve palsy. In one series, ten patients with an isolated axillary nerve palsy and an intact rotator cuff underwent transfer of a triceps branch of the radial nerve to the axillary nerve an average of 7.4 months after injury. At last follow-up, eight of the ten patients had regained M3 or better deltoid strength. No donor-site morbidity was noted.[12] Factors that have been shown to reduce the likelihood of a good outcome for triceps branch to axillary nerve transfer for isolated axillary nerve injury include increased time between injury and surgery, increasing body mass index, and increasing age.[19]

In addition, some consider the need for a long nerve graft to be an indication for nerve transfer rather than nerve graft repair. Wolfe et al. compared the outcome of long nerve grafts (>10 cm) with the outcome of triceps branch to axillary nerve transfer. They found that there was no significant difference between the two groups, with both groups achieving comparable deltoid function and range of motion.[17]

Overall, outcomes are generally favorable after surgical reconstruction of isolated axillary nerve palsy. Both nerve graft repair and nerve transfer are viable options for reconstruction. Whether time from injury and/or nerve graft length should be considered when determining whether to perform a nerve transfer rather than nerve graft repair remains unclear. The present data support the conclusion that good outcomes can be achieved both with long nerve grafts and with delayed nerve graft repair. Nonetheless, for optimal outcomes, time from injury to surgery should be minimized to 3 to 6 months when possible, and the shortest feasible nerve graft should be utilized in nerve graft repair.

References

1. Lee S, Saetia K, Saha S, Kline DG, Kim DH. Axillary nerve injury associated with sports. *Neurosurg Focus*. 2011;31:E10.
2. Payne MW, Doherty TJ, Sequeira KA, Miller TA. Peripheral nerve injury associated with shoulder trauma: a retrospective study and review of the literature. *J Clin Neuromuscul Dis*. 2002;4:1–6.
3. Visser CP, Coene LN, Brand R, Tavy DL. The incidence of nerve injury in anterior dislocation of the shoulder and its influence on functional recovery. A prospective clinical and EMG study. *J Bone Joint Surg Br*. 1999;81:679–685.
4. Gonzalez D, Lopez R. Concurrent rotator-cuff tear and brachial plexus palsy associated with anterior dislocation of the shoulder. A report of two cases. *J Bone Joint Surg Am*. 1991;73:620–621.
5. Guven O, Akbar Z, Yalcin S, Gundes H. Concomitant rotator cuff tear and brachial plexus injury in association with anterior shoulder dislocation: unhappy triad of the shoulder. *J Orthop Trauma*. 1994;8:429–430.
6. Brown TD, Newton PM, Steinmann SP, Levine WN, Bigliani LU. Rotator cuff tears and associated nerve injuries. *Orthopedics*. 2000;23:329–332.
7. Alnot JY, Liverneaux P, Silberman O. [Lesions to the axillary nerve]. *Rev Chir Orthop Reparatrice Appar Mot*. 1996;82:579–589.
8. Escamilla RF, Yamashiro K, Paulos L, Andrews JR. Shoulder muscle activity and function in common shoulder rehabilitation exercises. *Sports Med*. 2009;39:663–685.
9. Bertelli JA, Ghizoni MF. Nerve transfer from triceps medial head and anconeus to deltoid for axillary nerve palsy. *J Hand Surg Am*. 2014;39:940–947.
10. Sher JS, Uribe JW, Posada A, Murphy BJ, Zlatkin MB. Abnormal findings on magnetic resonance images of asymptomatic shoulders. *J Bone Joint Surg Am*. 1995;77:10–15.
11. Tempelhof S, Rupp S, Seil R. Age-related prevalence of rotator cuff tears in asymptomatic shoulders. *J Shoulder Elbow Surg*. 1999;8:296–299.

12. Wheelock M, Clark TA, Giuffre JL. Nerve transfers for treatment of isolated axillary nerve injuries. *Plast Surg (Oakv).* 2015;23:77–80.
13. Bonnard C, Anastakis DJ, van Melle G, Narakas AO. Isolated and combined lesions of the axillary nerve. A review of 146 cases. *J Bone Joint Surg Br.* 1999;81:212–217.
14. Moor BK, Haefeli M, Bouaicha S, Nagy L. Results after delayed axillary nerve reconstruction with interposition of sural nerve grafts. *J Shoulder Elbow Surg.* 2010;19:461–466.
15. Coene LN, Narakas AO. Operative management of lesions of the axillary nerve, isolated or combined with other nerve lesions. *Clin Neurol Neurosurg.* 1992;94:S64–S66.
16. Kline DG, Kim DH. Axillary nerve repair in 99 patients with 101 stretch injuries. *J Neurosurg.* 2003;99:630–636.
17. Wolfe SW, Johnsen PH, Lee SK, Feinberg JH. Long-nerve grafts and nerve transfers demonstrate comparable outcomes for axillary nerve injuries. *J Hand Surg Am.* 2014;39:1351–1357.
18. Ray WZ, Chang J, Hawasli A, Wilson TJ, Yang L. Motor nerve transfers: a comprehensive review. *Neurosurgery.* 2016;78:1–26.
19. Lee JY, Kircher MF, Spinner RJ, Bishop AT, Shin AY. Factors affecting outcome of triceps motor branch transfer for isolated axillary nerve injury. *J Hand Surg Am.* 2012;37:2350–2356.

Spinal Accessory Nerve Injury

Kevin Chan, Rishi Dihr, and Michael Fox

25

Case Presentation

A 30-year-old female presents with a 7-month history of persistent weakness and pain in the right shoulder after a lymph node biopsy from the right side of her neck under local anesthesia. She recalls experiencing sudden, severe pain during the procedure. On examination, there is a well-healed surgical scar in the posterior triangle of the neck. Percussion elicits a positive Tinel sign. There is obvious drooping of the right shoulder, wasting of the trapezius, and lateral scapular winging (Figure 25.1). The patient is unable to shrug her right shoulder. Active right shoulder abduction is approximately 60° (Figure 25.2) and forward elevation is approximately 100° (Figure 25.3).

Questions

1. What is the likely diagnosis?
2. What is the differential diagnosis?
3. What diagnostic test(s) can be ordered?

Assessment and Planning

Injury to the spinal accessory nerve (SAN) is suspected. A thorough history and physical examination, combined with an understanding of the anatomy of the SAN, are essential. The differential diagnosis includes both traumatic and atraumatic causes, including penetrating or blunt trauma to the neck, fracture malunion, glenohumeral instability, brachial neuritis, progressive neuromuscular disease, and cerebrovascular accident. However, the key to diagnosis is careful history taking, as the answer lies in the history of the presenting complaint. SAN injuries are historically iatrogenic. Surgeries in the posterior triangle of the neck that can injure the SAN include lymph node biopsies, excision of masses, or radical neck dissection for cancer. A high index of suspicion is needed, as the diagnosis is unfortunately frequently delayed. Average time to presentation of SAN injury is 6 months, and the outcomes for nerve repair are time-related.

If the history is not clear, radiographs of the cervical spine, chest, and shoulder can be obtained to rule out alternative causes. CT or MR imaging is needed if a mass is suspected. The most useful investigation is an electrodiagnostic test consisting of both nerve conduction studies (NCS) and electromyography (EMG). EMG can identify denervation changes in the sternocleidomastoid (SCM) muscle and/or trapezius

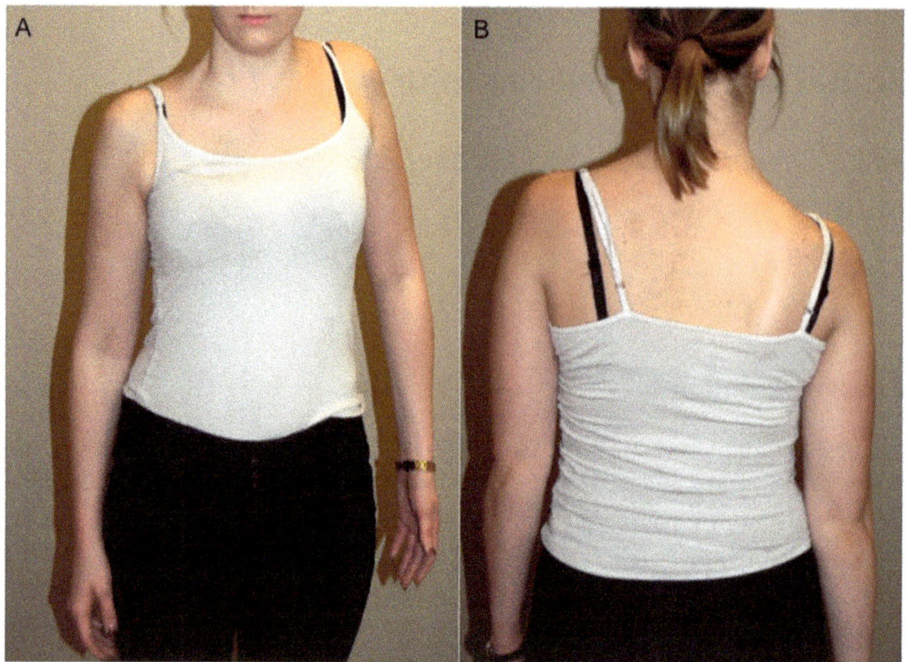

Figure 25.1. A and B, Photographs demonstrating clinical features of spinal accessory nerve palsy, including drooping of the affected shoulder, wasting of the trapezius, and lateral scapular winging.

muscle. After lymph node biopsy in the posterior triangle, SCM innervation will be normal, but the trapezius will show the fibrillations and positive sharp waves of denervated muscle. Serial electrodiagnostic tests can evaluate for signs of improvement if a neurapraxic injury was originally suspected. The majority of these injuries are neurotmesis or axonotmesis, and the surgeon should have a low threshold for exploration.

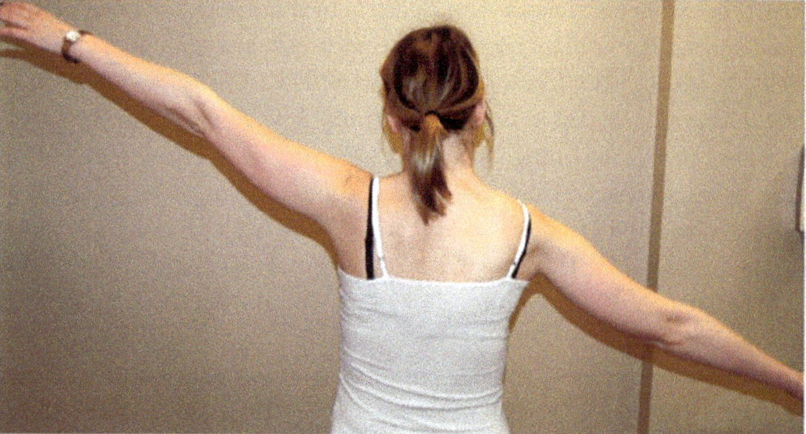

Figure 25.2. Patients with spinal accessory nerve palsy will have decreased shoulder abduction and subacromial impingement, because the paralyzed trapezius cannot rotate the scapula out of the way.

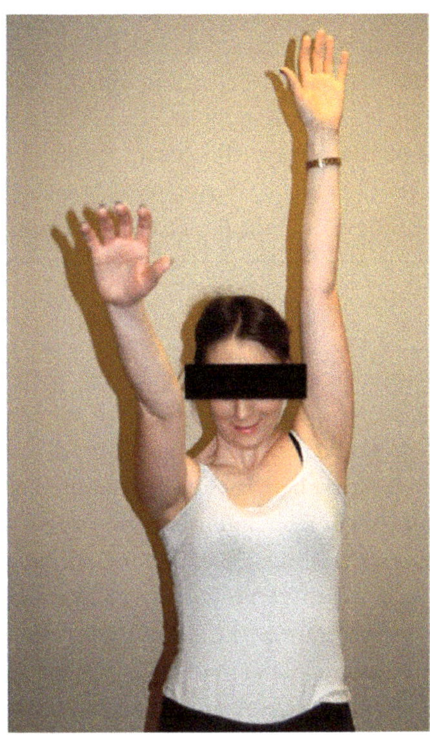

Figure 25.3. In spinal accessory nerve palsy, patients can generally achieve greater shoulder forward flexion than abduction due to compensation from surrounding muscles, including the anterior deltoid and the pectoralis major.

In the case presented, EMG shows active and chronic denervation of the right trapezius, with reduced motor recruitment and 2+ fibrillations. EMG of the right SCM is normal.

Oral Boards Review—Diagnostic Pearls

1. A meticulous history is mandatory. The examiner should elicit the nature of the dysfunction or disability, its onset, and its course to date. Every attempt should be made to elucidate the cause. Questions should be directed at identifying a history of trauma or neck surgery and its relation to the onset of symptoms, or any recent illnesses.
2. Paralysis of the trapezius results in characteristic physical exam findings:
   a. Asymmetry of the shoulder contour, with atrophy of the trapezius and drooping of the affected side.
   b. Lateral scapular winging, where the scapula drops down and away from the spine and posterior chest wall. The scapula is destabilized by the weight of the limb and is pulled forward by the unopposed serratus anterior. This contrasts with medial scapular winging caused by long thoracic nerve palsy.
   c. Inability to shrug the shoulder on the affected side.

d. An inability to abduct the affected shoulder beyond 90°, with an ability to forward flex to a greater level. This finding is due to compensation by surrounding muscles, including the anterior deltoid and the pectoralis major. In addition, the paralyzed trapezius results in an inability to rotate the scapula out of the way during shoulder abduction, leading to subacromial impingement, which may become symptomatic.

Decision-Making

As with all nerve injuries, management is dependent upon the type and severity. Nonoperative treatment is appropriate for neurapraxic injuries caused by traction on the upper limb. Serial electrodiagnostic tests and clinical examinations are used to follow these patients, starting with a baseline evaluation 3 to 6 weeks after injury, when denervation changes can be seen, followed by serial tests every 6 to 8 weeks until nerve recovery. Conservative treatment may also be indicated for patients with limited life expectancy or older patients with sedentary lifestyles or minimal symptoms.

Surgical indications include immediate deficits after penetrating trauma or surgery in the neck. In these situations, the probability of nerve laceration is high and the chance of spontaneous recovery is slim. The recommended approach is surgical exploration of the nerve and direct repair or nerve graft. Another surgical indication is the absence of clinical and electrodiagnostic improvements on serial examinations.

The critical time limit from date of injury to repair is unknown, but results are better if surgery is performed within 6 months of injury. Surgical options for chronic trapezius palsy in which the potential for muscle reinnervation has been lost include static and dynamic procedures. Static operations include scapulothoracic fusion or fasciodesis, in which fascial grafts stabilize the scapula to the vertebral spinous processes. These procedures have gradually fallen out of favor because results tended to deteriorate over time. Dynamic operations include the Eden-Lange muscle transfer, which involves the lateral transfer of the levator scapula, rhomboid minor, and rhomboid major muscles. Variations of this procedure exist, with recent modifications aimed at stabilization by attachment of the transferred muscles more laterally on the spine of the scapula, to better reproduce the function of the upper portion of the trapezius.

Questions

1. What are the anatomic landmarks for surgery?
2. Which structures should be noted to avoid perioperative morbidity?

Surgical Procedure

The SAN emerges from beneath the SCM about 5 to 10 mm cephalad to the point where the greater auricular nerve begins its upward course over the anterior face of the muscle (in the upper one half to one third of the distance from the sternum to the mastoid). After supplying the SCM, the nerve descends obliquely in the posterior triangle of the neck (bordered by the SCM anteriorly, trapezius posteriorly, and clavicle at the base) between the superficial and deep layers of the deep cervical fascia, where it is embedded in loose connective tissue and is in contact with the cervical lymph node chain. This is the most common site for iatrogenic injuries during lymph node biopsy. It is at this point that the SAN subtends its most superficial course. The nerve provides two or three branches to the upper part of the trapezius before passing under its anterior edge. It follows an oblique caudal course intramuscularly toward the middle and lower trapezius, giving branches to the muscle throughout its course.

Clinically, if the trapezius muscle is held between the surgeon's forefinger and thumb in a pinch grip, the anterior digit will accurately identify the entry point of the SAN into the muscle (Figure 25.4). This greatly helps in identification of the distal nerve, particularly in a scarred field. The patient should be positioned in a beach chair position or supine with a roll under the shoulders to encourage neck extension. The head can be turned to the contralateral side, as for a supraclavicular brachial plexus exploration. Excessive lateral rotation should be avoided. The neck, chest, and entire upper limb should be prepped and draped into the surgical field. Muscle relaxation is avoided to allow use of electrical stimulation to confirm identification of the SAN.

Surgical exposure can be approached by making a transverse incision about 2 cm above the clavicle. At times, however, exposure is completed by extending the original incision, because most cases of SAN palsy are iatrogenic. The platysma is divided in line with the skin incision, and subplatysmal flaps are bluntly developed to aid in exposure. The SAN is identified on the ventral surface of the trapezius. It can also be identified proximally as it emerges behind the SCM and traced distally. Primary treatment is neurolysis and/or primary repair or grafting of the nerve (Figure 25.5). Donor graft options can include the medial cutaneous nerve of the forearm, sural nerve, or supraclavicular nerve. A single or double supraclavicular nerve graft makes a good size match and lies within the surgical field, avoiding the need for further incisions. If

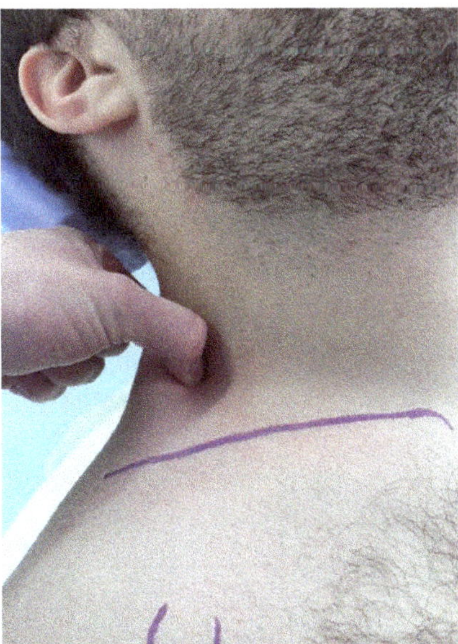

Figure 25.4. If the trapezius muscle is held between the surgeon's forefinger and thumb in a pinch grip, the anterior digit will accurately identify the entry point of the spinal accessory nerve into the muscle.

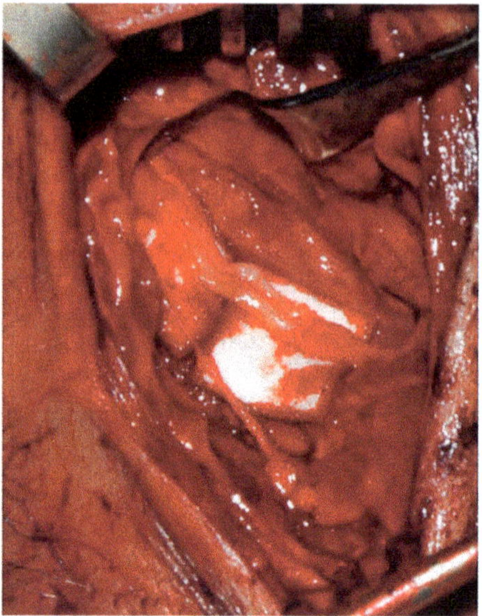

Figure 25.5. Intraoperative photograph demonstrating reconstruction of the spinal accessory nerve using supraclavicular nerves.

the defect is larger, the time interval is prejudicial, or the proximal stump cannot be reliably located, a nerve transfer is recommended, using the lateral pectoral nerve or fascicular transfer from the C7 trunk.

Aftercare

Patients should be placed in an appropriately sized soft collar for 4 weeks, followed by a gradual increase in activities and neck range of motion as tolerated. During this protected time, patients should also be instructed to avoid lateral neck rotation or flexion to the contralateral side to avoid excessive tension on the SAN, particularly when a repair or grafting procedure has been completed.

Oral Boards Review—Management Pearls

1. Time is muscle—earlier diagnosis and appropriate treatment are important to prevent irreversible loss of motor endplates and atrophy of the trapezius, which typically occur 12 to 18 months after injury.
2. Immediate deficits attributable to SAN injury after neck surgery or penetrating trauma are unlikely to recover spontaneously and should undergo surgical exploration and repair or grafting as necessary.
3. Pinch elevation of the trapezius helps with localization of the distal SAN.

Complications

General complications can include infection and injury to surrounding neurovascular structures. Preoperatively, it is important to discuss with the patient the possibility of incomplete symptom resolution, particularly the recovery of strength of the trapezius, when the diagnosis has been established on a delayed basis. The potential need for secondary reconstructive procedures should also be addressed.

Evidence and Outcomes

Large, prospective, controlled studies of the treatment of SAN palsy are lacking. Case series have generally documented improvements in pain and varying degrees of motor recovery. Poorer results have been reported when patients were more than 50 years old, when the palsy was due to a radical neck dissection or penetrating injury, and when the palsy was spontaneous.

References

1. Wiater JM, Bigliani LU. Spinal accessory nerve injury. *Clin Orthop Relat Res*. 1999;368:5–16.
2. Teboul F, Bizot P, Kakkar R, Sedel L. Surgical management of trapezius palsy. *J Bone Joint Surg Am*. 2005;87(suppl 1, pt 2):285–291.
3. Chandawarkar RY, Cervino AL, Pennington GA. Management of iatrogenic injury to the spinal accessory nerve. *Plast Reconstr Surg*. 2003;111(2):611–617.
4. Camp SJ, Birch R. Injuries to the spinal accessory nerve: a lesson to surgeons. *J Bone Joint Surg Br*. 2011;93(1):62–67.

Facial Nerve Injury

Mariano Socolovsky, Rafael Torino, and Leandro Pretto Flores

26

Case Presentation

A 38-year-old female teacher presented for an otology consultation complaining of hearing impairment in her left ear. She had first noticed the hearing defect 1 year earlier; however, at the time, her hearing loss seemed very slight, so she did not seek medical attention. The defect progressed slowly, ultimately leading to the current consultation. At the time of her first clinic visit, her neurologic examination was unremarkable. Audiometry and logo-audiometry were abnormal, demonstrating 70% and 80% decreases in hearing, respectively. MR imaging demonstrated a vestibular schwannoma in the left cerebellopontine angle (CPA). After an extensive discussion with the patient, resection via a suboccipital retrosigmoid approach was undertaken. During surgery, the facial nerve was monitored and preserved, and complete tumor excision was achieved. Complete (House-Brackmann grade VI) left-sided facial nerve palsy, affecting both the upper and lower face, was observed immediately postoperatively (Figure 26.1). No signs of clinical or electrophysiologic recovery were observed at 3-, 6-, or 9-month follow-up.

Questions

1. What is the likely diagnosis?
2. What is the appropriate timing for the diagnostic workup?
3. What is the appropriate time to stop rehabilitation and to plan a surgical procedure?

Assessment and Planning

The patient's medical history and, in some cases, physical examination play a principal role in determining the likely etiology of facial palsy, which in turn guides the therapeutic approach. Severe injury of the facial nerve in the CPA region was suspected in this case.

In patients with a history of head trauma, a lesion of the facial nerve at the petrous bone associated with a basilar skull fracture should be suspected. In such cases, conservative treatment is advocated. Most of the lesions recover partially or completely within months. A CT scan of the petrous bone is mandatory to determine the extent of the fracture. If no signs of recovery are seen within 12 months of the trauma, then surgical repair is indicated. In those surgical cases, the authors

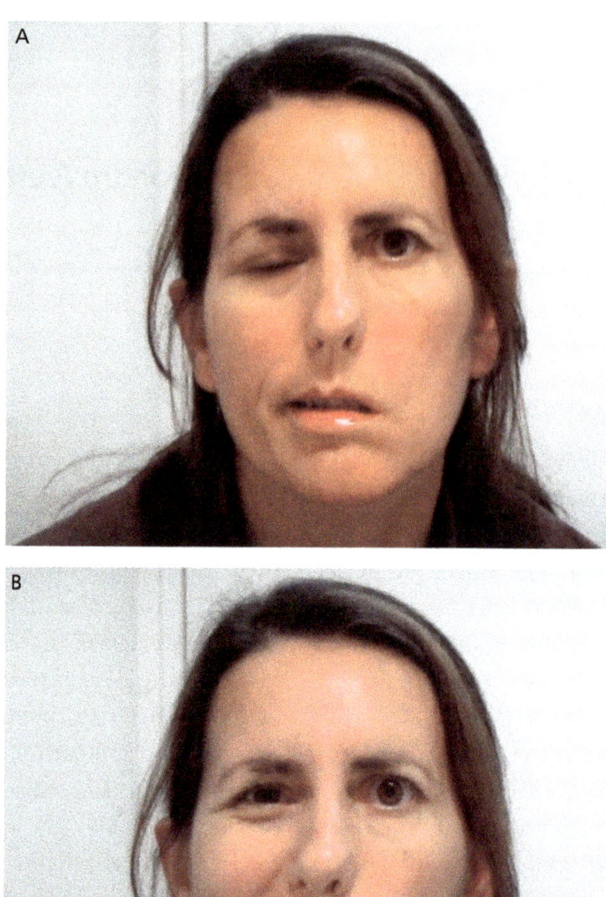

Figure 26.1. A, Complete left facial palsy after surgical resection of a vestibular schwannoma, with inability to close the eye. B, Smile asymmetry.

prefer to expose the facial nerve at the mastoid bone from the stylomastoid foramen through to the genu of the facial nerve. If a nerve injury is observed, the neuroma-in-continuity is resected and is replaced with a graft. If the injury is too proximal in the bone to allow adequate access to a good proximal facial nerve stump, then a nerve transfer is preferred, with partial hypoglossal and masseter nerves as the preferred donors.

In the case of sharp or blunt trauma to the parotid region, direct injury to the facial nerve distal to the stylomastoid foramen should be suspected. As in any case of penetrating trauma associated with a corresponding neurologic deficit, the nerve should be promptly explored and repaired. Most cases require the use of a nerve graft.

The ideal timing for the surgical procedure is 2 to 3 weeks after the injury, in order to allow time for the extent of injury to be clearly delineated in both nerve stumps. If preferred, immediate exploration after the trauma is acceptable, but care should be taken to excise all nerve tissue that was partially traumatized, in order to avoid delayed fibrous tissue formation at the suture site, which will prevent axons from regenerating. In cases of clean, sharp laceration, immediate exploration should be undertaken. The sural nerve or cervical branches available during exploration can serve as donors when nerve graft is necessary. In cases involving injury after the branching of the facial nerve at the parotid, adequate-caliber branches must be used. In all cases, facial nerve-to-facial nerve suture with or without interposed nerve grafts is the standard procedure for nerve repair. In selected cases, MR imaging of the facial nerve might help in visualizing the lesion.

When spontaneous palsy of the facial nerve occurs, an inflammatory neuropathy should be suspected (i.e., Bell's palsy). This is most commonly idiopathic but can be associated with varicella-zoster virus, herpes zoster virus, or *Borrelia burgdorferi* infection.[8] Acutely, treatment may include steroids and/or antivirals.[1–3] In some cases, facial nerve decompression is considered; however, these cases rarely require surgical repair of the nerve, because spontaneous recovery, or at least partial recovery, is the norm.[4]

As in the case presented, if the facial nerve palsy is associated with the resection of a CPA tumor, a direct nerve transfer should be planned. The same nerve donors mentioned above—partial hypoglossal and masseter—are also preferred here. The timing of surgery will depend upon the findings of the initial CPA tumor resection surgery: if it is known that the nerve was injured during the procedure and no direct repair was then feasible, a secondary repair should be scheduled after the resection surgery, allowing time for the patient to recover from the first procedure. If the nerve was preserved during surgery, then spontaneous recovery can be expected, but the surgeon should keep in mind that the results of nerve transfers for the facial nerve start to decay slightly 6 months after the injury and decay more pronouncedly 1 year after injury.

In some cases, a central etiology for facial nerve palsy should be considered. In cases where additional neurologic deficits are present, a central etiology is highly likely, although inflammatory neuropathies can affect the facial nerve and other peripheral nerves simultaneously. The physical examination can be helpful. Facial palsy that spares the forehead but affects the rest of the face suggests a central cause. A thorough neurologic examination should be performed, and CT and/or MR imaging can be extremely helpful in determining the diagnosis.

Questions

1. How do the clinical and radiologic findings influence surgical planning?
2. What is the most appropriate timing for intervention?
3. How should surgery be approached in a patient in whom no clear injury to the facial nerve is observed on radiologic exams?

Oral Boards Review—Diagnostic Pearls

1. A thorough and accurate medical history is crucial to determining the cause of facial palsy.
   a. In penetrating trauma to the facial nerve, a scar will clearly be seen affecting the parotid region (and is generally associated with complete palsies) or the face more medially (if so, expect partial palsy).
   b. When facial palsy occurs in a patient with a head injury, whether the injury is associated with signs of skull base trauma or not, a petrous bone fracture affecting the facial nerve should be suspected. Clinical examination and brain imaging studies are important to help differentiate this possibility from a central facial palsy.
   c. Spontaneous facial nerve palsy is not associated with a history of trauma. Vesicles in the external auditory canal are associated with a zoster-type infection, which generally has a worse prognosis for recovery than typical Bell's palsy, the latter being associated with complete recovery to baseline levels of function in most cases.
   d. In facial palsy after CPA tumor resection, it is key is to determine if the nerve was injured during tumor resection or if it was preserved both anatomically and functionally under monitoring. To determine this, the opinion of the surgeon who removed the tumor is most useful.
2. Neurophysiologic studies are needed.
3. Imaging can be useful in the evaluation of facial nerve palsy, although it does not always lead to a diagnosis.

Decision-Making

As in the case presented, which was a typical complete facial nerve palsy after resection of a vestibular schwannoma, the intraoperative scenario and the facial nerve condition guide decision-making. If the nerve is clearly injured or sectioned during surgery, direct repair of the facial nerve intraoperatively should be attempted. The repair may be difficult to undertake at that time, however, because the facial nerve may be deformed by the tumor, and the stumps, particularly the proximal stump at the apparent origin of the facial nerve in the pontomedullary sulcus, are generally unavailable or severely damaged. If direct repair is not feasible because the nerve has been injured at its proximal origin in the CPA, a facial nerve transfer is indicated.

If the facial nerve is preserved during surgery but complete facial nerve palsy develops after the procedure, spontaneous recovery can be expected, so the patient should be referred for postoperative rehabilitation a few weeks after the procedure. If no signs of recovery of the facial nerve are observed clinically or on electromyography (EMG) 10 to 11 months after the tumor resection procedure, then surgical repair of the palsy via nerve transfer is indicated. The interval between the onset of palsy and surgical repair should not exceed 1 year, since permanent facial impairment due to irreversible muscle atrophy would be expected. Some advocate surgery at 6 months postoperatively when there are no signs of clinical or EMG recovery.[5] Regardless, the decision for primary reconstructive surgery should be made within 1 year of the tumor resection.

Since there is a documented link between earlier nerve transfers and enhanced outcomes, electroneuromyography (ENMG) of the facial nerve may play an important role in some patients when a nerve transfer procedure is being considered. For example, in patients in whom the nerve is not damaged intraoperatively but complete facial palsy is observed postoperatively, facial ENMG performed during the first postoperative week that documents a motor response less than 10% of that on the contralateral (unaffected) side is associated with a very low rate of spontaneous recovery.[5,6] In this scenario, a nerve transfer procedure should not be delayed more than 2 to 3 months after tumor resection. On another note, serial EMG of the facial nerve that indicates reinnervation, even if it is not associated with clinical recovery, warrants consideration of conservative treatment, although never beyond 1 year postoperatively, as mentioned previously.

Given that no proximal stump of the facial nerve is available in cases similar to the one presented, the procedure of choice for reanimation is a nerve transfer. At present, the hypoglossal and masseter nerves are widely accepted motor axon donors for facial reinnervation. Contralateral cross-nerve reanimation using the healthy facial nerve is a third option, with some authors reporting good results in early cases (within a maximum of 2 months from the first surgery).[7–9] In cases like the patient presented, in whom the facial nerve was preserved during tumor resection but the palsy remained after 11 months, this surgical procedure is not recommended. The spinal accessory nerve, widely used as a motor axon source in brachial plexus surgery, has been abandoned for facial reanimation due to its association with uncomfortable dyskinesias. In very late cases (more than 24 months of palsy), surgical options include a free gracilis muscle transfer innervated by either the masseter or hypoglossal nerve or passive reconstruction (e.g., temporal muscle and tendon transfer to both the mouth and eye commissures).

Both hypoglossal and masseter nerve transfers have been shown to produce good results for facial reanimation. The classical complete section of the hypoglossal nerve followed by its direct suture to the facial nerve, described by Korte in 1903 and widely used until the 1990s, is associated with tongue atrophy and should be avoided.[10] Two techniques have been described to avoid tongue atrophy. The first utilizes mastoid dissection of the facial nerve and an interposed nerve jump graft between the facial and the hypoglossal nerves.[11] The second technique (simultaneously described by Sawamura, Ferraresi, and Atlas) utilizes a partial section of the hypoglossal nerve. After drilling the mastoid bone, a direct suture between the two nerves is performed.[12–15]

Masseter nerve transfers, described by Manktelow and Zuker, also provide good results.[9] The main advantage of this approach is that it is technically easier than a partial hypoglossal-to-facial nerve transfer, since there is no need to drill through the mastoid bone to achieve direct nerve coaptation. This spares the surgeon needing to be intimately familiar with the anatomy and surgical management of the temporal bone and shortens the procedure. A primary disadvantage of the masseter technique is denervation of the pterygoid and masseter muscles, which is usually well tolerated by the patient. Additionally, the masseter nerve has a smaller diameter than the facial nerve, so it is usually only possible to achieve good coaptation with a branch of the facial nerve, the buccal branch.[16,17] A recent report demonstrated that both techniques are adequate for facial reanimation, with the results of hypoglossal nerve transfer being slightly better when measured using a scale specifically developed to assess facial reanimation.[18] In the same study, use of an interposed graft to transfer the motor axons of a hemihypoglossal nerve to the facial nerve generated poorer results than either of the other two techniques.[18] The results with an interposed graft remain somewhat controversial, however, as others have reported results with the technique that were better than those reported above.[19]

Given that both hemihypoglossal-to-facial and masseter-to-facial nerve transfers are safe and produce excellent results, we believe that the personal preferences of the patient and surgeon are paramount. Currently, at our institution, we prefer to use the hypoglossal nerve as a donor, due to the slightly better results we have achieved with it. However, this preference remains a matter of discussion.

Questions

1. What is the importance of facial nerve preservation—or the inability to preserve it—during the surgical resection of a CPA tumor, in terms of the decision-making process if the patient develops complete facial nerve palsy?
2. Which nerve transfer techniques are most often used for facial reanimation? Which of them would be suitable for the present case?

Pivot Points

1. If the facial nerve is damaged during CPA tumor resection, a first attempt to repair it at the skull base should be made.
2. Because this is commonly not feasible, a nerve transfer procedure—scheduled as an elective procedure after the patient has completely recovered from the resection procedure—is mandatory. Hemihypoglossal, masseter, and cross-facial nerve transfers are the techniques most widely used.
3. When the facial nerve is preserved during surgery, but complete facial palsy develops afterward, postoperative rehabilitation should be started and continued for up to 1 year. If, however, facial palsy persists beyond 6 to 12 months, then the patient should be offered the option of a nerve transfer.

Surgical Procedure

For the case presented, we elected to perform a transfer of the hemihypoglossal nerve to the facial nerve. The surgical procedure is as follows. With the patient under general anesthesia and in a supine position on the operating table, the head is turned to the contralateral side. A semicircular retroauricular incision is created, extending 6 to 8 cm obliquely down the neck and cephalad 2 cm to just behind the mandibular angle. The tip of the mastoid process is exposed by removing muscle attachments and the periosteum with a periosteal elevator. Aided by the operating microscope, proximal dissection of the facial nerve is then performed by drilling the mastoid bone with a high-speed drill and diamond bur. A limited mastoidectomy, with a rectangular shape not exceeding 2 to 3 cm in width, is performed, opening the facial canal to expose the facial nerve from the external genu to the stylomastoid foramen. The nerve is then sectioned as proximally as possible and dissected from the mastoid bone. Distal extracranial dissection of the facial nerve at the stylomastoid foramen and the preauricular region up to the parotid gland is needed to complete nerve rerouting toward the neck and the hypoglossal nerve. Subsequently, the hypoglossal nerve is dissected at the most caudal portion of the cervical incision, where it is lying inferior and medial to the posterior belly of the digastric muscle. A standard nerve stimulator is used to confirm normal function of the hypoglossal nerve. The point where the mobilized facial nerve stump reaches the hypoglossal nerve defines the point of hypoglossal nerve section. Roughly one third to one half of the axial section of the hypoglossal nerve is transected. The facial nerve is coapted, without tension, directly to the proximal hypoglossal stump, using one or two stitches of 10-0 nylon interrupted suture, reinforced with fibrin sealant (Figure 26.2).

Oral Boards Review—Management Pearls

1. Adequate intramastoid facial nerve exposure from the external genu to the mastoid foramen is mandatory to avoid tension at the nerve suture site.
2. The proximal facial nerve stump should be skeletonized from the epineurium and dura mater, as the nerve width is much smaller than it seems without performance of this surgical maneuver.
3. The hypoglossal nerve should be sectioned only after the facial nerve is brought adjacent to it, so the exact amount of nerve that is needed for adequate coaptation can be calculated. Usually, about one third to one half of the hypoglossal nerve is enough to cover the facial nerve's width.
4. Given that neither nerve stump is covered by epineurium, one or two very superficial 10-0 or 11-0 nylon stitches should be placed to avoid stump injury.

Aftercare

Patients are generally discharged 24 to 48 hours after the nerve transfer procedure. Relative rest is indicated for 3 weeks with any nerve suture, to avoid tears or tension at the suture site.

Motor re-education and strengthening exercises should be initiated 3 weeks after surgery via a complete rehabilitation program, including daily exercises in front of a mirror. The first signs of reinnervation generally appear between 4 and 6 months after surgery. The patient will typically notice movement of the commissure while moving the tongue inside the mouth. Further re-education exercises allow the patient to achieve complete symmetry at rest and dynamic movement of the face upon speaking, although it is difficult to attain a spontaneous smile or independent movement of each facial muscle (Figure 26.3).

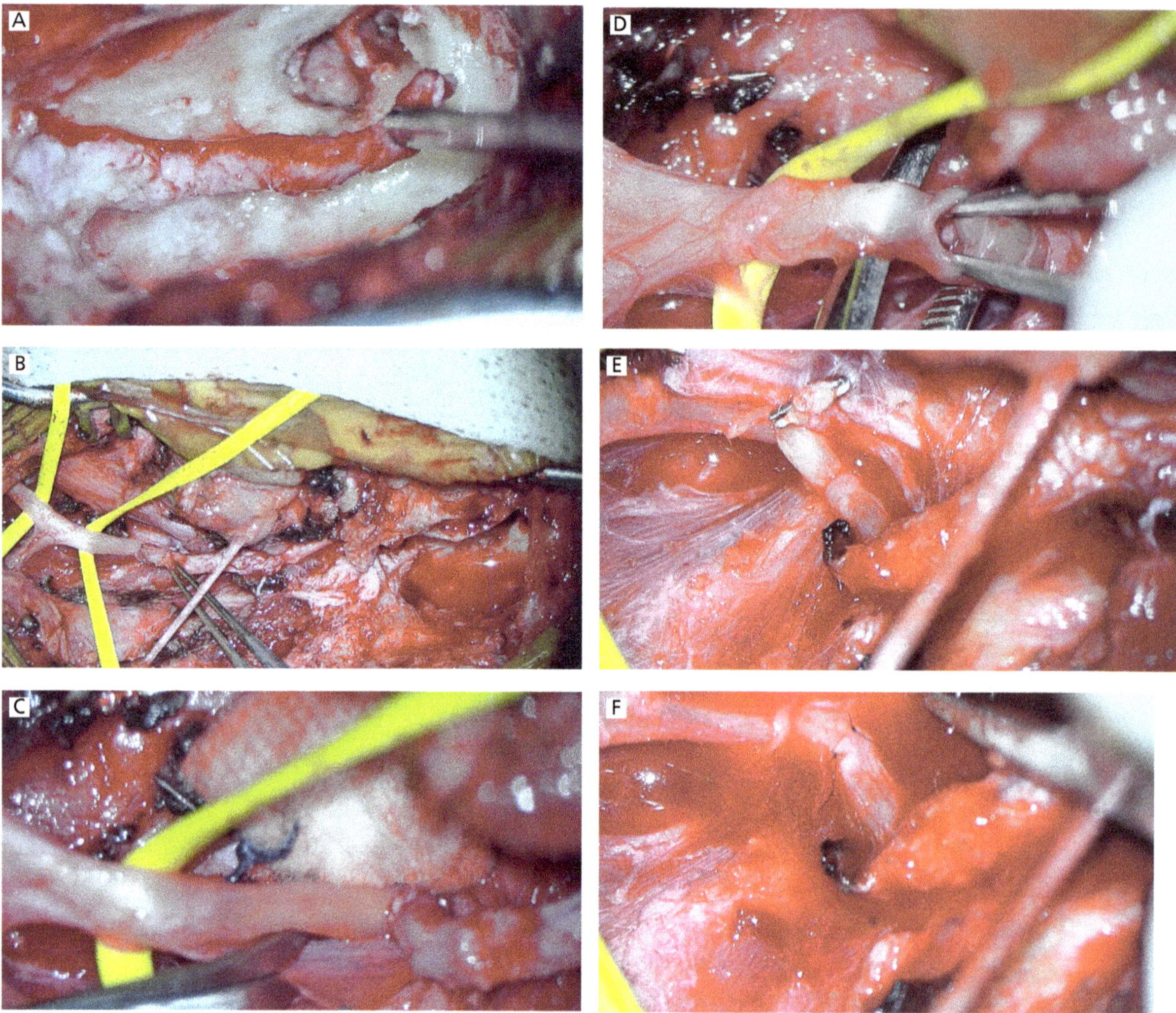

Figure 26.2. A, Facial nerve exposed after drilling of the mastoid bone. B, The hypoglossal nerve (left of figure, yellow loops) is exposed at the upper neck region, and the mastoid portion of the facial nerve (right of figure, held by forceps) is rerouted toward the hypoglossal nerve. C, An epineuriotomy is performed in the hypoglossal nerve. D, The hypoglossal nerve is opened with interfascicular dissection, and half of it is sectioned. E, The nerve stumps of the facial nerve and half of the hypoglossal nerve, which have a similar size, are approximated without tension. F, One or two 10-0 nylon stitches are placed to support the coaptation.

Complications and Management

A cervical hematoma is a rare complication, but the possibility always exists. Consequently, adequate hemostasis is of paramount importance prior to wound closure. Some patients may notice slight clumsiness of their tongue when they pronounce certain words, particularly those containing the letters *d* and *r*, but this will invariably disappear after a maximum of 2 months. Slight tongue atrophy can be seen in some patients after surgery, but this generally improves quickly once the patients commence rehabilitation.

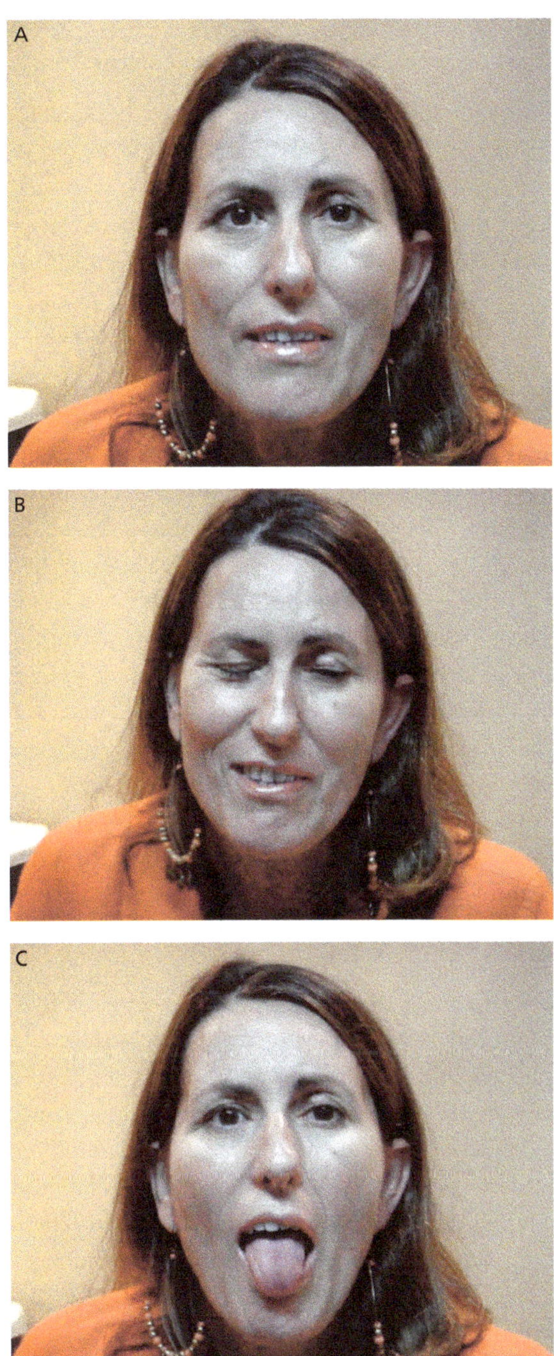

Figure 26.3. A, Postoperative image of facial symmetry 18 months after the nerve transfer procedure. B, Good eye closure. C, Good tongue preservation.

Oral Boards Review—Complication Pearls

1. Adequate hemostasis is mandatory to avoid a cervical hematoma.
2. Some signs of hemitongue dysfunction can be expected, although they tend to be transient and disappear after the rehabilitation program is initiated.
3. Mastoid drilling should be performed carefully to avoid facial nerve injury.
4. During cervical dissection, extreme caution is warranted to avoid accidental injury to important vascular structures.

Evidence and Outcomes

The literature contains abundant retrospective data on the outcomes achieved with the various reinnervation techniques. To date, it seems that the best results can be obtained with hypoglossal and masseter nerve transfers. Some surgeons claim that cross-facial anastomosis can restore spontaneous movements of the face (e.g., spontaneous blinking or smiling), but these claims require further verification, because the results seem to be aleatory and highly dependent upon surgical timing.

In our own series, hemihypoglossal transfer without a graft outperformed the same procedure with a graft and also masseter transfer. Masseter transfer results were also satisfactory. These data argue against the use of an interpositional graft with hemihypoglossal transfer.[18] The satisfactory results of both hemihypoglossal and masseter transfer make these nerves our preferred donors, although given its slightly better results in our hands, we prefer hemihypoglossal transfer when possible. Early signs of recovery can be expected around 6 months postoperatively when masseter transfer is utilized and approximately 11 months postoperatively when hemihypoglossal transfer is utilized.[5]

In cases where direct repair of the facial nerve or repair with a graft are technically feasible, these procedures should be preferentially performed rather than nerve transfer, as the results for direct repair with or without a graft exceed those for nerve transfer.[6] The repair should be performed in a tension-free manner, but when possible, direct repair should be performed due to its superior results compared to repair with a graft.[6] In one study, House-Brackmann grade III or better results at 24 months postoperatively were achieved in 85% of patients with end-to-end repair of the facial nerve, 56% of patients who had repair with a cabled interposition graft, and 25% who underwent hypoglossal-facial nerve transfer.[6]

Intraoperatively recognized injuries to the facial nerve during surgery in the CPA should be repaired at that time, whenever proximal and distal stumps can be identified. In one study, 45% of patients had good recovery of facial function with intraoperative facial nerve repair using interposition grafts, 36% had fair recovery, and 18% had minimal or no recovery. In that study, graft length did not correlate with recovery.[20] In another study, 68% of patients achieved House-Brackmann grade III facial function.[7]

While outcomes are certainly improved with shorter duration from palsy onset to surgery and whenever possible surgery should be undertaken 12 months or less from palsy onset, hemihypoglossal-to-facial nerve transfer has been performed in patients with longstanding facial nerve palsy (more than 24 months) with satisfactory results.[15,21]

Every effort should be made to perform reanimation as soon as lack of spontaneous recovery is confirmed, but reanimation can be considered even in longstanding facial palsy. Recent data suggest that lack of clinical and electromyographic recovery at 6 months after injury essentially rules out satisfactory spontaneous recovery. As a result, earlier surgery can be considered when patients do not show signs of recovery by 6 months.[5]

References

1. Arican P, Dundar NO, Gencpinar P, Cavusoglu D. Efficacy of low-dose corticosteroid therapy versus high-dose corticosteroid therapy in Bell's palsy in children. *J Child Neurol.* 2017;32:72–75.
2. Khedr EM, Badry R, Ali AM, et al. Steroid/antiviral for the treatment of Bell's palsy: double blind randomized clinical trial. *Restor Neurol Neurosci.* 2016;34:897–905.
3. Sullivan F, Daly F, Gagyor I. Antiviral agents added to corticosteroids for early treatment of adults with acute idiopathic facial nerve paralysis (Bell palsy). *JAMA.* 2016;316:874–875.
4. Socolovsky M, Paez MD, Masi GD, Molina G, Fernandez E. Bell's palsy and partial hypoglossal to facial nerve transfer: case presentation and literature review. *Surg Neurol Int.* 2012;3:46.
5. Albathi M, Oyer S, Ishii LE, Byrne P, Ishii M, Boahene KO. Early nerve grafting for facial paralysis after cerebellopontine angle tumor resection with preserved facial nerve continuity. *JAMA Facial Plast Surg.* 2016;18:54–60.
6. Malik TH, Kelly G, Ahmed A, Saeed SR, Ramsden RT. A comparison of surgical techniques used in dynamic reanimation of the paralyzed face. *Otol Neurotol.* 2005;26:284–291.
7. Ozmen OA, Falcioni M, Lauda L, Sanna M. Outcomes of facial nerve grafting in 155 cases: predictive value of history and preoperative function. *Otol Neurotol.* 2011;32:1341–1346.
8. Stephanian E, Sekhar LN, Janecka IP, Hirsch B. Facial nerve repair by interposition nerve graft: results in 22 patients. *Neurosurgery.* 1992;31:73–76, discussion 77.
9. Zuker RM, Manktelow RT. A smile for the Mobius' syndrome patient. *Ann Plast Surg.* 1989;22:188–194.
10. Korte W. Ein Fall von Nervenpfropfung: des Nervus facialis auf den Nervus hypoglossus. *Deutsche med Wohnschr.* 1903;17:293–295.
11. May M, Sobol SM, Mester SJ. Hypoglossal-facial nerve interpositional-jump graft for facial reanimation without tongue atrophy. *Otolaryngol Head Neck Surg.* 1991;104:818–825.
12. Atlas MD, Lowinger DS. A new technique for hypoglossal-facial nerve repair. *Laryngoscope.* 1997;107:984–991.
13. Ferraresi S, Garozzo D, Migliorini V, Buffatti P. End-to-side intrapetrous hypoglossal-facial anastomosis for reanimation of the face. Technical note. *J Neurosurg.* 2006;104:457–460.
14. Martins RS, Socolovsky M, Siqueira MG, Campero A. Hemihypoglossal-facial neurorrhaphy after mastoid dissection of the facial nerve: results in 24 patients and comparison with the classic technique. *Neurosurgery.* 2008;63:310–316, discussion 317.
15. Sawamura Y, Abe H. Hypoglossal-facial nerve side-to-end anastomosis for preservation of hypoglossal function: results of delayed treatment with a new technique. *J Neurosurg.* 1997;86:203–206.

16. Borschel GH, Kawamura DH, Kasukurthi R, Hunter DA, Zuker RM, Woo AS. The motor nerve to the masseter muscle: an anatomic and histomorphometric study to facilitate its use in facial reanimation. *J Plast Reconstr Aesthetic Surg*. 2012;65:363–366.
17. Coombs CJ, Ek EW, Wu T, Cleland H, Leung MK. Masseteric-facial nerve coaptation—an alternative technique for facial nerve reinnervation. *J Plast Reconstr Aesthetic Surg*. 2009;62:1580–1588.
18. Socolovsky M, Martins RS, di Masi G, Bonilla G, Siqueira M. Treatment of complete facial palsy in adults: comparative study between direct hemihypoglossal-facial neurorrhaphy, hemihypoglossal-facial neurorrhaphy with grafts, and masseter to facial nerve transfer. *Acta Neurochir (Wien)*. 2016;158:945–957, discussion 957.
19. Flores LP. Surgical results of the hypoglossal-facial nerve jump graft technique. *Acta Neurochir (Wien)*. 2007;149:1205–1210, discussion 1210.
20. Henkel K, Lange P, Eiffert H, Nau R, Spreer A. Infections in the differential diagnosis of Bell's palsy: a plea for performing CSF analysis. *Infection*. 2017;45:147–155.
21. Yetiser S, Karapinar U. Hypoglossal-facial nerve anastomosis: a meta-analytic study. *Ann Otol Rhinol Laryngol*. 2007;116:542–549.

Emergent Nerve Injury

Amgad S. Hanna, Lisa M. Block, and A. Neil Salyapongse

27

Case Presentation

A 21-year-old woman presented to the emergency department (ED) with a deep laceration to her left proximal volar forearm after she fell through a plate glass window. Arterial bleeding was noted from the laceration, which was approximately 10 cm long and was located just distal and radial to the antecubital fossa. ED staff placed a tourniquet on the patient's proximal arm upon her arrival. The patient was in hemorrhagic shock, which limited initial evaluation of her hand. She was resuscitated and was taken emergently to the operating room by the trauma surgery team. Exploration revealed intact brachial, radial, and ulnar arteries, with lacerated superficial veins and a small arterial branch. The laceration was noted to extend deep to the muscle bellies. No other damaged structures were noted. The lacerated vascular structures were ligated, and the tourniquet was released 110 minutes after placement. On postoperative day 1, the patient was found to have left hand weakness, as well as numbness over the lateral volar forearm and dorsal hand. Consultation with a nerve surgeon was obtained, and detailed examination revealed weak finger extension, wrist extension, and thumb extension and abduction and diminished sensation over the dorsal thumb, dorsal radial hand, and lateral volar forearm. The remainder of the neurologic examination was normal, including elbow flexion, elbow extension, brachioradialis function, wrist flexion, and median- and ulnar-innervated hand intrinsics. Three days after injury, the patient showed no improvement.

Questions

1. What structures are most likely damaged?
2. What are the possible mechanisms of injury in this patient?
3. What other workup should be done, if any?
4. What is the appropriate timing for the diagnostic workup?

Assessment and Planning

The nerve surgeon suspects injury to the radial nerve just proximal to its division into the superficial sensory radial nerve and posterior interosseous nerve (PIN) as well as injury to the lateral antebrachial cutaneous (LABC) nerve.

Detailed analysis of the patient's history will provide the first clues in diagnosing a nerve injury. Specific motor function and sensory deficits will often indicate which structures are damaged. Acute injuries may involve muscle, tendon, and/or vascular structures in addition to nerves, which can confound the initial evaluation. Consideration of the mechanism of injury can be beneficial in determining the type and degree of nerve injury. Stretch, compression, or crush injuries can result in neurapraxia (focal conduction block due to myelin damage with intact axons) or axonotmesis (axonal disruption with preservation of the nerve sheaths), whereas lacerations and penetrating injuries more often lead to partial or complete neurotmesis (complete transection of axons and all supporting tissue).[1]

Physical examination is the core diagnostic modality when evaluating acute nerve injuries. The location and depth of injury are major clues as to the possible nerve(s) injured. Precise and thorough testing of motor strength and cutaneous sensation will provide detailed information regarding which nerve functions are intact and which are absent or diminished. Careful evaluation of the open injury should be undertaken as soon as possible in a safe and clean manner. Visual inspection with good lighting and loupe magnification with gentle irrigation and probing can be safely conducted in the ED, provided that the patient is medically stable and can undergo such examination and that it is performed by an experienced examiner in order to minimize further trauma to the injured tissues. This inspection can yield valuable information about which structures may be damaged in the acute laceration. Care should be taken when controlling bleeding vessels in the wound in order to avoid iatrogenic nerve injury, as small vessels may run adjacent to important nerves. Indiscriminate clamping or ligation of these vessels may result in additional nerve trauma. In a life-threatening situation, control of bleeding comes first, but one should always be mindful of nearby structures in order to minimize secondary damage.

Although physical examination remains the principal means of diagnosing acute nerve injury, additional modalities may prove useful in some circumstances. Nerve conduction studies (NCS) and electromyography (EMG) provide valuable information about nerve function, but their utility is often limited in diagnosing acute nerve injuries, as it is difficult to distinguish between neurapraxia and axonotmesis/neurotmesis and between partial and complete transection in the first 10 to 14 days after injury. Serial NCS and EMG are critical when paired with serial physical examinations in following chronic and recovering nerve injuries.

Ultrasound and MR imaging are the imaging modalities most often used for nerves. Ultrasound is inexpensive, fast, and safe; it can accurately image nerve edema, neuroma formation, and partial versus complete lacerations. MR neurography and tractography can provide more accurate assessment of nerve continuity. However, the clinical utility of MR imaging is often limited in the setting of acute nerve injury due to its additional expense, the lengthy time needed to obtain the study, and the relative sufficiency of physical examination.

In the patient described here, the differential diagnosis included laceration injury, compression/ischemic injury from the tourniquet, and intraoperative iatrogenic injury, including transection, clip ligation, or thermal injury. The patient sustained a deep laceration injury from falling through a plate glass window, which mechanistically would produce a clean, sharp laceration. The tourniquet in this case was a medical grade pneumatic tourniquet placed by a medical professional in a controlled setting and was released in under 2 hours. Tourniquets that are placed in the field, by laypersons, or by improvising with nonmedical equipment have a higher rate of nerve compression injury.[2–4] Additionally, tourniquets that are left in place for more than 120 minutes have increasing risk of nerve injury, due to both compression injury and nerve ischemia.[2] However, even when placed in a controlled setting, with precise pressure settings, and when deflated within recommended time limits, tourniquets can still cause transient or permanent nerve injury. Finally, the initial exploration and management were performed by a trauma surgeon, and the operative report mentioned ligation of multiple bleeding intramuscular vessels. This raises the possibility of iatrogenic damage during clamping or ligation of the bleeding vessels.

It is very important to establish a neurologic baseline as soon after trauma as it is safe to do so. Traumatic nerve injuries should have maximal deficits immediately after trauma. Delayed onset or progressive neurologic deficits should raise the possibility of an etiology other than direct trauma, such as the development of a compressive hematoma or compartment syndrome. It is important not to attribute delayed onset or progressive neurologic deficits to trauma, to investigate the deficits further, and to intervene if an additional source of injury is found.

Oral Boards Review—Diagnostic Pearls

1. ABCs. Any trauma evaluation should start with evaluation and management of the airway, breathing, and circulation. Such management takes precedence over any neurologic injuries or considerations.
2. Physical examination is the cornerstone in diagnosing acute nerve injuries.
   a. Evaluate location and depth of injury in relation to location of nerves.
   b. Perform precise motor function testing, with special attention to the muscle groups whose innervation is distal to the injury.
   c. Perform detailed sensory testing, noting areas of tingling, diminished sensation, and absent sensation. Also note the presence of any Tinel sign, particularly near the injury.
   d. Knowing the mechanism of injury (e.g., crush, laceration, or penetrating trauma) can help estimate the type and degree of nerve injury.
3. NCS and EMG are more useful in the setting of delayed presentation, after nerve repair, or with chronic injury. It is difficult to accurately diagnose acute nerve injuries (within 10 to 14 days) using these modalities, and some injuries, such as partial lacerations, may be missed altogether.
4. Ultrasound and MR imaging are the modalities of choice when radiographic studies are desired. These studies can demonstrate nerve swelling, neuroma formation, and partial- versus full-thickness lacerations. Imaging often is not required when the history and physical examination provide clear indication of which structures are damaged.

Questions

1. How do the physical examination findings influence treatment planning in this patient?
2. What is the preferred therapeutic intervention for this type of injury?
3. What is the most appropriate timing for intervention in this patient?

Decision-Making

The presumed mechanism of injury and overall stability of the patient are the two most important factors in determining management. A rough rule that can be applied is the rule of threes: clean, sharp lacerations should be repaired within 3 days; dirty, ragged transections should be repaired at approximately 3 weeks; and closed injuries should be considered for repair at 3 months. As in this case, in a trauma situation where thorough neurologic examination is often not feasible at presentation and when interventions happen quickly, it can be difficult to establish the temporal relationship between the onset of neurologic deficits and their proximate cause. When a laceration is present over an area with a suspected nerve injury, the nerve should be considered transected until proven otherwise. Assuming the patient is medically stable, when a nerve laceration is suspected, repair should be performed as expediently as possible, because the best results are obtained when repair is performed within 3 days. The longer the time interval from injury to repair, the greater the degree of nerve retraction due to elastic recoil and the greater the degree of fibrosis within the injured nerve ends, which decreases overall nerve health and capacity for optimal coaptation.

Direct repair of a clean nerve laceration in a tension-free manner remains the ideal method of nerve repair, when possible. This type of repair is indicated in cases of sharp nerve transection, with minimal gap between the nerve ends, and with clean, viable soft tissue coverage. Minimal nerve resection of less than 1 mm is required to optimize the nerve ends for repair. Mobilization of the proximal and distal stumps may help gain length and minimize gapping. Simple direct repair is performed in an end-to-end manner when possible, utilizing 8-0 or 9-0 nylon suture under microscope or loupe magnification.

In the event of a ragged laceration, often the result of a crush/shear type injury or laceration with a dull object, the nerve ends should be considered an evolving zone of injury. Typical management involves tagging the nerve ends with a metal surgical clip in the acute period to allow later localization and suturing them to a fixed, local structure, such as muscle fascia, in order to prevent significant retraction. Time is then allowed for the full extent of the injury to be demarcated, typically a period of 3 weeks. At that time, repair is undertaken and the damaged nerve ends are resected back to the point of healthy nerve. If the resulting gap exceeds 3 cm, typically a nerve graft will be required to achieve a tension-free repair. Alternatively, if the nerve ends are not severely damaged, the repair can be performed acutely. This will require resection of the nerve ends to the level of normal, well-aligned architecture in order to optimize nerve regeneration across the repair site. This resection should be performed incrementally in order to preserve as much length as possible, and it should be carried to the level where discrete bleeding fascicles can be visualized. The gap between the nerve ends will determine whether a nerve graft is required. Regardless, in these cases, exploration should be undertaken acutely, with severely damaged nerve ends tagged for later repair and with nerve ends with minor injury repaired with or without a graft.

The management of dirty lacerations should include expedient washout, ideally in the operating room, but if the patient is medically unstable or otherwise unable to undergo surgery, washout should occur as soon as possible either in the ED or at the bedside. Washout should employ high-volume, low-pressure sterile irrigant in order to avoid additional trauma to delicate structures. Nerve repair can occur in the same operative encounter as washout if the surgeon is convinced that the wound is truly clean and the nerve ends are not severely damaged. In the case of highly contaminated wounds, such as agricultural injuries, or in delayed presentation where inflammation or infection is already present in the wound bed, the nerve endings should be tagged and definitive repair should be deferred until the wound is clean and free of infection (2 to 3 weeks).

In closed injuries, the nerve should not be presumed to be transected. Conservative management should be implemented initially to allow time for spontaneous recovery. The patient should be followed clinically and with serial electrodiagnostic studies. If no spontaneous recovery is demonstrated by 3 months, consideration should be given to operative exploration with intraoperative electrophysiologic testing. Operative management depends on the findings, but it could include neurolysis alone, resection of a neuroma-in-continuity with primary or graft repair, or nerve transfer. Details of these management decisions are the topic for another chapter.

Regardless of the mechanism of injury, when definitive repair is undertaken and the gap between the nerve ends is greater than 3 cm or when the ends are unable to be coapted without tension, direct repair should not be performed. In these cases, bridging the gap with a nerve conduit, processed allograft, or autologous nerve graft is required. At this point, the gold standard for substantial segmental gaps, especially when greater than 3 cm, is autologous nerve grafting, although the data supporting this are limited to animal models.[5–8] Pure sensory nerves are most often harvested for autologous grafting in order to avoid the motor deficits that would occur with harvesting a combined motor-sensory nerve or a pure motor nerve. Autologous grafts require two neurorrhaphies, potentially a second operative site, increased operative time, and inevitably some donor-site morbidity, even if it is only isolated sensory loss. Nerve conduits are an alternative that may be appropriate in some circumstances. Nerve conduits provide an enclosed, optimal environment for linking the two nerve ends in order to facilitate the pathway of axon regeneration. Benefits of this approach include the avoidance of donor-site morbidity from harvesting a nerve graft, as well as prevention of axonal "wandering." Allografts are now available as an alternative for gaps less than 5 cm to avoid donor-site morbidity. Sensory outcomes for short gaps bridged with processed allografts seem to be equivalent to outcomes for autografts and superior to outcomes for synthetic nerve conduits.[7,9]

Questions

1. How are ragged lacerations managed differently than clean lacerations?
2. What is the optimal management of a large segmental gap?
3. What are the trade-offs when deciding between immediate and delayed nerve repair in a dirty wound?

Surgical Procedure

Nerve repair should be performed under general anesthesia, whenever possible, given the potential lengthy nature of the operation as well as the possibility of harvesting a nerve graft from another limb. Paralytics should be avoided to allow intraoperative nerve stimulation. The patient should be positioned so that the affected extremity is easily accessible. A tourniquet is optional, but the authors prefer its use. When a tourniquet is used, it should be placed high on the injured extremity to allow for precise dissection and neurorrhaphy in a bloodless field. Exposure should be generous, to allow full visualization of the damaged structures. The existing laceration should be incorporated into the surgical incision and may need to be extended. When anatomy is severely distorted, the exposure may need to be extended proximally to allow identification of normal anatomy and thereby facilitate proper identification of injured structures. Nerve dissection and repair should be performed under microscope or loupe magnification to allow for precise operative technique. Depending on the size of the nerve, 6-0 and 7-0 nylon are appropriate for epineurial suturing, whereas 8-0, 9-0, or 10-0 nylon should be used for perineurial suturing or nerve grafting. Neurorrhaphies are supplemented with fibrin glue and can be wrapped with a nerve wrap.

In the case presented, the existing laceration was re-opened over the proximal volar forearm (Figure 27.1). A radial sensory nerve (RSN) branch was found to be lacerated at the level of the proximal forearm, three branches of the PIN were found to be lacerated distal to the initial branch point, and the LABC was noted to be completely transected (Figure 27.2). Microsurgical repairs of the RSN branch

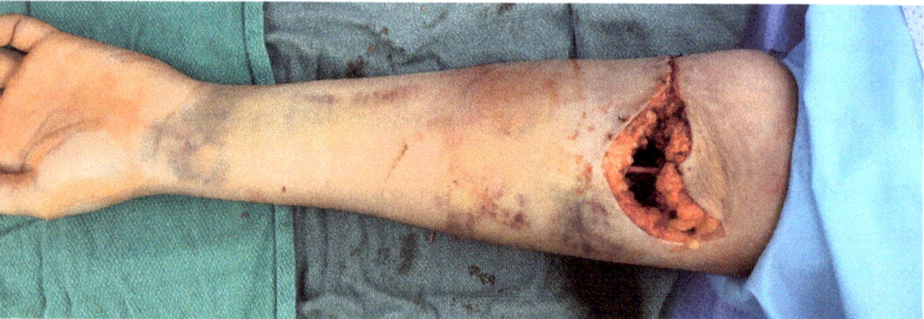

Figure 27.1. Existing laceration re-opened over the proximal volar forearm to expose underlying injured structures.

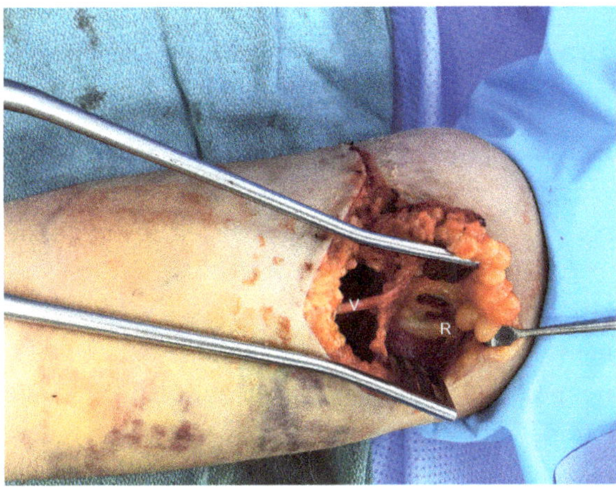

Figure 27.2. Surgical exploration revealed lacerations to radial nerve branches (R). V = superficial vein.

and three motor branches of the PIN were performed using cable grafts from the transected LABC nerve (Figure 27.3). The neurorrhaphies were performed with 9-0 nylon and were reinforced with nerve wrap. After nerve repair was complete, the wound was irrigated, the skin was closed, and the patient was placed in a bulky postoperative splint.

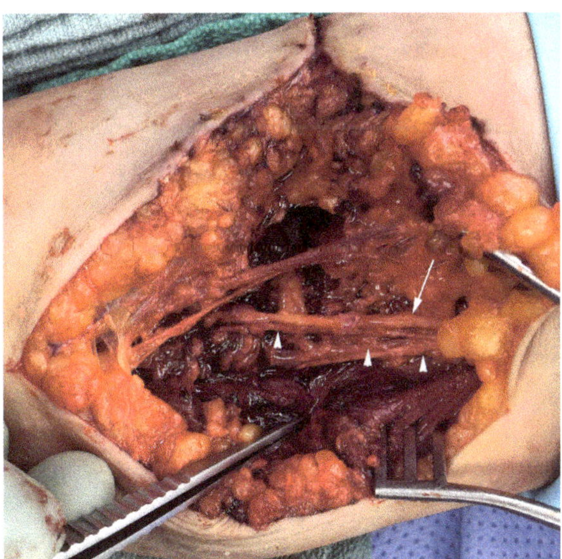

Figure 27.3. Superficial radial nerve (arrow) and three posterior interosseous nerve branches (arrowheads) are each repaired with interposition grafting using a segment of the transected lateral antebrachial cutaneous nerve. Each neurorrhaphy was performed with fine nylon sutures and was reinforced with allograft nerve wrap.

Oral Boards Review—Management Pearls

1. Direct, tension-free repair of sharply lacerated nerves in a clean wound bed with viable soft tissue coverage is the ideal nerve repair, when possible.
2. Resection of ragged nerve ends is indicated when the injury has resulted in tattered nerve endings. Resection of the shortest amount of nerve possible to produce clean nerve ends with discernable bundles and nerve architecture should be performed.
3. When the injury or indicated resection results in a gap that makes tension-free repair not possible, nerve conduit or nerve grafting is indicated.
   a. Nerve grafting with autologous nerve interposition graft is the gold standard for treating segmental nerve defects. Sensory nerves, such as sural nerve, are most commonly used.

Pivot Points

1. Even with a clean, sharp mechanism of injury, if the nerve ends are found to be ragged or in poor condition, they must be resected until normal bleeding fascicular architecture is visualized. If this results in a segmental gap that is unable to be repaired directly without tension, harvest an autologous nerve graft or bridge the gap with a nerve conduit. Prior to the operation, the surgeon should obtain the patient's informed consent for autograft, if the procedure is not emergent, and sterilely prep and drape an area for potential nerve harvest, such as the contralateral sural nerve.
2. If the wound bed is grossly contaminated or acutely inflamed, the surgeon should be prepared to thoroughly irrigate the wound and to defer definitive nerve repair until the wound bed is amenable to healthy tissue healing. Tagging the lacerated nerve ends with a visible, permanent suture, such as Prolene and/or a metal surgical clip, will help identify the nerve ends when repair can be undertaken.

Aftercare

The patient should be placed in a sling or a splint in a neutral position that allows protection of the nerve, avoidance of tension on the suture line, and prevention of secondary problems (such as development of acute carpal tunnel syndrome if the wrist is splinted in extreme flexion or equinus deformity if the ankle is splinted in extreme plantar flexion). Generally, a single dose of perioperative antibiotics is sufficient for an acute injury that undergoes prompt washout. However, if gross contamination or acute infection is present, longer antibiotic regimens may be justifiable. The splint should remain in place until the first follow-up visit, which should occur within 1 week of surgery. The patient should be counseled to elevate the extremity as much as possible to minimize swelling around the repaired nerve and to seek medical attention if there is extreme pain, which could indicate development of compartment syndrome.

Patients should also be counseled that return of function is a slow and arduous process, with nerve regeneration occurring at a rate of approximately 1 mm per day. Patients will need to be active participants in their recovery by engaging consistently in therapy to maintain supple joint range of motion while slowly improving strength. They may also need to comply with serial splinting while motor strength returns.

Complications and Management

One of the most worrisome complications of nerve repair is failure of nerve regeneration and subsequent permanent loss of function. This can result in loss of protective sensation, leading to an increased risk of thermal or physical injury. Loss of motor function leads to irreversible atrophy beginning within 18 months of denervation, which ultimately results in limb imbalance and loss of function. These chronic deficits may eventually require tendon transfers in order to regain some function in the affected limb.

Neuropathic pain is a rare but potentially severely debilitating complication after properly repaired nerve injury. It is difficult to manage for both patient and surgeon and requires close collaboration with an occupational therapist and pain specialist. Treatment modalities include medications, massage, transcutaneous electrical nerve stimulation (TENS), percussion, active limb use and mobilization, and neuromodulation with spinal cord or nerve stimulation. Neuroma is a different entity that will develop if the axons in the regenerating proximal stump are not able to re-enter the distal stump. Neuromas can subsequently become painful if they are subjected to repeated mechanical stimulation, such as when the neuroma is located superficially on an extremity. Treatment with surgical excision and nerve stump wrapping or burying in muscle is usually the last resort in treating painful neuromas.

Cold intolerance is a common outcome of even technically perfect nerve repair. It can result in serious consequences to the patient, including inability to return to work.[10,11]

Oral Boards Review—Complications Pearls

1. Failure of nerve repair can have serious long-term effects on limb function, ultimately resulting in loss of protective sensation and/or motor function. These late complications may require treatment with tendon or nerve transfer.
2. Pain related to nerve injury, including cold sensitivity, neuropathic pain, and painful neuromas, can be difficult to manage. Usually, pain management requires a multidisciplinary approach.

Evidence and Outcomes

Success of nerve repair is dependent on multiple factors: the age of the patient (younger patients have better outcomes after nerve repair), the nature of the nerve injury (clean, sharp lacerations have a better prognosis than dirty, ragged lacerations), the time to repair of the injury (delayed repair results in worse outcomes than expedient repair), the level of the lesion (more distal lesions generally have more successful outcomes), and the associated damage to the limb (extremities with concomitant severe injuries have overall worse function than those with isolated nerve lacerations).[12–20] Evidence shows that the best results occur in patients who are young and healthy and who sustained isolated clean and sharp nerve lacerations that are repaired immediately by an experienced nerve surgeon with direct, tension-free repair.

The nerve involved in the injury is also an important predictor of outcome. In the upper extremity, radial and median nerve injuries at comparable levels appear to have similar outcomes, while ulnar nerve outcomes at similar levels are much poorer. This is likely secondary to the fact that the radial and median nerves innervate primarily proximal muscles, while the ulnar nerve innervates primarily distal muscles. Primary suture for all three nerves leads to the best outcomes, surpassing both secondary suture and nerve graft repair. Following sharp laceration, 56% to 91% of patients can be expected to achieve Louisiana State University Health Sciences Center (LSU) grade 3 or better recovery, with the outcome dependent on the nerve involved, level of injury, and technique utilized for repair.[21]

With ballistic injuries, gunshot wounds on average have a more favorable outcome than shrapnel injuries. Neuropathic pain is a particular problem in these patients. Worse outcomes with shrapnel injury appear to be related to foreign particles remaining postoperatively. The best outcomes for both gunshot wounds and shrapnel injuries relative to neuropathic pain appear to be achieved with early surgical intervention (< 2 months) with neuroma resection and nerve graft repair rather than neurolysis alone.[22] Similar to sharp lacerations, ulnar nerve ballistic injuries have worse outcomes than radial or median nerve ballistic injuries. Secondary repair techniques, such as tendon transfer, are often needed in the case of ulnar nerve ballistic injuries. Outcomes are particularly poor when the median and ulnar nerves are both injured simultaneously.[23]

Similar factors affect outcomes for lower extremity nerve lacerations. The level of injury and nerve involved both appear to be particularly important. More distal injuries have better outcomes than more proximal injuries, and injuries to the tibial nerve have better outcomes than injuries to the common peroneal nerve. Primary repair also has better outcomes than secondary suture or nerve graft repair. The best outcomes have been observed for tibial nerve transections at the knee, where nearly 100% of patients recovered to at least LSU grade 3. The worst outcomes have been observed for common peroneal nerve injury at the buttock level, where only 30% of patients recovered to LSU grade 3 or better.[24]

References

1. Seddon HJ. A classification of nerve injuries. *Br Med J.* 1942;2:237–239.
2. Dayan L, Zinmann C, Stahl S, Norman D. Complications associated with prolonged tourniquet application on the battlefield. *Mil Med.* 2008;173:63–66.
3. Kragh JF Jr, Walters TJ, Baer DG, et al. Practical use of emergency tourniquets to stop bleeding in major limb trauma. *J Trauma.* 2008;64:S38–S49, discussion S49–S50.

4. Scerbo MH, Mumm JP, Gates K, et al. Safety and appropriateness of tourniquets in 105 civilians. *Prehosp Emerg Care*. 2016;20:712–722.
5. Longo MV, Marques de Faria JC, Isaac C, Nepomuceno AC, Teixeira NH, Gemperli R. Comparisons of the results of peripheral nerve defect repair with fibrin conduit and autologous nerve graft: an experimental study in rats. *Microsurgery*. 2016;36:59–65.
6. Sahakyants T, Lee JY, Friedrich PF, Bishop AT, Shin AY. Return of motor function after repair of a 3-cm gap in a rabbit peroneal nerve: a comparison of autograft, collagen conduit, and conduit filled with collagen-GAG matrix. *J Bone Joint Surg Am*. 2013;95:1952–1958.
7. Whitlock EL, Tuffaha SH, Luciano JP, et al. Processed allografts and type I collagen conduits for repair of peripheral nerve gaps. *Muscle Nerve*. 2009;39:787–799.
8. Wu R, Wang L, Chen F, et al. Evaluation of artificial nerve conduit and autografts in peripheral nerve repair in the rat model of sciatic nerve injury. *Neurol Res*. 2016;38:461–466.
9. Rinker BD, Ingari JV, Greenberg JA, Thayer WP, Safa B, Buncke GM. Outcomes of short-gap sensory nerve injuries reconstructed with processed nerve allografts from a multicenter registry study. *J Reconstr Microsurg*. 2015;31:384–390.
10. Novak CB, Anastakis DJ, Beaton DE, Mackinnon SE, Katz J. Cold intolerance after brachial plexus nerve injury. *Hand (N Y)*. 2012;7:66–71.
11. Novak CB, Mackinnon SE. Evaluation of cold sensitivity, pain, and quality of life after upper extremity nerve injury. *Hand (N Y)*. 2016;11:173–176.
12. Birch R, Raji AR. Repair of median and ulnar nerves. Primary suture is best. *J Bone Joint Surg Br*. 1991;73:154–157.
13. Ertem K, Denizhan Y, Yologlu S, Bora A. [The effect of injury level, associated injuries, the type of nerve repair, and age on the prognosis of patients with median and ulnar nerve injuries]. *Acta Orthop Traumatol Turc*. 2005;39:322–327.
14. Johnson EO, Zoubos AB, Soucacos PN. Regeneration and repair of peripheral nerves. *Injury*. 2005;36(suppl 4):24–29.
15. Kalomiri DE, Soucacos PN, Beris AE. Nerve grafting in peripheral nerve microsurgery of the upper extremity. *Microsurgery*. 1994;15:506–511.
16. Millesi H. Factors affecting the outcome of peripheral nerve surgery. *Microsurgery*. 2006;26:295–302.
17. Noaman HH. Management and functional outcomes of combined injuries of flexor tendons, nerves, and vessels at the wrist. *Microsurgery*. 2007;27:536–543.
18. Ruijs AC, Jaquet JB, Kalmijn S, Giele H, Hovius SE. Median and ulnar nerve injuries: a meta-analysis of predictors of motor and sensory recovery after modern microsurgical nerve repair. *Plast Reconstr Surg*. 2005;116:484–494, discussion 495–486.
19. Secer HI, Daneyemez M, Gonul E, Izci Y. Surgical repair of ulnar nerve lesions caused by gunshot and shrapnel: results in 407 lesions. *J Neurosurg*. 2007;107:776–783.
20. Siemionow M, Brzezicki G. Chapter 8: current techniques and concepts in peripheral nerve repair. *Int Rev Neurobiol*. 2009;87:141–172.
21. Murovic JA. Upper-extremity peripheral nerve injuries: a Louisiana State University Health Sciences Center literature review with comparison of the operative outcomes of 1837 Louisiana State University Health Sciences Center median, radial, and ulnar nerve lesions. *Neurosurgery*. 2009;65:A11–A17.

22. Rochkind S, Strauss I, Shlitner Z, Alon M, Reider E, Graif M. Clinical aspects of ballistic peripheral nerve injury: shrapnel versus gunshot. *Acta Neurochir (Wien)*. 2014;156:1567–1575.
23. Taha A, Taha J. Results of suture of the radial, median, and ulnar nerves after missile injury below the axilla. *J Trauma*. 1998;45:335–339.
24. Murovic JA. Lower-extremity peripheral nerve injuries: a Louisiana State University Health Sciences Center literature review with comparison of the operative outcomes of 806 Louisiana State University Health Sciences Center sciatic, common peroneal, and tibial nerve lesions. *Neurosurgery*. 2009;65:A18–A23.

Iatrogenic Peripheral Nerve Injury

Christian Heinen and Thomas Kretschmer

28

Case Presentation

A 63-year-old, obese woman suffered a complex fracture of the humerus. Initial treatment consisted of plate osteosynthesis via a ventromedial approach. Immediately after surgery the patient reported wrist and finger drop, along with pain and sensory deficits in the radial dorsal portion of the hand, including the tips of the thumb and index finger. The surgeon suspected a retraction/pressure injury to the radial nerve and informed the patient that surgery went as planned and the radial nerve was intact, giving her a good prospect for spontaneous recovery. She was informed that nerve recovery occurs slowly and may take 2 to 3 years. Physiotherapy was initiated, but no further investigations were considered to be necessary. As the patient saw no improvement, she referred herself to a neurologist, who then referred her to a nerve surgeon 3.5 months after her operation. Clinical exam revealed absent extension of the wrist and metacarpophalangeal joints, as well as absent thumb abduction. Latissimus dorsi, shoulder abduction, external rotation, elbow flexion/extension, and wrist and finger flexion were full strength.

Questions

1. What is the working diagnosis? Which nerve is affected?
2. What is the presumed anatomic level of injury?
3. What diagnostic testing can support the working diagnosis?
4. What is the appropriate diagnostic workup, treatment, and timing?

Assessment and Planning

General Considerations

In the patient described, the working diagnosis was iatrogenic injury of the radial nerve at the level of the upper arm, distal to the triceps branches. The hallmark of iatrogenic nerve injury is a new sensorimotor deficit and/or neuropathic pain apparent directly after surgery. Establishing the timeline is crucial in working through the differential diagnosis, which includes Parsonage-Turner syndrome, postoperative hematoma, and traumatic nerve injury (not iatrogenic). In the case of iatrogenic injury, the neurologic deficits should be maximal immediately postoperatively, whereas in postoperative Parsonage-Turner syndrome, the patient typically awakens without any deficit and then with variable timing develops pain followed by weakness. Similarly, postoperative hematoma should be considered when the patient awakens without deficits but then in the postoperative period develops progressive neurologic deficits. In the case of traumatic nerve injury, the deficits should have been already present and maximal preoperatively, although with multisystem trauma this can sometimes be difficult to establish.

With iatrogenic nerve injury, the crucial question is whether the severity of the lesion will allow spontaneous recovery or requires surgery. As timing for nerve repair is critical to obtain good functional results, this question needs to be answered as soon as possible. In evaluating the potential for spontaneous recovery, lesion mechanism, functional status (complete versus incomplete), level of the lesion, and the nerve affected are all considered. Therefore, meticulous assessment of the clinical history and physical examination are fundamental. Most of the time, the patient can give a clear account of the timeline of deficits and potential improvement. Distinguishing primary traumatic nerve injury from iatrogenic injury is important with regard to the mechanism of injury but not for timing. Unfortunately, iatrogenic injury is more prone to delay in nerve repair because of unrealistic expectations for spontaneous recovery.

Operative and medical reports may give hints about the level of the lesion, extent, and potential mechanism. Common mechanisms for iatrogenic nerve injury that should be considered include complete and partial nerve transection, compression injury related to positioning, retraction, or tourniquet, thermal injury related to cautery, and compression injury related to surgical instrumentation. Identifying the most likely mechanism of injury is important in determining the likelihood of spontaneous recovery and optimal management.

In this particular case, a pure radial nerve injury has to be differentiated from a more proximal posterior cord lesion. On thorough physical examination, intact triceps, latissimus dorsi, and deltoid muscles (all innervated by the posterior cord) exclude a more proximal (i.e., axillary/infraclavicular) level of the lesion. Also, in the case of injuries located in the upper arm, concomitant median and/or ulnar nerve involvement needs to be ruled out.

Following traumatic nerve injury, iatrogenic or otherwise, it is important to observe for signs of incomplete injury and spontaneous recovery. For radial nerve injuries in the upper arm (distal to the triceps branches), the brachioradialis is an indicator muscle for ongoing regeneration. Spontaneous recovery of the brachioradialis is often overlooked in patients with a complete wrist and finger drop. Functional integrity of the superficial sensory branch also needs to be tested. The next diagnostic step consists of imaging and electrodiagnostics. Nerve conduction studies (NCS) and electromyography (EMG) help to unravel the functional state of nerve and muscle. Although they are not useful in the immediate postinjury period, NCS and EMG can help identify the extent and nature of injury 2 to 3 weeks after injury and can also be used in a serial fashion to follow recovery. Increasing intentional motor activity of dependent muscles on serial electrodiagnostics is a major sign of ongoing regeneration.

In recent years, imaging with high-frequency neurosonography has evolved to be a major tool for decision-making. Complete and partial nerve disruption, as well as major neuroma formation, can be sonographically visualized in most cases, eliminating the need for ongoing observation. Neurosonography allows detailed imaging of the nerve and its surrounding tissue, including muscle quality.[1] High-frequency, 12- to

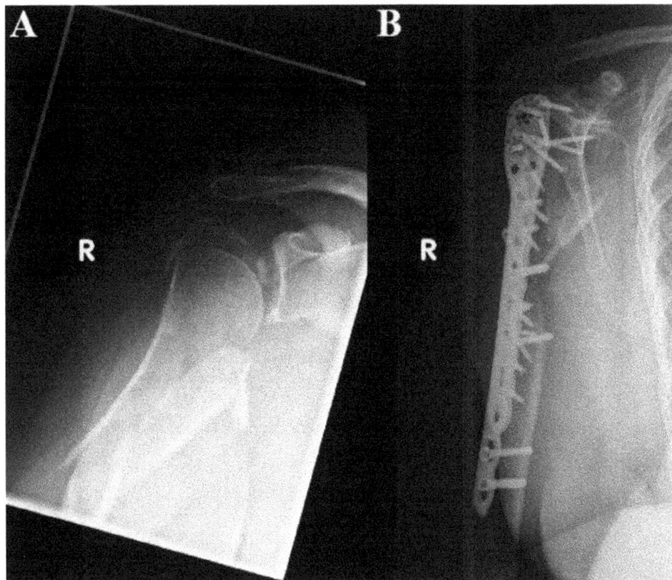

Figure 28.1. A, X-ray of fractured humerus. B, X-ray of fractured humerus after osteosynthesis.

17-MHz probes and compound imaging techniques are necessary. Discontinuities, epi- and intraneural scarring, and the relationship of major nerves to surgical instrumentation (e.g., plates, screws) can be detected. Ultrasound is easy to use, although results are dependent on the skill and experience of the operator and is readily available. The quality of high-frequency ultrasound, however, drops significantly with increasing anatomic depth (e.g., sciatic nerve at the gluteal level).

Dedicated MR imaging can assess nerves along their course and also can assess surrounding tissue with high anatomic resolution. MR imaging is also able to detect neuroma formation, caliber changes in the nerve, and discontinuity of deeper nerve lesions. Imaging of muscle quality (e.g., "denervation edema" and/or fatty atrophy), vessel depiction, detection of hematomas, and identification of scar are other useful features of MR imaging. However, in patients with metal artifact, MR imaging may have limitations in nerve visualization. CT and X-rays are important modalities for imaging bone and surgical instrumentation. Both may have a potential role in preparation for nerve surgery (Figure 28.1).

Case-Related Findings

According to the patient, neurologic deficits, including pain and wrist/finger drop, occurred maximally immediately after surgery and were not present primarily after trauma. The operative report described an "intact radial nerve, which was carefully dissected and spared within the visible field." Physical examination revealed intact triceps function but complete paralysis of the muscles innervated by the distal radial nerve (brachioradialis, supinator, extensor carpi radialis and ulnaris, extensor digitorum communis, extensor pollicis longus and brevis, extensor indicis, and abductor pollicis longus). In addition, complete numbness was found in the distribution of the superficial radial nerve branch. Nerve conduction studies showed no potential in the radial nerve and EMG showed pathologic spontaneous activity but no voluntary motor function for the muscles innervated by the distal radial nerve. On ultrasound, the radial nerve could be seen within the cubital fossa. When the nerve was followed proximally toward the plate, it ended in scar tissue close to the plate. Due to the patient's obesity, high-frequency ultrasound was limited.

Oral Boards Review—Diagnostic Pearls

1. Detailed history and physical examination are crucial/pivotal.
2. A wrist/finger drop with intact triceps function and a sensory deficit in the distribution of the superficial radial nerve are typical for radial nerve lesions after humeral fracture and/or internal fixation of the humerus.
3. Finger extension in the proximal and distal interphalangeal joints is mediated by the lumbricals (median and ulnar nerve-innervated) and not by the radial nerve (so-called "trick movement" mimicking radial function).
4. Nerve imaging should be performed as early as possible and consists of high-frequency neurosonography and/or MR imaging, with the latter being more susceptible to limitation by metal artifacts.
5. If the nerve is found to be in discontinuity or deeply damaged, there is no need to wait for spontaneous regeneration and early surgery should be considered.
6. Electrophysiologic studies should be carried out early and, in unclear cases, may be repeated over time in order to monitor for possible regeneration.

Questions

1. How do the clinical, electrophysiologic, and radiologic findings affect treatment?
2. How should treatment be timed?
3. What has to be taken into account when considering surgery?

Decision-Making

Common Clinical Scenarios for Iatrogenic Nerve Injury

If nerve transection or injury secondary to surgical instrumentation is suspected, immediate surgical exploration should be undertaken. In cases where nerve transection, complete or partial, is recognized intraoperatively, primary repair in a tension-free manner should be undertaken in the same operative setting when possible. In cases where tension-free repair is not possible, nerve graft repair should be performed in the same operative setting. Early, tension-free, primary repair offers the best hope for recovery.

While iatrogenic nerve injury can occur with any operation, there are some well-described clinical scenarios associated with iatrogenic nerve injury. In these situations, at least limited data exist to aid in decision-making regarding management, timing of any potential intervention, and likely outcomes.

Hip arthroplasty and other surgical procedures near the hip place a myriad of nerves at risk for iatrogenic injury, including the femoral nerve, sciatic nerve, and lateral femoral cutaneous nerve. In one series, 25% of sciatic nerve lesions and 60% of femoral nerve lesions that required treatment were iatrogenic.[2] The incidence of iatrogenic nerve damage with total hip arthroplasty is reportedly as high as approximately 7%, with approximately 50% recovering by 2 years postoperatively.[3,4] Risk of iatrogenic nerve injury appears to be higher with revision surgery.[3] A variety of etiologies have been proposed, including retraction injury, positioning/stretch injury related to extreme lateral rotation of the leg or hyperextension, cement extravasation, thermal injury related to cement, direct nerve injury, significant leg lengthening, and postoperative hematoma. Reported risk factors other than revision surgery include younger age, female sex, longer operative time, and posterior (versus anterior) approach.[5]

With sciatic nerve injury related to total hip arthroplasty, the peroneal division seems to be more susceptible to injury. Retraction weight seems to be the biggest risk factor for sciatic nerve injury.[6] Not only is the sciatic nerve at risk intraoperatively, but also delayed sciatic nerve palsy can occur related to hardware irritation, component failure, or wear-related pseudotumor formation.[7] Approximately 50% of patients who develop common peroneal-predominant sciatic palsy can expect to make a full recovery, with the average time to recovery being approximately 1 year for partial lesions and 1.5 years for complete lesions. The only factor that has been identified that adversely affects recovery is obesity.[8] There are some data to suggest that outcomes are better when sciatic neurolysis is performed. In these cases, surgery should not be delayed beyond 12 months.[9,10] Other centers have performed distal decompression of the peroneal nerve at the fibular tunnel. Early evidences suggests this may also be an effective strategy, with positive predictors of postoperative recovery including motor unit action potentials in the tibialis anterior or peroneus longus on preoperative electromyography.[11]

The reported incidence of femoral neuropathy after total hip arthroplasty ranges from 0.1% to 2.4%.[12] With a posterior approach, the common position of the retractors places both the femoral and obturator nerves at risk of retraction injury.[13] There is no consensus regarding management of these injuries. An initial period of conservative management is warranted, but the duration is unclear. Due to metal artifacts and deeply situated lesions, imaging is limited in this area. However, if MR imaging or ultrasound depicts a severe lesion, surgery should be scheduled. If spontaneous recovery is lacking, options include neurolysis, neuroma resection with graft repair, and obturator to femoral nerve transfer, although there are no data that determine the best course of treatment.[14–16]

Injury to the lateral femoral cutaneous nerve is the most common iatrogenic nerve injury in total hip arthroplasty, with related symptoms reported in up to 67% of patients.[17] Hip resurfacing may have an even higher incidence.[17] Hypesthesia in the distribution of the lateral femoral cutaneous nerve is more common than paresthesias, but, nonetheless, injury to this nerve has been associated with reduced quality of life.[18] Most symptoms spontaneously resolve by 2 years.[19] Given that the majority of patients experience spontaneous symptom resolution, a period of conservative management or management with neuropathic pain medications is justified. Optimal management of the minority of patients who have persistent symptoms is unclear, but nerve exploration with either neurolysis or neurectomy is probably warranted in these patients.

Both the saphenous nerve and common peroneal nerve are at risk in total knee arthroplasty. Risk factors for common peroneal nerve injury include younger age and obesity. The majority of common peroneal nerve palsies are incomplete. Approximately 75% of incomplete nerve palsies recover fully, while complete palsies rarely recover fully.[20] This suggests conservative management should be employed for incomplete palsies, but early surgical exploration may be warranted for complete palsies.

Injury to the saphenous nerve, particularly the infrapatellar branch, is common in total knee arthroplasty, with some series reporting that up to 84% of patients sustain injury to the infrapatellar branch.[21] Saphenous neurectomy can be effective and beneficial, with high rates of patient satisfaction.[22] The natural history and likelihood of spontaneous recovery are unclear. One center has implemented a protocol to determine candidacy for surgical denervation that includes pain lasting at least 1 year, failure of conservative and pharmacologic management, positive Tinel sign along the course of the saphenous nerve/infrapatellar branch, and a positive response to nerve block with 1% lidocaine.[22]

In the upper extremity, shoulder surgery, clavicular fractures and repairs, and humeral fractures and repairs are among the most commonly encountered scenarios for iatrogenic nerve injury.[23,24] Due to its course passing the spiral groove adjacent to the bone and returning to the medial aspect of the arm in the cubital fossa, the radial nerve is especially prone not only to traumatic injury but also to iatrogenic injury during open reduction and plate fusion of humeral fractures. The risk of iatrogenic injury during open surgical repair of a diaphyseal humeral fracture is approximately 7%, while the rate of radial nerve injury from the initial trauma and fracture is approximately 20%.[25] Exposure type is significantly associated with radial nerve risk, with lateral exposure having the highest risk and anterolateral exposure having the lowest risk.[25] The radial nerve tends to recover well both spontaneously and after surgical repair.

Spinal accessory nerve injury complicates 3% to 6% of cervical lymph node biopsies, predominantly Zone 1 biopsies.[26,27] The most common presenting symptom of spinal accessory nerve injury is pain, likely secondary to scapulohumeral dysfunction. Most patients do not notice a limitation in abduction; rather, the most common presenting sign is the inability to sustain abduction.[27] If neurologic injury is suspected, surgery should not be delayed. The outcomes of surgical exploration are excellent. Surgery should involve exploration of the nerve with nerve action potential (NAP) recordings if the nerve is found to be in continuity. If NAPs are present across the lesion, neurolysis alone should be performed. If the nerve is transected or NAPs are absent across the lesion, direct suture or graft repair should be undertaken. The majority of patients recover grade 3 or better function and have improvement in pain.[27–29]

C5 palsy after cervical decompression is a well-known complication. Most series report the incidence to be approximately 5% to 9%.[30–33] The majority (80% to 90%) of patients fully recover by 2 years postoperatively.[30,31] Negative prognostic indicators include severe palsy (motor grade 2 or less) and injury encompassing more than just C5 (typically C5-C6 or C5-C6-C7).[30,31] Median time to full recovery falls between

6 months and 1 year.[31] For these patients, a period of conservative management should be undertaken, as most patients will recover spontaneously. If no recovery is evident by 6 to 12 months, consideration can be given to reconstruction using nerve transfers or tendon transfers.

Case-Specific Decision-Making

Usually the radial nerve is one of the best-regenerating nerves in the human body. In the literature, spontaneous recovery rates of up to 92% have been reported, with better rates for closed fractures.[34] Unfortunately, this reputation for spontaneous recovery is one of the reasons why necessary repair is often neglected or unnecessarily delayed. Partial injury or partial recovery does not exclude the need for surgery. In cases of partial but substantial nerve injury, surgery might be necessary to regain function or ease pain. Furthermore, one key factor for successful treatment is timing. If nerve damage requiring surgery is detected, there is no need for a "wait and see" approach. Earlier operative intervention is associated with improved outcomes. Thus, the authors strongly recommend early intervention when necessary and possible. Late referral is a major and frequent obstacle to optimal recovery. The surgeon responsible for the iatrogenic injury may minimize the extent of nerve damage and raise unrealistically high hopes for spontaneous recovery.

In the case presented here, 3.5 months after surgery, there were no signs of improvement, with a complete clinical lesion of the radial nerve distal to the triceps branches. In addition, EMG showed pathologic activity only, and ultrasound revealed a lesion in discontinuity with massive scar. Thus, there was a clear indication for surgery. Patients always need to be prepared for and counseled about potential graft repair, but they also should be counseled regarding other options that may be necessary, including tendon transfer. In cases where there is suspected injury related to surgical instrumentation, it may be necessary to enlist other surgical colleagues to aid in surgery so that surgical instrumentation can be appropriately managed.

Questions

1. What is the best surgical approach?
2. How should the patient be positioned and why?
3. What are the possible surgical techniques?
4. What are the steps to surgical exposure?
5. What surgical instruments should be available?

Surgical Procedure

General Considerations

Surgery is performed under general anesthesia, without the use of long-acting muscle relaxants to allow for intraoperative nerve stimulation and electrophysiologic testing. The authors prefer totally intravenous anesthesia (TIVA). A surgical microscope, microsurgical instruments, intraoperative high-frequency ultrasound, and intraoperative electrophysiological monitoring (EMG of wrist and finger extensors and possible recording of NAPs) are essential surgical tools. Other instruments that should be available include screwdrivers and pliers in case there is a need for plate removal. The surgeon should keep in mind that, in some cases, multiple approaches are needed. Positioning, surgical preparation, and draping should take this into consideration.

Positioning

In surgery to address iatrogenic radial nerve injury, patients are positioned supine, with the impaired arm abducted 90° on a broad armrest or hand table. Care should be taken to ensure all pressure points are appropriately padded. Surgical access to the cubital fossa/proximal radial portion of the forearm, the lateral aspect of the upper arm, and the axillary and infraclavicular part of the brachial plexus in cases of proximal lesions should be possible. One leg is prepared for potential harvesting of the sural nerve for use as nerve graft.

Surgical Considerations

The radial nerve is the larger of two terminal branches of the posterior cord and passes through the triangular interval to enter the posterior compartment of the arm. The triceps branches usually leave the nerve in the axilla before the main trunk takes its lateral course around and directly adjacent to the humerus to the cubital fossa. In the cubital fossa, the nerve slopes medially to run between the biceps/brachialis and brachioradialis muscles. The goal of initial dissection is to identify the healthy portions of the nerve proximal and distal to the lesion. Thus, the dissection is begun in the cubital fossa, with identification of the distal, presumably intact, radial nerve. The nerve is approached via a ventral, mid to lateral incision in the proximal lower arm. The nerve can then be followed proximally toward the lesion. Identification of the intact portion of the nerve proximally can be more challenging, and sometimes access through a separate incision in the medial upper arm is required. Once the lesion is isolated, a decision about the proper surgical measure can be made (i.e., neurolysis versus graft repair versus split repair).

In cases of discontinuity, nerve graft repair can be undertaken, using sural nerve as graft. The neuromatous proximal and distal nerve ends are resected back to healthy nerve with normal fascicular architecture. The number of grafts is determined by the cross-sectional size of the radial nerve and by the available length of graft. The nerve graft is then coapted proximally and distally in a tension-free manner with suture (we prefer 10-0) augmented with fibrin glue. For long lesions, it is sometimes necessary to graft from the medial proximal arm at the level of the axilla to the distal posterolateral arm. Use of two incisions with tunnelling of grafts is effective in such cases. Rerouting the grafts on the ventral (brachialis) side of the humerus allows graft length to be spared (2–3 cm).

For lesions in continuity, decision-making is more difficult. A combination of palpation and microscopic visualization, direct nerve stimulation, recording of NAPs, and high-frequency ultrasound is utilized to decide between full-segment resection and graft repair, partial neuroma resection and split-graft repair, and/or internal versus external microscopic neurolysis. If the nerve has been screwed, pinned, or plated or has undergone cerclage, removal of the osteosynthetic material might be necessary.

Therefore, it is essential to obtain a preoperative orthopedic consultation regarding whether the material can be safely removed without replacement or will need to be replaced, and in some cases, intraoperative collaboration with orthopedic surgery colleagues may be necessary.

Surgery

For the patient presented here, we started with an incision in the cubital fossa, allowing identification of the distal intact nerve as described above. As the nerve was followed proximally, the nerve was found to be screwed underneath the plate. We then extended the skin incision along the lateral aspect of the humerus. Dissection of the nerve further proximally allowed exclusion of a double crush lesion. After identifying the intact proximal nerve portion, we followed it down to the point where the nerve was screwed underneath the plate. Scar tissue was removed and external neurolysis was performed. With clear discontinuity of the nerve and a gap spanning approximately 5 cm, the right sural nerve was harvested via a mini-incision using a nerve stripper and was prepared for grafting. Because the grafts would pass directly on the plate, a pedicled autologous fat flap was dissected and was placed underneath the sural nerve grafts. Under microscopic view, both stumps were resected back to healthy nerve, the grafts were positioned and then coapted in a tension-free manner using 10-0 suture augmented with fibrin glue (Figure 28.2A-G). The wound was then copiously irrigated and closed in layers. An arm sling was applied to prevent rupturing of the coaptations.

Oral Boards Review—Management Pearls

1. Positioning and draping should allow for surgical access to the radial nerve throughout its anatomic course and also should allow nerve graft harvesting.
2. Complete dissection of the lesion as well as the proximal and distal intact nerve portions is mandatory.
3. In cases of a lesion in continuity, aside from anatomic criteria, such as intraneural scarring, intraoperative electrophysiologic and ultrasound exams facilitate decision-making.
4. In grafting, resection back to intact, healthy nerve for both the proximal and distal stumps is crucial, with a tension-free coaptation of the nerve graft.

Pivot Points

1. Careful and early workup of postoperative radial nerve lesions will help discern which patients require nerve surgery.
2. If the severity of the lesion impedes spontaneous recovery, nerve surgery should be scheduled.
3. Late referral is one of most important barriers to maximizing recovery.

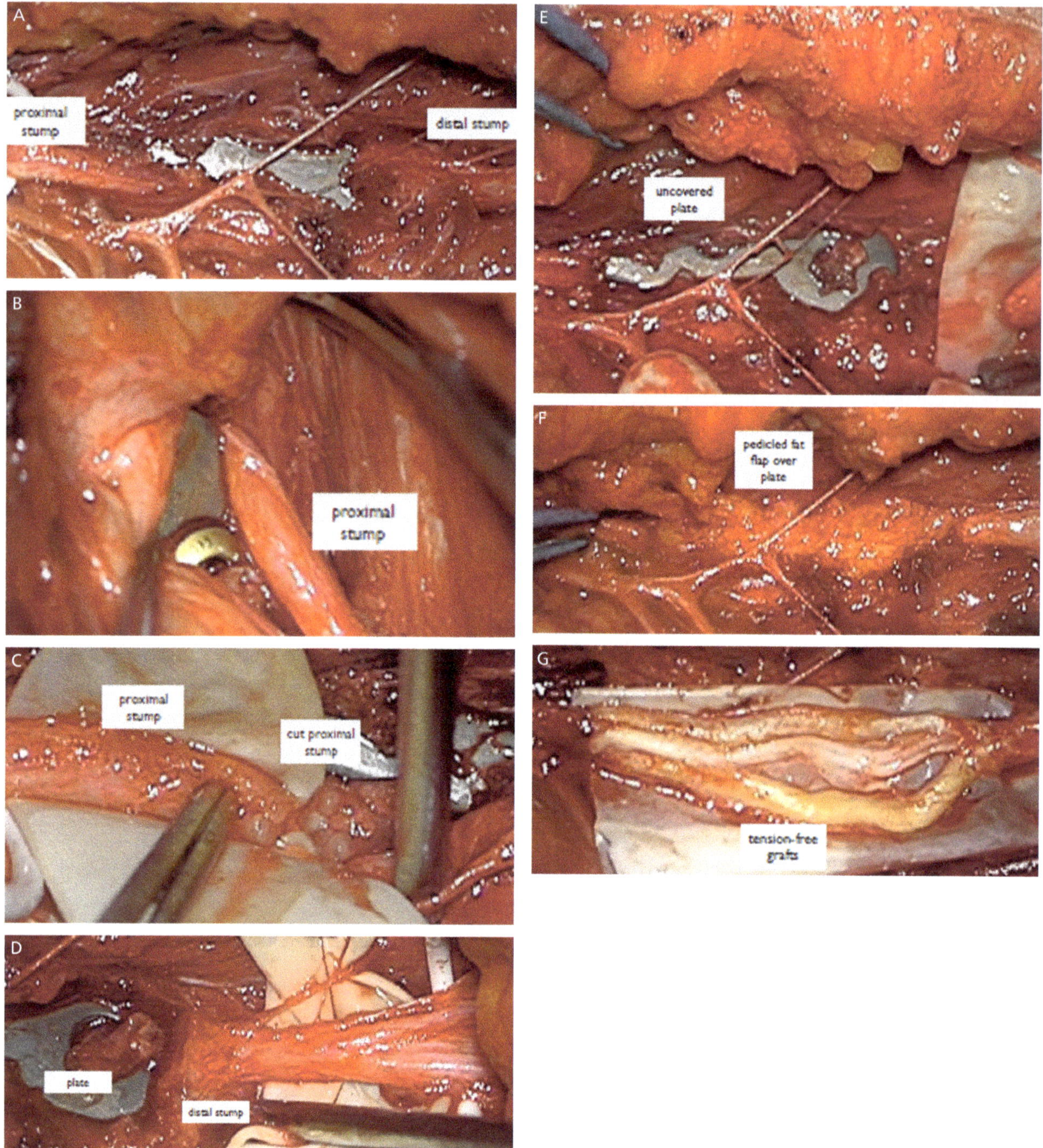

Figure 28.2. Intraoperative photographs. A, Exposure of the normal proximal and distal portions of the radial nerve. B, Magnified view of the proximal nerve beneath the plate. C, Resection of the proximal stump of the nerve back to healthy, nonscarred nerve. D, Distal nerve stump beneath the plate. E, View after cutting of the proximal and distal nerve stumps. F, Plate covered by a pedicled fat flap. G, Tension-free nerve grafts.

Aftercare

After graft repair, patients are moderately immobilized to prevent disruption of the coaptation sites. Patients usually are told not to flex/extend the adjacent joints more than 30° each for 2 to 3 weeks in order not to jeopardize the coaptations. First follow-up is scheduled 6 months after surgery for clinical evaluation and electrophysiologic examination and then is continued every 6 months for at least 3 years. After decompression and neurolysis, we allow mobilization immediately postoperatively and follow-up at 3 months, as regeneration can be expected earlier. Subsequently, follow-up occurs at 6-month intervals for up to 3 years. We evaluate clinically and with electrophysiologic assessment. All patients should undergo regular (i.e., 2 to 3 times per week) and long-term physiotherapy.

Complications and Management

Severe complications are infrequent in operations on the lateral aspect of the humerus. In proximal lesions requiring axillary or infraclavicular access, brachial plexus structures and especially the vessels have to be spared. A set of vascular instruments and the correct vessel sutures should be available in the operating room. Attention has to be paid to the triceps branches by using a nerve stimulator for detection. If the branches are inadvertently cut, immediate repair by direct suture is mandatory.

Sensory branches of the posterior brachial cutaneous nerve can be harmed. Focused, tissue-sparing dissection in anatomic planes and avoidance of muscle transection prevents bleeding and edema. Osteosynthetic material and surgical instrumentation have to be removed very cautiously. Further orthopedic operations following nerve repair harbor the risk of new nerve damage. As a consequence, nerve surgery should be the last in the chronologic order but within a time frame of 2 to 6 months to maximize the potential for recovery.

Evidence and Outcomes

Approximately 10% to 20% of humeral fractures are associated with radial nerve injuries.[25,35,36] The radial nerve itself is considered one of the best-recovering nerves, with useful function recovering in approximately 98% of patients after nerve graft repair.[37] Earlier intervention is clearly correlated with improved outcomes.[38] Success rates drop with more proximal injuries and with concomitant injuries, such as vessel or plexus laceration.[39,40]

All mechanisms of intraoperative trauma have been reported, including complete and partial nerve transection, stretch injury related to retraction, thermal damage due to cautery or bone cement, ischemic injury/compression secondary to a tourniquet, and malpositioning. One major barrier is late referral, as surgeons tend to neglect such complications and patients are consoled with vague statements regarding the damage and its prognosis, often with unrealistic expectations for spontaneous recovery. Taking all this into account with the individual pattern of damage, prognosis may differ significantly from patient to patient.

References

1. Koenig RW, Pedro MT, Heinen CP, et al. High-resolution ultrasonography in evaluating peripheral nerve entrapment and trauma. *Neurosurg Focus*. 2009;26:E13.
2. Antoniadis G, Kretschmer T, Pedro MT, Konig RW, Heinen CP, Richter HP. Iatrogenic nerve injuries: prevalence, diagnosis and treatment. *Dtsch Arztebl Int*. 2014;111:273–279.
3. Brown GD, Swanson EA, Nercessian OA. Neurologic injuries after total hip arthroplasty. *Am J Orthop (Belle Mead NJ)*. 2008;37:191–197.
4. Zappe B, Glauser PM, Majewski M, Stockli HR, Ochsner PE. Long-term prognosis of nerve palsy after total hip arthroplasty: results of two-year-follow-ups and long-term results after a mean time of 8 years. *Arch Orthop Trauma Surg*. 2014;134:1477–1482.
5. Jacob AK, Mantilla CB, Sviggum HP, Schroeder DR, Pagnano MW, Hebl JR. Perioperative nerve injury after total hip arthroplasty: regional anesthesia risk during a 20-year cohort study. *Anesthesiology*. 2011;115:1172–1178.
6. Telleria JJ, Safran MR, Harris AH, Gardi JN, Glick JM. Risk of sciatic nerve traction injury during hip arthroscopy—is it the amount or duration? An intraoperative nerve monitoring study. *J Bone Joint Surg Am*. 2012;94:2025–2032.
7. Xu LW, Veeravagu A, Azad TD, Harraher C, Ratliff JK. Delayed presentation of sciatic nerve injury after total hip arthroplasty: neurosurgical considerations, diagnosis, and management. *J Neurol Surg Rep*. 2016;77:e134–138.
8. Park JH, Hozack B, Kim P, et al. Common peroneal nerve palsy following total hip arthroplasty: prognostic factors for recovery. *J Bone Joint Surg Am*. 2013;95:e55.
9. Chughtai M, Khlopas A, Gwam CU, et al. Nerve decompression surgery after total hip arthroplasty: what are the outcomes? *J Arthroplasty*. 2017;32:1335–1339.
10. Regev GJ, Drexler M, Sever R, et al. Neurolysis for the treatment of sciatic nerve palsy associated with total hip arthroplasty. *Bone Joint J*. 2015;97-B:1345–1349.
11. Wilson TJ, Kleiber GM, Nunley RM, Mackinnon SE, Spinner RJ. Distal peroneal nerve decompression after sciatic nerve injury secondary to total hip arthroplasty. *J Neurosurg*. 2018 Feb 2:1–5. doi:10.3171/2017.8.JNS171260. [Epub ahead of print]. PMID: 29393761.
12. Fox AJ, Bedi A, Wanivenhaus F, Sculco TP, Fox JS. Femoral neuropathy following total hip arthroplasty: review and management guidelines. *Acta Orthop Belg*. 2012;78:145–151.
13. McConaghie FA, Payne AP, Kinninmonth AW. The role of retraction in direct nerve injury in total hip replacement: an anatomical study. *Bone Joint Res*. 2014;3:212–216.
14. Campbell AA, Eckhauser FE, Belzberg A, Campbell JN. Obturator nerve transfer as an option for femoral nerve repair: case report. *Neurosurgery*. 2010;66:375, discussion 375.
15. Goubier JN, Teboul F, Yeo S. Transfer of two motor branches of the anterior obturator nerve to the motor portion of the femoral nerve: an anatomical feasibility study. *Microsurgery*. 2012;32:463–465.
16. Inaba N, Sato K, Suzuki T, et al. Partial obturator nerve transfer for femoral nerve injury: a case report. *J Orthop Sci*. 2018;23:202–204.
17. Goulding K, Beaule PE, Kim PR, Fazekas A. Incidence of lateral femoral cutaneous nerve neurapraxia after anterior approach hip arthroplasty. *Clin Orthop Relat Res*. 2010;468:2397–2404.
18. Homma Y, Baba T, Sano K, et al. Lateral femoral cutaneous nerve injury with the direct anterior approach for total hip arthroplasty. *Int Orthop*. 2016;40:1587–1593.
19. Bhargava T, Goytia RN, Jones LC, Hungerford MW. Lateral femoral cutaneous nerve impairment after direct anterior approach for total hip arthroplasty. *Orthopedics*. 2010;33:472.

20. Park JH, Restrepo C, Norton R, Mandel S, Sharkey PF, Parvizi J. Common peroneal nerve palsy following total knee arthroplasty: prognostic factors and course of recovery. *J Arthroplasty.* 2013;28:1538–1542.
21. Henningsen MH, Jaeger P, Hilsted KL, Dahl JB. Prevalence of saphenous nerve injury after adductor-canal-blockade in patients receiving total knee arthroplasty. *Acta Anaesthesiol Scand.* 2013;57:112–117.
22. Nahabedian MY, Johnson CA. Operative management of neuromatous knee pain: patient selection and outcome. *Ann Plast Surg.* 2001;46:15–22.
23. Carofino BC, Brogan DM, Kircher MF, et al. Iatrogenic nerve injuries during shoulder surgery. *J Bone Joint Surg Am.* 2013;95:1667–1674.
24. Thavarajah D, Scadden J. Iatrogenic postoperative brachial plexus compression secondary to hypertrophic non-union of a clavicle fracture. *Ann R Coll Surg Engl.* 2013;95:e55–57.
25. Claessen FM, Peters RM, Verbeek DO, Helfet DL, Ring D. Factors associated with radial nerve palsy after operative treatment of diaphyseal humeral shaft fractures. *J Shoulder Elbow Surg.* 2015;24:e307–311.
26. Cesmebasi A, Spinner RJ. An anatomic-based approach to the iatrogenic spinal accessory nerve injury in the posterior cervical triangle: how to avoid and treat it. *Clin Anat.* 2015;28:761–766.
27. Park SH, Esquenazi Y, Kline DG, Kim DH. Surgical outcomes of 156 spinal accessory nerve injuries caused by lymph node biopsy procedures. *J Neurosurg Spine.* 2015;23:518–525.
28. Goransson H, Leppanen OV, Vastamaki M. Patient outcome after surgical management of the spinal accessory nerve injury: a long-term follow-up study. *SAGE Open Med.* 2016;4:2050312116645731.
29. Kim DH, Cho YJ, Tiel RL, Kline DG. Surgical outcomes of 111 spinal accessory nerve injuries. *Neurosurgery.* 2003;53:1106–1112, discussion 1102–1103.
30. Lim CH, Roh SW, Rhim SC, Jeon SR. Clinical analysis of C5 palsy after cervical decompression surgery: relationship between recovery duration and clinical and radiological factors. *Eur Spine J.* 2016;26:1101–1110.
31. Macki M, Alam R, Kerezoudis P, Gokaslan Z, Bydon A, Bydon M. Manual muscle test at C5 palsy onset predicts the likelihood of and time to C5 palsy resolution. *J Clin Neurosci.* 2016;24:112–116.
32. Nassr A, Eck JC, Ponnappan RK, Zanoun RR, Donaldson WF III, Kang JD. The incidence of C5 palsy after multilevel cervical decompression procedures: a review of 750 consecutive cases. *Spine (Phila Pa 1976).* 2012;37:174–178.
33. Shou F, Li Z, Wang H, Yan C, Liu Q, Xiao C. Prevalence of C5 nerve root palsy after cervical decompressive surgery: a meta-analysis. *Eur Spine J.* 2015;24:2724–2734.
34. Korompilias AV, Lykissas MG, Kostas-Agnantis IP, Vekris MD, Soucacos PN, Beris AE. Approach to radial nerve palsy caused by humerus shaft fracture: is primary exploration necessary? *Injury.* 2013;44:323–326.
35. Kretschmer T, Heinen CW, Antoniadis G, Richter HP, Konig RW. Iatrogenic nerve injuries. *Neurosurg Clin N Am.* 2009;20:73–90, vii.
36. Noble J, Munro CA, Prasad VS, Midha R. Analysis of upper and lower extremity peripheral nerve injuries in a population of patients with multiple injuries. *J Trauma.* 1998;45:116–122.
37. Roganovic Z, Pavlicevic G. Difference in recovery potential of peripheral nerves after graft repairs. *Neurosurgery.* 2006;59:621–633.

38. Kretschmer T, Antoniadis G, Braun V, Rath SA, Richter HP. Evaluation of iatrogenic lesions in 722 surgically treated cases of peripheral nerve trauma. *J Neurosurg.* 2001;94:905–912.

39. Birch R. The treatment and prognosis of major nerve injury in the adult upper limb. *Current Orthopaedics.* 1999;13:9–19.

40. Venouziou AI, Dailiana ZH, Varitimidis SE, Hantes ME, Gougoulias NE, Malizos KN. Radial nerve palsy associated with humeral shaft fracture. Is the energy of trauma a prognostic factor? *Injury.* 2011;42:1289–1293.

Nerve Transfers for Spinal Cord Injury

Daniel Hafez, Adam Bevan, and Wilson Z. Ray

29

Case Presentation

A 56-year-old, right-handed man presented in a delayed fashion to a neurosurgeon with a complete (ASIA-A) spinal cord injury at the level of C6. Fifteen months earlier, he had been a driver in a motor vehicle collision, and he sustained a closed fracture and dislocation of the cervical spine at C5-C7. He underwent a C5-C7 anterior cervical discectomy and fusion (ACDF) and a posterior cervical laminectomy and fusion at a separate facility. In addition, he had fractured his right humerus and right wrist, both of which were surgically repaired. He had a prolonged recovery at a rehabilitation hospital and presented for consideration of peripheral nerve transfers. On physical exam, mental status and cranial nerves were intact. He had 5/5 strength in his deltoids and biceps bilaterally. He had good supination, pronation, and wrist extension. He had 0/5 strength in his triceps, finger flexors, and hand intrinsic muscles bilaterally. He had good passive range of motion in both his proximal and distal interphalangeal joints, with mild fixed flexion that he used to augment his wrist extension tenodesis. He had good passive range of motion with wrist flexion at the previous fracture site. Sensation was absent below the C6 level. The patient had no interval change in his motor or sensory exam for the preceding 13 months.

Assessment and Planning

In spinal cord injury, early work with peripheral nerve transfers has demonstrated promising results. In the case presented, the patient had a compete injury at C6, and it appeared that he could benefit from multiple peripheral nerve transfers. The goals of nerve transfer in patients with spinal cord injury differ significantly from the goals in patients with brachial plexus injury. In adult patients with brachial plexus injury, the primary goals of reconstruction are elbow flexion, shoulder abduction, and external rotation. Patients with spinal cord injury differ in that they typically have preserved proximal function and more distal deficits. The goal in reconstruction is to restore movement needed for specific activities. Major movements that have been targeted for restoration include elbow extension (to allow the patient to assist in transfers) and pinch, grasp, and release, which can aid in controlling a motorized wheelchair as well as in feeding oneself. Other major goals are hand sensation and diaphragm reinnervation to allow ventilator weaning and spontaneous respiration.

A variety of nerve transfer strategies may be available to accomplish these goals, depending on the level of injury. Commonly employed nerve transfers for restoration of elbow extension include axillary nerve branch to triceps branch and teres minor branch to triceps branch.[1–5] Restoration of grasp typically involves reinnervation of the anterior interosseous nerve (AIN). Commonly employed strategies include brachialis branch to AIN, brachioradialis branch to AIN, extensor carpi radialis brevis (ECRB) branch to flexor pollicis longus (FPL) branch, and supinator branch to AIN.[6–12] The functionality of grasp is increased if the patient also has voluntary release, which is typically accomplished by reinnervation of the posterior interosseous nerve (PIN). The most commonly described nerve transfer option is supinator branch to PIN.[5,14–16] Similarly, hand function is improved with sensation. Recently, two nerve transfer strategies have been described for restoration of hand sensation: median nerve cutaneous branches to the ulnar proper digital nerve of the little finger and lateral antebrachial cutaneous nerve to medial antebrachial cutaneous nerve.[17] Finally, high cervical spinal cord injuries can result in loss of voluntary diaphragmatic control due to loss of phrenic innervation. The spinal accessory nerve (SAN) has been used to reinnervate the phrenic nerve.[17–20]

Electromyography (EMG) and nerve conduction studies (NCS) are essential to help determine whether peripheral nerve transfers would be possible and appropriately utilized. These studies are particularly useful in distinguishing upper motor neuron (UMN), lower motor neuron (LMN), and mixed injuries (especially around the level of injury). When LMN injury is evident, as with typical peripheral nerve injuries, reinnervation should occur within 6 to 12 months of injury in order to prevent irrecoverable damage to the neuromuscular junctions (NMJ). In muscles with only UMN injury, the window for reinnervation seems indefinitely open due to persistence of a healthy NMJ. Operative intervention should be reserved for patients with a stable neurologic exam for at least 6 to 12 months, although some authors advocate for 24 months of preoperative neurologic stability. This ensures that no viable muscles capable of regeneration or spontaneous recovery are included in the treatment plan, and typically it makes only those segments with UMN dysfunction viable targets for reinnervation.

Decision-Making

The EMG and NCS findings for the patient are summarized in Tables 29.1 and 29.2. He had UMN dysfunction in his median and ulnar distribution, with mixed UMN and LMN dysfunction in the radial distribution. EMG findings of severe denervation with relative sparing of sensory nerve action potentials (SNAPs) denoted primarily preganglionic lesions (roots or anterior horn cells). Functional electrical stimulation (FES) can be useful in distinguishing UMN lesions from LMN injuries. Muscles with UMN dysfunction (Figure 29.1) with intact anterior horn cells below the zone of injury stimulate strongly, while muscles with a mixed injury pattern will stimulate weakly or not at all. FES used in conjunction with EMG and NCS can help differentiate pure UMN dysfunction from mixed upper and LMN injury. In this patient, that became particularly relevant during evaluation of the triceps and PIN for reinnervation. Last, it is often difficult to clearly discern a superimposed median/ulnar

Table 29.1.
Summary of Nerve Conduction Studies[a]

Nerve	CMAP	Motor Latency	SNAP	Sensory Velocity
Left median	Normal	Normal	Slightly diminished	Normal
Right median	Normal	Prolonged 5.3 msec	Small	Normal
Left ulnar	Normal	Prolonged 5.7 msec	Small	Normal
Right ulnar	Normal	Normal	Small	Normal
Left radial	Reduced	Prolonged 5.3 msec	Slightly diminished	Delayed
Right radial	Reduced	Prolonged 6.4 msec	Small	Delayed

[a]Findings for the size of the compound motor action potential (CMAP) and the sensory nerve action potential (SNAP), as well as their respective velocities.

entrapment, which is not infrequently identified on the neurodiagnostics and may or may not have clinical relevance.

Based on clinical exam, EMG, NCS, and FES, the surgeon can identify potential available donors for nerve transfer and can prioritize the functional needs of the patient to identify targets for nerve transfer. Combining these results allows the surgeon to devise a comprehensive reconstruction strategy, which may consist of a combination of nerve transfer, tendon transfer, and/or advanced prosthetic augmentation. The goal of nerve transfers in the setting of spinal cord injury is to transfer healthy nerves innervated by the rostral, uninjured spinal cord to intact distal nerves below the zone of injury (Figure 29.1). In the setting of a C6 spinal cord injury, the brachialis nerve from uninjured C5 can readily be transferred to the AIN/flexor digitorum superficialis (FDS; C8). Based on preoperative FES findings, other potential transfers for this patient included posterior deltoid/teres minor to triceps (using a prone posterior approach) and supinator branch to PIN (via a separate forearm incision).

Surgical Procedure

Although some generalities apply, specific surgical details depend on the reconstructive strategy and the specific nerve transfers to be performed. The brachialis to AIN nerve transfer is used here as an example. The procedure is performed under general anesthesia without the use of long-acting paralytics, which would interfere with intraoperative stimulation. Intraoperative motor mapping is used to identify both recipients and donors. In contrast to LMN injuries, such as with brachial plexus or peripheral lesions, in spinal cord/UMN injuries, the nerve recipients can be precisely identified based on intraoperative activation prior to neurotization. The patient is positioned with the arm abducted on a table so that the axilla and medial surface of the arm are accessible to the surgeon. The arm is prepped so that all muscles are exposed and visible during stimulation. A tourniquet is typically not used, because it may interfere with intraoperative nerve stimulation. The incision is made

Table 29.2.
Summary of Electromyography Findings[a]

Muscle	Side	Fibs	PSW	MUP	Recruit	Activate
Deltoid	Right	–	–	+	Mildly reduced	Normal
	Left	–	–	+	Normal	Normal
Biceps brachii	Right	–	–	+	Normal	Normal
	Left	–	–	+	Normal	Normal
Triceps brachii	Right	2+	2+	–	None	Normal
	Left	2+	2+	–	None	Normal
Brachioradialis	Right	–	–	+	Severely reduced	Normal
	Left	–	–	+	Moderately reduced	Normal
Pronator teres	Right	–	–	+	Mildly reduced	Normal
	Left	–	–	+	Mildly reduced	Normal
Extensor digitorum communis	Right	2+	2+	–	None	None
	Left	2+	2+	–	None	None
Flexor digitorum superficialis	Right	2+	2+	–	None	None
	Left	2+	2+	–	None	None
Dorsal interosseous	Right	2+	2+	–	None	None
	Left	2+	2+	–	None	None
Abductor Pollicis brevis	Right	2+	2+	–	None	None
	Left	2+	2+	–	None	None
Flexor pollicis longus	Right	2+	2+	–	None	None
	Left	2+	2+	–	None	None

[a]Plus (+) and minus (–) signs denote presence and absence, respectively, of fibrillations (Fibs), positive sharp waves (PSW), volitional motor unit potentials (MUP) or reinnervation MUP, and neurogenic potentials (long duration and large amplitude).

in the medial aspect of the arm in the bicipital cleft. Careful dissection is used to sequentially identify the neural elements. After dissection, intraoperative stimulation can be used to precisely identify both donor and recipient fascicles. In the case of the donor nerve, the nerve fascicles should be dissected as distally as possible. The recipient nerve requires careful dissection to isolate the nerve/fascicles of interest and to prevent reinnervation of muscles with LMN dysfunction. Knowledge of the internal and external topography of each nerve is important. For example, for brachialis to AIN transfer, the AIN fascicle is located in the posteromedial portion

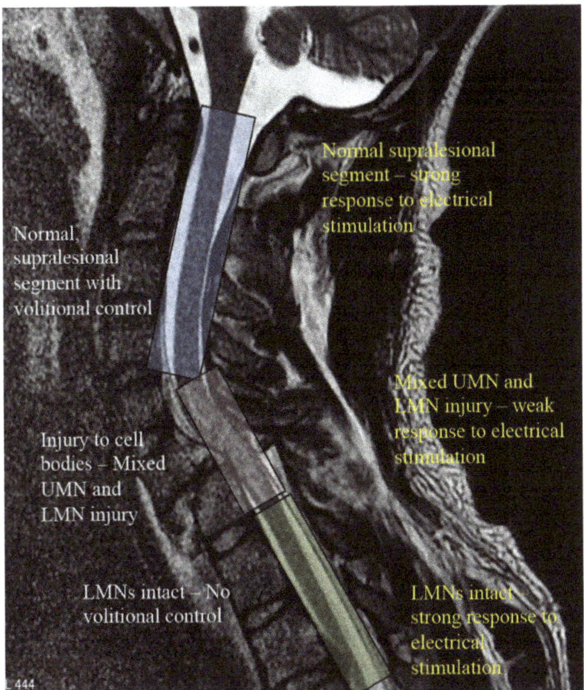

Figure 29.1. T2-weighted, sagittal MR image demonstrating the zones of injury. Shown in blue is the normal intact supralesional segment (with normal volitional control), which serves as the origin of potential donor nerves. The gray area is the zone of injury, which typically includes both lower motor neuron (LMN) and upper motor neuron (UMN) dysfunction. Nerves originating from this zone typically respond weakly or not at all to functional electrical stimulation (FES). The green area is below the zone of injury, with intact anterior horn cells and viable recipients for reinnervation. Nerves originating from this zone respond strongly to FES.

of the median nerve and the brachialis branch will be distal to the biceps branch of the musculocutaneous nerve. Vessel loops are helpful to tag/identify nerves. After correct identification, the recipient nerve is transected as proximally as possible. This allows the donor nerve to maximally span the distance to the recipient for a tension-free repair. Tension reduces vascular supply to the nerve and transmission velocity and increases microscarring. However, redundant donor length will prolong the duration of time required for reinnervation. Nerve coaptation should be performed in an end-to-end fashion. The epineuriums of the donor and recipient nerves are sewn together using 9-0 or 10-0 microsuture, followed by fibrin glue. In addition to the AIN/FDS reinnervation that can be achieved through this approach, the exposure allows the triceps branch to be directly stimulated if any question remains about the state of the NMJ. In the setting of a gap between donor and recipient nerves, nerve autograft can be used. Most studies demonstrate higher success rates if a graft can be avoided. Commonly used donor grafts include sural nerve (which requires a separate incision) or the medial antebrachial cutaneous nerve, which can be taken without a separate incision.

Oral Boards Review—Management Pearls

1. No long-acting paralytics should be used, to allow intraoperative stimulation.
2. Drape the entire extremity into the surgical field to allow visualization of all muscles during electrical stimulation.
3. Isolation of the specific recipient nerve/fascicle is important in order to prevent reinnervation of functioning muscles or muscles with LMN injury.
4. Avoid tension at the repair site while still ensuring well-opposed epineurium.

Pivot Points

1. If a gap > 3 cm between donor and recipient exists, nerve autograft will typically be required to achieve a tension-free coaptation.
2. Intraoperative direct stimulation can be used to verify viable NMJs.

Aftercare

Depending on the site of transfer, the limb is placed in a soft splint for 1 week to prevent excessive movement and disruption of the repair site. Range-of-motion exercises are used early postoperatively to prevent scarring around the coaptation. Physical therapy is a critical component for motor re-education. Co-contraction of donor and recipient territories is the core of eventual independent control. Therapy can begin 4 to 6 weeks postoperatively. Routine follow-up visits are scheduled to evaluate for reinnervation. Regeneration of the nerve is revealed by an advancing Tinel sign. Signs of reinnervation appear 3 to 9 months after surgery, with improvements continuing 18 to 24 months postoperatively.

Complications and Management

Postoperative complications of nerve transfer can be classified as immediate or late. Immediate surgical complications include bleeding, infection, poor wound healing, and injury to adjacent nerves. Intraoperatively, if donor and recipient nerves are not adjacent to one another, a gap may exist that requires use of a graft to span the distance. The graft may be an autograft from another site, increasing the morbidity of the surgery, or it may be a synthetic allograft, which may be less effective and increase the risk of surgical failure.

The main late complication is failure to achieve meaningful functional recovery. While only a few case series describe clinical outcomes of nerve transfers in the setting of spinal cord injury, existing case reports suggest one should expect results comparable to results one would expect for traditional nerve transfers for brachial plexus injuries.

Oral Boards Review—Complication Pearls

1. Intraoperative complications can be reduced by focused exploration and dissection to expose donor and recipient nerves.
2. Success of the transfer is affected by a variety of factors: nerve tension, epineurium opposition, vascular supply, and scar formation postoperatively.

Evidence and Outcomes

There are an increasing number of case reports and case series demonstrating the successful use of nerve transfers for spinal cord injury/tetraplegia. Few large studies and no randomized controlled trials currently exist.

In the largest study examining elbow extension recovery for patients with midcervical spinal cord injuries, branches of the axillary nerve were used to reinnervate the triceps in 13 limbs in seven patients. M4 elbow extension recovery was achieved in 11 limbs and M3 in the remaining two limbs.[14]

The largest study examining restoration of finger flexion included a cohort of nine patients and 17 limbs. Nerve transfers utilized in the study included brachialis branch to AIN, brachialis branch to median nerve, brachioradialis branch to AIN, and ECRB branch to AIN. Finger flexion was restored in four of eight limbs utilizing the brachialis to AIN transfer (three with M3 function and one with M4). ECRB branch to AIN seemed to work the best, with all five of five limbs achieving M4 strength.[6]

Data regarding finger extension are even more limited. One study evaluated seven patients. Surgical procedures performed included either supinator branch to PIN or free transfer of gracilis muscle innervated by the supinator branch. No patients receiving a free muscle transfer recovered greater than M2 strength. Supinator branch to PIN nerve transfer led to recovery of M3 strength in three limbs.[13] In another study of 13 limbs where supinator branch to PIN nerve transfer was utilized, thumb extension recovered to M4 strength in eight limbs and M3 in four limbs, while finger extension recovered to M4 in 12 limbs.[14]

The largest study available examining diaphragm reinnervation via the phrenic nerve utilized spinal accessory to phrenic nerve transfer with simultaneous placement of a diaphragmatic pacemaker in 14 patients. EMG activity in the diaphragm was detected in 13 of 14 patients after nerve transfer. More importantly, however, eight of the 13 patients were able to achieve periods of ventilator independence, with a mean duration of 10 hours. Two of the patients regained spontaneous respiratory control.[18]

The use of nerve transfers in the setting of spinal cord injury is a relatively new field of study, and clinical studies to evaluate the success of transfers and long-term function may take many years. As the field matures, more data will become available about the outcomes of the various transfers. Currently, many of the largest available studies come from a single center. It remains to be seen if the results reported will be similar across centers and also with larger numbers of patients. As surgeons gain more experience with nerve transfers for tetraplegia, a combined reconstruction strategy using both nerve and tendon transfers will likely yield the most favorable functional improvements.[21]

References

1. Bertelli JA, Ghizoni MF, Tacca CP. Transfer of the teres minor motor branch for triceps reinnervation in tetraplegia. *J Neurosurg*. 2011;114:1457–1460.
2. Bertelli JA, Tacca CP, Winkelmann Duarte EC, Ghizoni MF, Duarte H. Transfer of axillary nerve branches to reconstruct elbow extension in tetraplegics: a laboratory investigation of surgical feasibility. *Microsurgery*. 2011;31:376–381.
3. Fox IK, Davidge KM, Novak CB, et al. Nerve transfers to restore upper extremity function in cervical spinal cord injury: update and preliminary outcomes. *Plast Reconstr Surg*. 2015;136:780–792.
4. Fox IK, Davidge KM, Novak CB, et al. Use of peripheral nerve transfers in tetraplegia: evaluation of feasibility and morbidity. *Hand (N Y)*. 2015;10:60–67.
5. van Zyl N, Hahn JB, Cooper CA, Weymouth MD, Flood SJ, Galea MP. Upper limb reinnervation in C6 tetraplegia using a triple nerve transfer: case report. *J Hand Surg Am*. 2014;39:1779–1783.
6. Bertelli JA, Ghizoni MF. Nerve transfers for restoration of finger flexion in patients with tetraplegia. *J Neurosurg Spine*. 2016;1–7.
7. Bertelli JA, Mendes Lehm VL, Tacca CP, Winkelmann Duarte EC, Ghizoni MF, Duarte H. Transfer of the distal terminal motor branch of the extensor carpi radialis brevis to the nerve of the flexor pollicis longus: an anatomic study and clinical application in a tetraplegic patient. *Neurosurgery*. 2012;70:1011–1016, discussion 1016.
8. Brown JM. Nerve transfers in tetraplegia I: background and technique. *Surg Neurol Int*. 2011;2:121.
9. Brown JM, Mackinnon SE. Nerve transfers in the forearm and hand. *Hand Clin*. 2008;24:319–340, v.
10. Hawasli AH, Chang J, Reynolds MR, Ray WZ. Transfer of the brachialis to the anterior interosseous nerve as a treatment strategy for cervical spinal cord injury: technical note. *Global Spine J*. 2015;5:110–117.
11. Hsiao EC, Fox IK, Tung TH, Mackinnon SE. Motor nerve transfers to restore extrinsic median nerve function: case report. *Hand (N Y)*. 2009;4:92–97.
12. Mackinnon SE, Yee A, Ray WZ. Nerve transfers for the restoration of hand function after spinal cord injury. *J Neurosurg*. 2012;117:176–185.
13. Bertelli JA, Ghizoni MF. Nerve and free gracilis muscle transfers for thumb and finger extension reconstruction in long-standing tetraplegia. *J Hand Surg Am*. 2016;41:e411–e416.
14. Bertelli JA, Ghizoni MF. Nerve transfers for elbow and finger extension reconstruction in midcervical spinal cord injuries. *J Neurosurg*. 2015;122:121–127.
15. Bertelli JA, Tacca CP, Ghizoni MF, Kechele PR, Santos MA. Transfer of supinator motor branches to the posterior interosseous nerve to reconstruct thumb and finger extension in tetraplegia: case report. *J Hand Surg Am*. 2010;35:1647–1651.

16. Hahn J, Cooper C, Flood S, Weymouth M, van Zyl N. Rehabilitation of supinator nerve to posterior interosseous nerve transfer in individuals with tetraplegia. *Arch Phys Med Rehabil.* 2016;97:S160–168.
17. Bertelli JA, Ghizoni MF. Nerve transfer for sensory reconstruction of C8-T1 dermatomes in tetraplegia. *Microsurgery.* 2016;36:637–641.
18. Kaufman MR, Elkwood AI, Aboharb F, et al. Diaphragmatic reinnervation in ventilator-dependent patients with cervical spinal cord injury and concomitant phrenic nerve lesions using simultaneous nerve transfers and implantable neurostimulators. *J Reconstr Microsurg.* 2015;31:391–395.
19. Ray WZ, Chang J, Hawasli A, Wilson TJ, Yang L. Motor nerve transfers: a comprehensive review. *Neurosurgery.* 2016;78:1–26.
20. Wang C, Zhang Y, Nicholas T, et al. Neurotization of the phrenic nerve with accessory nerve for high cervical spinal cord injury with respiratory distress: an anatomic study. *Turk Neurosurg.* 2014;24:478–483.
21. Bertelli JA, Ghizoni MF. Single-stage surgery combining nerve and tendon transfers for bilateral upper limb reconstruction in a tetraplegic patient: case report. *J Hand Surg Am.* 2013;38:1366–1369.

Index

Tables and figures are indicated by an italic *t* and *f* following the page number.

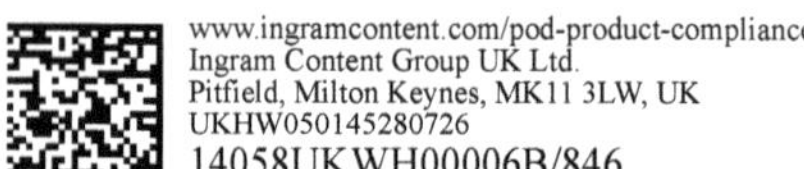

www.ingramcontent.com/pod-product-compliance
Ingram Content Group UK Ltd.
Pitfield, Milton Keynes, MK11 3LW, UK
UKHW050145280726
14058UKWH00006B/846

9 780190 617127